Gambling Problems in Youth

Theoretical and
Applied Perspectives

Gambling Problems in Youth
Theoretical and Applied Perspectives

Edited by

Jeffrey L. Derevensky
McGill University
Montreal, Quebec, Canada

and

Rina Gupta
McGill University
Montreal, Quebec, Canada

Kluwer Academic / Plenum Publishers
New York, Boston, Dordrecht, London, Moscow

Library of Congress Cataloging-in-Publication Data

Gambling problems in youth: theoretical and applied perspectives/edited by Jeffrey L. Derevensky and Rina Gupta.
    p. cm.
    Includes bibliographical references and index.
    ISBN 0-306-48585-0
      1. Teenage gamblers—Psychology. 2. Teenage gamblers—Social conditions. 3. Adolescent psychology. I. Derevensky, Jeffrey L. II. Gupta, Rina.

HV6710.G35 2004
363.4'2'0835—dc22

2004042179

ISBN: 0-306-48585-0

eISBN: 0-306-48586-9

©2004 Kluwer Academic / Plenum Publishers, New York
233 Spring Street, New York, N.Y. 10013

http://www.wkap.nl/

10 9 8 7 6 5 4 3 2 1

A C.I.P. record for this book is available from the Library of Congress

Permissions for books published in Europe: *permissions@wkap.nl*
Permissions for books published in the United States of America: *permissions@wkap.com*

Printed in the United States of America

distribution, determinants and natural course of these risky behaviors among
young people. The epidemiology of gambling helps us to understand who
is doing what kind of gambling and where. More focused research with
young people helps us to understand how risky behaviors begin, are sustained, and then transformed into patterns that are more mature and
entrenched—both healthy and unhealthy. Because the vast majority of young
people already have gambled by time they reach their last year in high school,
it is vital to learn about the risk and protective factors that increase or decrease
the likelihood that they will develop a gambling-related problem.

Gambling studies hold enormous potential to improve the human condition. For example, the study of gambling disorders in general and youthful gambling in particular holds the potential to teach us more about addictive behaviors (e.g., drug use disorders) than these substance use disorders
can teach us about intemperate gambling. In its pure state, gambling is
unfettered by intoxicant use. Consequently, it becomes possible to study
the development, maintenance and resolution of addiction without the con-
taminating effects of psychoactive drug use. Although excessive gamblers
often use alcohol and other psychoactive drugs, it is possible to study those
who do not imbibe—particularly among youth. Recently, in a series of very
important studies, neuroscientists have shown that central nervous system
reward circuits for winning money parallel the reward mechanisms associated with the anticipation of cocaine use or the appreciation of female
beauty by males. In addition, some gamblers experience blackouts while
in action; some experience withdrawal when they try to stop gambling. All
of this growing evidence seems to show that gambling has the capacity to
mimic the subjective effects of ingesting psychoactive drugs and that this
experience can change important characteristics of the central nervous system. Young people are most vulnerable to these changes because aspects
of their neurobiology remain immature until about age 18. Powerful
emotional experiences have the capacity to impact adversely a developing
central nervous system. Consequently, we have a special duty to understand and protect young people from experiences that can compromise
their development. After all, young people represent the future of society.

At first glance, the advances in neuroscience research amaze onlook-
ers who are surprised to learn that gambling holds the potential to produce
such powerful effects. Upon further inspection, however, it seems to me
that the more interesting observation is that gambling might be informing us that traditional models of addiction have been less than accurate.
Perhaps drugs are not as responsible for addiction as many once thought.
If gambling can become an addictive pattern in the absence of drug use,
with all of the sequalae typically associated with drug dependence, then
maybe addiction does not simply rest upon the action of psychoactive drugs.

More likely, addiction emerges from an extraordinary relationship between a vulnerable user and the objects of interest in their environment. When this relationship stimulates a subjective shift that is sufficiently robust, reliable and desirable, the roots of addiction are propagated.

Research on the growth of knowledge reveals that, during the second half of the 20th century, as legalized gambling expanded around the world, gambling studies also exploded. For example, between 1999 and 2002, one third of all the gambling-related scholarly citations ever published were released in academic publications. It is remarkable indeed to think that much of what we know about gambling behavior has been learned during just the past five yea

This confusion derives from the fact that gambling is a proxy for many other activities and circumstances. For example, people who gamble tend to take more risks, in general, than people who do not gamble. Excessive and disordered gamblers have a disproportionate number of psychological and social problems—both before and after their gambling. Casual observers often think that gambling causes criminal activity; however, do criminals gamble or do gamblers become criminals? Does gambling lead to depression, or do depressed people find respite in gambling? Only prospective longitudinal research can answer these questions accurately—anything less is speculation.

As the field of gambling studies prepares to address these and other fundamental questions by conducting new and more theoretically driven research, even more central questions emerge. Does understanding adult gambling inform us about youthful gambling? Youthful gambling problems might be qualitatively different from adult problems. Our knowledge of adult gambling might not apply to young people. For example, treatments for young people need to consider their immature neurobiology as well as their developing personalities and cognitive skills. It is possible, then, that gambling and gambling disorders are different constructs for young people compared to their adult counterparts. If this is so, then we might not have an accurate index of the prevalence of youthful gambling. Like drug taking, the reported lifetime prevalence of adverse gambling-related activities tends to go down; this of course is impossible since the lifetime prevalence of any pattern can only increase as people age. Something important happens to the meaning of previous life events and experiences as people mature; the end result is uncertainty about the value of lifetime prevalence rates. President John F. Kennedy once noted that, "The great enemy of the truth is very often not the lie—deliberate, contrived, and dishonest—but the myth—persistent, persuasive, and unrealistic."

Without an accurate understanding of youthful gambling, we risk accepting premature truths. Historical time and place influence the nature of "truth" and its associated repository of facts. In large measure, the social setting determines conventional wisdom; in turn, ideological conventions shape the social setting. To illustrate, during the 1930s, it was widely thought that dance music (i.e., jazz), in general, and dance music on the radio in particular were objects of addiction; listening to jazz was responsible for the demise of young people and their American families. One front-page headline in the 1932 Oregonian warned, "The Great American Narcotic . . . The Great American Brain-Killer is Dance Music." Another headline cautioned, "Jazz has Invaded College Life." Still another claimed, "Radio, Rum, Jazz Blamed for Insanity." These headlines serve to remind us that objects of "addiction" wax and wane. Each has its time; each has its cultural context. Gambling is now in the midst of a remarkable run of popularity that is fueling its expansion. However, as it has in the past, gambling opportunities eventually will recede—but, likely never disappear.

Careful study is required to determine which activities hold addiction risk because of novelty effects and which activities represent more enduring threats. For young people, both kinds of threats are very real and important, but derive from different sources. Similar to the trepidation surrounding youth, jazz and the radio, social observers now tout fears with respect to the influence of computers, video games and the Internet. Just as the development of the continuous still changed the manufacturing of gin and role of alcohol in society, the introduction of the hypodermic needle represented new technology that adversely shifted the use and effects of opioids during the 19th century. Similarly, contemporary technological advances might be shifting social priorities and, as a result, introducing new health risks, particularly to young people. However, it also might be that after a period of adaptation, people will learn to use these tools more responsibly—like the radio. Just as the English gradually adjusted to the gin craze of the 18th century, there is some evidence that young people in Nevada have adapted to their gambling surroundings and experience less than average levels of gambling-related problems. With every technological change, the important public policy issue to consider is whether a society can afford to wait for the inevitable adaptation—learning to enjoy jazz in moderation—or must intervene formally—like the 18th century Gin Acts.

These considerations lead to the matter of prevention. Any discussion of youthful gambling is incomplete without thinking about prevention. Preventing youthful risk taking is different from preventing adult risk taking. Therefore, education and awareness programs must target youth in a way that is effective and engaging. Effective messages that attract and influence adults can repel young people who might wonder what all the hollering is about, leaving them to do just the opposite of what the message intended. This book will stimulate many additional and equally important questions;

it also will help readers begin to formulate answers. In an effort to "do good," I urge that potential answers be carefully evaluated so that, despite good intentions, we "do no harm."

Avoiding harm is a tricky matter. And this brings us back to the beginning. Gambling-related public policy must protect the young, elderly, and otherwise vulnerable. Some people would develop policy that would prohibit all gambling. I wonder if the absence of all gambling would make the world a better place, where people would be less susceptible to harm. Temptation can stimulate character development. Learning to say no to enticing opportunities is an important part of human development and identity formation. Young people need temptation to fully develop character and facilitate the growth of a mature central nervous system. If all risks and temptation were absent, character development might be compromised or, at least, take a different direction yielding difficult to imagine consequences.

These kinds of considerations lead to my final thoughts. Too often, the fundamental issues of human experience become political footballs. Gambling is no different. Currently, gambling opponents and proponents argue about the value of gambling. Both need gambling to sustain their interests and activities. Both groups tend to select from the small but rapidly growing body of scientific research only those results that support their position. We should expect this kind of bias from stakeholders and advocates in a political debate. As scientists and health care providers, however, we must assure that our young people are guided by balanced, even handed information.

As I mentioned earlier, the scientific literature is growing rapidly. Judging the quality of research results is another matter. To make use of science, scientists, public policy makers and casual observers alike must classify the strength of the evidence. Science has a tendency to undo itself. New findings advance our understanding and change the way we view previous research. This is how science and scientific knowledge evolves. Many years ago, for example, my research (and others) revealed that college students experienced gambling-related problems at a considerably higher rate than their adult counterparts from the general population. More than twenty years later, my new research (and others) shows that college students are gambling at about the same rate as their adult counterparts and, contrary to my expectations, likely experiencing similar rates of gambling disorders. What has changed? Perhaps the rate of gambling has shifted among young people (e.g., a period effect or a cohort effect). Perhaps the way we study young people has changed. Perhaps young people's interest has shifted. Perhaps we aren't really studying gambling at all but something more complex for which gambling serves as a proxy. Only more research will reveal the answers to these questions.

This book represents one of the very first building blocks upon which future gambling research and understanding will rest. There are many mysteries to solve and discoveries to make. It is likely that the keys to these puzzles are embedded in the discussions that are included in, and will be stimulated by, this book. Let us be certain that these discussions are open, honest and thorough. Young people deserve our best effort to prevent or correct any gambling-related harms that might befall them.

Editors

Jeffrey L. Derevensky, Ph.D. is Professor of School/Applied Child Psychology, Department of Educational and Counseling Psychology, McGill University; and Associate Professor, Department of Psychiatry, McGill University. He is Co-Director of the McGill University Youth Gambling Research & Treatment Clinic and the International Centre for Youth Gambling Problems and High-Risk Behaviors. He is a child psychologist who has published widely, is an Associate Editor of the *Journal of Gambling Studies;* and is on the editorial board of several journals. He is a member of the National Network on Gambling Issues and Research, Canadian Centre on Substance Abuse; Centre d'Excellence, Université Laval; is an International Associate of the Centre for the Study of the Social Impact of Gambling, University of Plymouth, England; and is a member of the Program Advisory Board, Institute for Research on Pathological Gambling and Related Disorders, Division on Addictions, Harvard Medical School.

Rina Gupta, Ph.D. is a child psychologist and Assistant Professor (part-time) of School/Applied Child Psychology at McGill University. Her research has been focused on youth gambling problems. She is on the editorial board of the *Journal of Gambling Studies* and is Co-Director of the McGill University Youth Gambling Research & Treatment Clinic and the International Centre for Youth Gambling Problems and High-Risk Behaviors. She has provided more than 100 clinical and research presentations at national and international conferences and meetings, has published widely, and has provided expert testimony before a number of government committees and national and international commissions.

Contributors

Nicole (Nikki) Arthur, M.A., is a licensed marriage and family counselor. Her clinical interests include youth with impulse disorders and the impact of addiction on marriage.

Alexander (Alex) Blaszczynski, Ph.D., is Professor of Psychology, School of Psychology, University of Sydney; Head of the Department of Medical Psychology, Westmead Hospital, Sydney; and Co-Director of the University of Sydney's Gambling Research Unit. Together with Professor Neil McConaghy, he established the first hospital based gambling treatment program in Sydney, Australia. Dr. Blaszczynski has published extensively in the field of gambling, has been actively involved in gambling treatment and clinical research, is author of a self-help book, *Overcoming Problem Gambling*, and has conducted numerous training workshops. He was chairman of the Working Party for the Australian Psychological Society and committee member of the Australian Medical Association's position papers on problem gambling. He is a founding member of the Australian National Council for Problem Gambling, the National Association for Gambling Studies, and a foundation director of the Australian Institute of Gambling Studies. He is on the Advisory Board of the International Centre for Youth Gambling Problems and High-Risk Behaviors, McGill University, Canada; editorial board member of the *International Gambling Studies;* and International Advisory Committee member for the *Electronic Journal of Gambling Issues.* In 1995, Professor Blaszczynski was a co-recipient of the American Council of Problem Gambling Directors Award for his contributions to research in the field of pathological gambling.

Andria Botzet, M.A., helps administer several research projects at the University of Minnesota that explore the role of early delinquency and drug abuse on functioning in young adulthood.

R. Andrew Chambers, M.D., is Director of the Laboratory for Translational Neuroscience of Dual Diagnosis Disorders and Assistant Professor of Psychiatry in the Indiana University School of Medicine. His research interests concern the neurobiolgical basis for substance use disorder vulnerability across psychiatric disorders and in adolescence and young adulthood. Dr. Chambers has been the recipient of a National Alliance for Research in Schizophrenia and Depression (NARSAD) Young investigator Award and a National Institute of Drug Abuse (NIDA) Physician Scientist Training Program grant both focused on characterizing an animal model of dual diagnosis schizophrenia.

Anne-Elyse Deguire, M.Sc., currently heads the prevention initiatives at the International Centre for Youth Gambling Problems and High-Risk Behaviors at McGill University after having obtained her master's degree in psycho-education at the Université de Montréal. She has been involved in multiple prevention efforts with both elementary and secondary school students. She remains actively involved in the development, training, implementation, and evaluation of the Centre's prevention initiatives and has presented her work at national and international conferences.

Janine C. Delahanty, M.A., earned her Master's degree in Clinical Psychology from Loyola College in Maryland. She is currently a doctoral candidate in the Human Services Psychology program, specializing in Behavioral Medicine at the University of Maryland, Baltimore County. She is interested in intentional behavior change, both the promotion of positive health behaviors (i.e., dietary changes) and the cessation of negative health habits (i.e., smoking). Additionally, she has diverse research interests in the area of addictive behaviors, particularly smoking and club drugs.

Carlo C. DiClemente, Ph.D., is Professor and Chair, Department of Psychology at the University of Maryland, Baltimore County. Dr. DiClemente is the author of numerous scientific articles and book chapters on motivation and behavior change and the application of this model to a variety of problem behaviors. His most recent book is *Addiction and Change: How Addictions Develop and Addicted People Recover* was published in 2003. Dr. DiClemente is also co-author of a self-help book based on this model of change, *Changing for Good,* and several professional books including *The Transtheoretical Model, Substance Abuse Treatment and the Stages of Change,* and *Group Treatment for Substance Abuse: A Stages of Change Therapy Manual.* His current research interests include smoking initiation and cessation, alcoholism and substance abuse treatment, dual diagnosis, early intervention with problem drinkers, pregnancy smoking cessation, college drinking and gambling, and initiation of health protection and health threatening behaviors.

Laurie Dickson, M.A., is a doctoral student in School/Applied Child Psychology at McGill University. She has been involved in gambling research at the Center for Addiction and Mental Health in Toronto and McGill University's International Centre for Youth Gambling Problems and High-Risk Behaviors. Her interests include the study of resiliency, risk taking, and prevention of adolescent high-risk behaviors and the development and evaluation of science-based prevention programs for children and adolescents.

Meredith Gillespie, B.A., is a MA student in School/Applied Child Psychology at McGill University. She has been involved in research at McGill's International Centre for Youth Gambling Problems and High-Risk Behaviors and with The Teen Relationships Project at Queen's University. Her interests include the study of aggression/victimization, delinquency, media influences, and the prevention of adolescent high-risk behaviors.

Jon E. Grant, J.D., M.D., M.P.H., is an Assistant Professor of Psychiatry and Human Behavior at Brown Medical School and is the Director of the Impulse Control Disorders Clinic at Butler Hospital in Providence, Rhode Island. Dr. Grant is the author of *Stop Me Because I Can't Stop Myself*, a book on impulse control disorders published by McGraw-Hill (2002), and co-editor, with Marc Potenza, of *Pathological Gambling: A Clinical Guide to Treatment* published by the American Psychiatric Association (June, 2004). Dr. Grant is also the current Editor of the *Journal of Gambling Studies*. His major areas of research are the phenomenology and pharmacological management of impulse control disorders, in particular pathological gambling and kleptomania.

Mark Griffiths, Ph.D., is Professor of Gambling Studies, Nottingham Trent University (UK). A chartered psychologist, he has established an international reputation in the area of gambling and gaming addictions. He was the recipient of the John Rosecrance Research Prize and three other International awards for outstanding scholarly contributions to the field of gambling research. He has published over 120 refereed research papers, books, and book chapters and has over 350 other non-refereed publications. He has served as a member on a number of national committees and was until very recently the U.K. National Chair of Gamcare (National Association on Gambling).

Durand F. Jacobs, Ph.D., ABPP, is a Diplomate in Clinical Psychology and Professor of Medicine (Psychiatry and Behavioral Sciences) at Loma Linda University Medical School. He has been directly involved in treatment, training of health professionals, and research on addictive behaviors over the past 40 years. In 1972 he assisted in establishing the first inpatient treatment program for compulsive gamblers. In 1982 he published *The General Theory of Addictions*, a new model for understanding and treating addictions. His studies were the first to describe the extent and nature of gambling among high school age youth, and to document the special vulnerability of children whose parents gambled excessively. He has lectured and published extensively. He has been the recipient of awards from the National Council on Problem Gambling, Harvard Medical School's Division on Addictions, the Institute for the Study of Gambling and Commercial Gaming, American Psychological Association and the International Centre for the Youth Gambling Problems and High-Risk Behaviors for lifetime contributions to the field of gambling.

Jennifer Langhinrichsen-Rohling, Ph.D., is a Professor in the Department of Psychology at the University of South Alabama. She is also a licensed clinical psychologist. Her research and clinical interests include adolescent risk behaviors (e.g., gambling, suicide proneness, delinquency, family-of-origin violence). She has published extensively on these topics with more than 50 articles appearing in peer-reviewed journals. Dr. Langhinrichsen-Rohling received her Ph.D. from the University of Oregon in 1990. She completed her internship at the Palo Alto VA and Stanford Medical Center. In 1999, Dr. Langhinrichsen-Rohling was the recipient of a new investigator award from the National Center for Responsible Gaming. Results from this grant have been published in the *Journal of Gambling Studies*.

Willa Leitten, M.Ed., is currently a project manager for several pharmacotherapy studies projects at the University of Minnesota, including studies to reduce urges for impulse-related behavioral problems.

Carmen Messerlian, M.Sc., is Director of Program Development and Communications at the International Centre for Youth Gambling Problems and High-Risk Behaviors at McGill University. Carmen obtained her Master of Science in Health Promotion from the London School of Hygiene and Tropical Medicine in England. Bringing experience in public health, she has been instrumental in developing and applying health promotion models and theories to youth gambling. She has presented her work at national and international conferences.

Lia Nower, J.D., Ph.D., is an Assistant Professor, School of Social Welfare, and a research fellow at the Center for International Studies at the University of Missouri-St. Louis. She is a former Fulbright Scholar and National

Institute of Mental Health research fellow and research intern at the National Research Council in Washington, D.C. A licensed attorney and former criminal prosecutor, Dr. Nower provides evaluation and consultation for government, industry and corporate clients and gambling-related expert witness testimony. A nationally certified compulsive gambling counselor and clinical supervisor for the National Council on Problem Gambling, she conducts national and international trainings for gambling counselors. Dr. Nower also serves as a member of the editorial board of *Electronic Journal of Gambling Issues*, a reviewer for several journals, and a visiting research scholar at the Gambling Research Unit, University of Sydney. She publishes in the areas of youth and adult gambling.

Marc N. Potenza, M.D., Ph.D., is Director, Problem Gambling Clinic; Director, Women and Addictive Disorders Core, Women's Health Research at Yale; and Assistant Professor of Psychiatry, Yale University School of Medicine. His major research interest is in the field of addiction psychiatry. In particular, his work focuses on the relationship between pathological gambling and drug use disorders. He is applying a variety of techniques to investigate the characteristics of pathological gamblers, ranging from clinical investigations into the characteristics, consequences, and treatment of problem and pathological gambling to functional magnetic resonance imaging studies exploring regional brain activities underlying gambling urges in pathological gamblers. Recent awards include a Young Investigator Award from the National Alliance for Research on Schizophrenia and Depression, a Neuroscience Research Award from the National Center for Responsible Gaming, and the early Career Award from the National Center for Responsible Gaming. He has also been the recipient of the Drug Abuse Research Scholar Program in Psychiatry Award from the National Institute on Drug Abuse and the American Psychiatric Association.

Debra L. Schlundt, B.S., is a second-year graduate student in the Human Services Psychology Program, specializing in clinical psychology and behavioral medicine at the University of Maryland, Baltimore County. She obtained her bachelors in psychology and sociology from Towson University. Her clinical and research interests include both dual diagnoses, particularly with addictive behaviors, and college binge drinking.

Howard Jeffrey Shaffer, Ph.D., C.A.S., is an Associate Professor and Director of the Division on Addictions at Harvard Medical School and The Cambridge Hospital. He is also the founder of the American Academy of Health Care Providers in the Addictive Disorders, the first international credentialing body for clinicians working in the addictive disorders.

His newest project is the establishment of the Institute for Research on Pathological Gambling and Related Disorders within the Division on Addictions at Harvard Medical School. A clinical psychologist licensed in the Commonwealth of Mass., he maintains an active private practice and consults internationally to a variety of organizations in business, education, human services, and government. Currently, he is the incoming editor of *The Psychology of Addictive Behaviors* and serves on the editorial boards of many other publications. Dr. Shaffer is the past editor of the *Journal of Gambling Studies*. In addition to his more than 150 professional articles, he has published 10 books and monographs, including *Quitting Cocaine: The Struggle Against Impulse* (with Dr. Stephanie Jones), *Compulsive Gambling: Theory, Research and Practice*, edited with Dr. Blase Gambino, Sharon Stein, and Thomas Cummings, and *Youth, Gambling, and Society: Futures at Stake*, edited with Matthew Hall, Joni Vander Bilt and Elizabeth George. Dr. Shaffer's work has helped to shape how people understand the full range of addictive behaviors.

Randy Stinchfield, Ph.D., is a licensed clinical psychologist, Assistant Professor, and Associate Director, Center for Adolescent Substance Abuse Research, Department of Psychiatry, University of Minnesota Medical School. He is a consulting psychologist to a number of treatment and research agencies. After receiving his Ph.D. in clinical psychology from Brigham Young University he completed an internship at the Minneapolis VA Medical Center. Dr. Stinchfield has conducted a number of clinical studies and surveys in the area of problem gambling with both adult and youth samples which has been published in several journals. Dr. Stinchfield was the recipient of the National Council on Problem Gambling's 2002 Research Award. He currently serves on the editorial boards of the *Journal of Gambling Studies* and the *Electronic Journal of Gambling Issues*.

Ken C. Winters, Ph.D., is Director of the Center for Adolescent Substance Abuse Research and Professor of Psychiatry at the University of Minnesota. His research interests include adolescent drug abuse and problem gambling. He has published numerous assessment tools and research articles in these areas and has been the recipient of several research grants in the field of addictions. He is on the editorial board of the *Journal of Child and Adolescent Substance Abuse* and is an associate editor for the *Psychology of Addictive Behaviors* and the *Journal of Gambling Studies*. He is a consultant to numerous organizations, including the Hazelden Foundation, National Institute on Drug Abuse, Center for Substance Abuse Treatment, World Health Organization, and the Mentor Foundation.

Richard Wood, Ph.D., is currently a senior psychology lecturer and researcher at Nottingham Trent University. He recently worked as a Post-Doctoral Research Fellow at the International Centre for Youth Gambling Problems and High-Risk behaviors at McGill University, where he undertook various research projects examining problem gambling. His main research focus is upon understanding risky behaviors of adolescents. His most recent research examines the development and impact of technology in relation to gambling behavior. Dr. Wood has published papers in a variety of journals and presented his findings at numerous international and national conferences. His consultancies include work for the Association of European Lotteries.

Preface[1]

Gambling and games of chance have been popular throughout history. While the globalization of gambling has passed through a number of cycles, its current status, in most cultures, as a socially acceptable form of entertainment suggests its continued growth and expansion. Gambling has undergone a profound transformation during the past two decades. Throughout the world more and more countries have begun to realize the enormous revenues generated from legalized gaming. This newfound source of revenue and its general acceptance by the public has fueled its expansion and massive growth.

Most individuals gamble for enjoyment and entertainment, to socialize, and tempt their luck without many negative repercussions. However, a small percentage of individuals have difficulty controlling their gambling participation, resulting in significant disruptions to many parts of their lives. For such individuals, their inability to set and maintain reasonable limits, their preoccupation with gambling, their apparent need to seek the action and excitement associated with their playing patterns, and their inability to stop in spite of their desire to do so results in serious harm to the individual, family members, peers and employers.

While the realization that certain individuals may suffer the negative consequences associated with excessive gambling is not new, the awareness that this could afflict young people in their teens has been largely ignored. The study of issues pertaining to youth problem gambling began in earnest in the early 1980's; concentrating primarily on the prevalence rates of gambling and the types of activities in which youth were engaged. These early studies were followed by research examining the correlates

---

1. We would like to thank the staff at the International Centre for Youth Gambling Problems and High-Risk Behaviors for their many contributions. In particular, we would like to thank Dr. Tanya Bergevin and Meredith Gillespie who provided outstanding assistance in helping bring this project to fruition.

associated with youth gambling and problem gambling and their relationship to other high-risk behaviors and addictive disorders. This type of research continued into the mid 1990's when researchers began reaching farther into uncovering the etiology and risk factors involved in the development of gambling problems among young people. These studies expanded what was currently known about the correlates of gambling problems and researchers began to try to integrate this knowledge into some basic theoretical frameworks. Concomitant with the knowledge that youth were not only gambling but that some were experiencing a number of significant negative gambling-related problems, a number of clinical researchers began trying to provide therapeutic interventions using alternative models predicated upon their beliefs as to the underlying issues surrounding disordered gambling. Simultaneously, prevention initiatives, although limited, were being developed and implemented in order to help prevent gambling-related problems from arising.

The focus on youth remains very important for a multitude of reasons. As young minds are forming from childhood through the teen years, important developmental stages are crystallizing. Healthy childhood development increases the likelihood that these individuals will mature into well-adjusted adults in their personal, social, and professional lives. Constructs such as one's identity, sense of self, social skills, personality, and vision for the future are partially formed through experiences during one's childhood and adolescent years. The consequences for youth who are side-tracked by any number of major traumatic events, addictive behaviors, or repeated negative experiences that interfere with this development can be long-lasting.

Gambling participation falls on both ends of the spectrum, from healthy, normal levels of involvement, to more problematic levels. Most adolescents will engage in gambling activities as part of their normal behavior and will not be adversely affected. However, those adolescents who are preoccupied with gambling and who perceive themselves as incapable of controlling their gambling often experience long-lasting negative consequences in terms of their academic standing, interpersonal relationships, their psychological development, general mental health, as well as the consequences often arising from criminal behaviors. While the actual prevalence rates of youth with significant gambling problems are somewhat contentious, there remains a need to explore ways to best protect and minimize the harm that can result from excessive playing.

Over the past decade the adversarial relationship once apparent between the gambling/gaming industry and researchers and treatment providers has dissipated. The industry has now begun to accept that with widespread proliferation of gambling a number of individuals will experience negative problems. Similarly, many professionals have come to realize that in spite of the industry's desire to maximize profits, they have begun working in earnest together to help minimize problems associated with youth gambling problems. Such examples include staff training, the development of joint public service announcements, the prohibition of specific licensed products attractive to youth, and the sponsorship of school-based curriculum and research.

Recent national commissions held in many countries have concluded that adolescents and young adults remain particularly high-risk and vulnerable to new gaming-related technologies and to developing gambling-related problems. Together, governmental regulators, the industry, researchers and treatment providers have begun to explore ways of minimizing the harm resulting from excessive gambling. Such collaborative efforts have provided a solid platform for the development of responsible social policies and standards of care that will serve to minimize the occurrence of gambling problems and better address the needs of those who gamble excessively.

The past decade has seen a surge in research in the field of youth gambling, yet our knowledge still remains in its infancy. Large sample, longitudinal studies are non-existent. Many questions remain unanswered. Yet, following models linked to adolescent risky behaviors, resiliency, risk-taking, risk and protective factors, and knowledge acquired from research on other addictions, great strides have been accomplished in our understanding of adolescent gambling behavior and problem gambling. Clearly, many of our ideas, programs and initiatives need careful scientific evaluation. We have yet to reach the standards associated with *Best Practice* set forth in treatment and prevention efficacy studies. Yet, as a discipline we need to be held to the highest scientific standards.

Gambling has recently been viewed from a public health perspective. The use of a public health lens remains important in addressing the multiplicity of issues related to youth problem gambling as it recognizes the severity of the problem and helps to mobilize community and governmental resources in its process. The potential mental health, economic, social, legal and physical problems associated with excessive gambling require the development of responsible social polices and a concerted effort by professionals. More knowledge is needed, and ongoing research is imperative to address issues such as developmental trajectories through longitudinal designs, safety standards that would best protect our young populations, neurological bases of gambling addictions, treatment and prevention efficacy, and the development of instruments to best identify those at-risk as well as those who are pathological gamblers.

There is substantial reason to suggest that disordered gambling amongst youth, similar to other addictive behaviors, is a multidimensional condition involving bio-psycho-social determinants including a physiological predisposition, environmental stressors, social and familial influences, psychological processes, and individual personality characteristics. This book provides the most current empirical findings and theoretical frameworks in the field of youth gambling and serves as a comprehensive resource for those wishing to better understand the current state of knowledge concerning youth gambling problems. The contributing authors will challenge some beliefs, provide recommendations and directions for future basic and applied research, and raise provocative questions surrounding some of our current practices.

We anticipate that the information provided will help to inspire future research, the refinement and development of new screening tools, and promote more science-based treatment, prevention, and social policy efforts. Yet in our search for the Holy Grail, let us not underestimate the accomplishments made to date. Our current research and knowledge must guide our understanding and the development of responsible social policies. Such concerns cannot be overstated as we have a generation of youth that will spend their entire lives in state owned and/or regulated gambling. Should the prevailing adolescent prevalence rates continue into adulthood, serious social consequences will ensue.

JEFFREY L. DEREVENSKY
RINA GUPTA

Contents

PART V: TREATMENT

PART VI: PREVENTION

PART VII: SOCIAL POLICY ISSUES

Part I

Chapter 1

Youth Gambling in North America
Long-term Trends and Future Prospects

Durand F. Jacobs

There now exists a broad, fairly representative, and empirically derived database that describes in considerable detail the parameters of juvenile gambling in North America. Collectively, the 26 studies included in this review highlight the relationship between juvenile gambling and attending factors attributable to personal, family, peer, school, and broader community influences. The prevalence surveys have provided disturbing new insights into the surprisingly early age of onset for gambling among our children; about where, with whom, on what, and how much juveniles gamble; as well as their self reports on the short term negative consequences some youth experience as a result of their gambling. Several studies have also examined the underlying motives that lead juveniles to gamble, and identified the psychological correlates of those with gambling-related problems. These latter findings suggest new directions for future inquiries about the predisposing causes, probable course, and treatment of problematic gambling.

Prevalence of Juvenile Gambling in the United States and Canada (1984–2002)

Trends

The frequently voiced impression that the involvement of middle school and high school age youth in gambling has tended to increase over the years

1

finds strong support from the findings of sixteen independent studies conducted in the United States between 1984 and 2002 (see Tables 1 and 2). Table 1 covers the period 1984 through 1988, when the first five pioneering studies on juvenile gambling were completed (Jacobs, 1989a). The median level of participation by middle and high school age students having gambled during the previous 12 month period was 45% with a range of between 20 and 86%. During the period 1989 to 2002, the median level of participation in gambling was 65%, with a range between 49 and 86% (see Table 2). This leaves little doubt that juvenile gambling throughout the United States has increased significantly over the past decade and a half.

Ten studies completed in Canada between 1988 and 2001 revealed that past prevalence rates for juvenile gambling ranged from 60 to 91%, with a median participation level of 67%, suggesting comparable U.S. findings for the same period. Thus, the dominant trend has been an increase in juvenile gambling throughout North America between 1984 and 2002. Based on these combined findings, one can reasonably project that 70% of middle and high-school students throughout North America will have gambled for money during the past year.

Games Played by Juvenile Gamblers

A consistent finding across the studies of juvenile gambling is that adolescents (12–17 years of age) have managed to penetrate and participate, to

Table 1. Early Studies of Juvenile Gambling in the United States (1984–1988)

Investigator(s)	Lesieur & Klein (N=892)	Jacobs et al. (N=843)	Jacobs et al. (N=257)	Kuley & Jacobs (N=212)	Steinberg (N=573)	Median Prevalence Level
Year survey completed	1984	1985a	1987	1987	1988	
Gambled for money in past 12 months	86%	20%	45%	40%	60%	45%
Age of onset for gambling						
before 11 years old	a	41%	30%	39%	27%	35%
11–15 years old	a	40%	58%	48%	43%	46%
after 15 years old	a	9%	12%	13%	31%	16%
State	NJ b	CA	CA b	VA	CT	

[a] not reported
[b] lottery operating at time of survey

Table 2. Later Studies of Juvenile Gambling in the United States (1989–2002)

Investigator(s)	Kuley & Jacobs (N=147)	Winters et al. (N=1,095)	Wallisch (N=924)	Volberg (N=1,054)	Shaffer et al. (N=856)	Wallisch (N=3,079)	Volberg (N=1,007)	Westphal et al. (N=11,736)	Proimos et al. (N=16,948)	Volberg & Moore (N=1,000)	Volberg (N=1,004)	Median Level
Year survey completed	1989	1990	1993	1993	1994	1995	1996	1998	1998	1999	2002	
Gambled for money in past 12 months	58%	52%	66%	71%	70%	67%	53%	86%	53%	65%	49%	65%
Mean age of onset of gambling	12 years	11 years	12 years	12 years	a	13 years	13 years	11 years	a	12 years	13 years	12 years
State	VA b	MN	TX	WA b	MA b	TX b	GA b	LA b	VT b	WA b	NV	

[a] not reported

[b] lottery operating at time of study

some degree, in every form of social, government sanctioned, and illegal gambling available in their homes, communities and in places where they travel. To the casual observer the range of these activities is quite startling. It includes cards, dice, and board games with family and friends; betting with peers on games of personal skill, such as pool and bowling; arcade or video games for money; buying raffle tickets; sports betting with friends or at off-track satellite betting parlors; wagering at horse and dog race tracks, and at cock fights; gambling in bingo and card rooms; betting on Jai-Alai; playing slot machines and table games in casinos; buying pull tabs and lottery tickets; playing on video lottery terminals; playing the stock market; wagering on the Internet, and placing bets with a bookmaker. Naturally, the local availability of games and gambling outlets differ. Some may have readily accessible casinos, others may have lotteries, still others may have nearby race tracks, etc.

Notwithstanding the availability of gambling opportunities, the four most popular games that emerge repeatedly among youth include: cards, dice and board games with family and friends; games of personal skill with peers; sports betting (usually with peers, but also with a bookmaker); and bingo. However, wherever a state or provincial lottery had been operative before the prevalence study was completed, these government-promoted lottery games typically become favored by juvenile gamblers. Indeed, introduction of state or provincial lotteries invariably produces an increase in the numbers of both adults and juveniles who gamble in that jurisdiction, especially when pull-tabs, scratch cards, and other games that offer instant reinforcement are accessible.

After completing the first national study on gambling in America, Kallick, Suits, Dielman and Hybels (1976) concluded that when a state promotes one form of gambling, all forms of gambling—both legal and illegal—tend to increase. In an interesting study examining lottery playing on juvenile gambling, Jacobs (1994) reported that (a) post-lottery prevalence rates for juvenile gambling had increased significantly from pre-lottery levels, (b) the lottery had become a favored form of wagering, and (c) expenditures on other forms of gambling had increased from pre-lottery levels. Jacobs (1994) called this combination of factors the *Pied Piper Effect*.

In Tables 1–3, a notation designates the state or province where a lottery had been operating for some time *prior* to the conduct of the survey on juvenile gambling. This was the case in ten states between 1984 and 2002, where the prevalence rates for juveniles who had gambled for money in the past 12 months was between 45 and 86%, with a median level of 65%. Between 1984 and 2002 in the six states where surveys were completed before the lottery had become fully operative, the median level of youth who reported having gambled in the previous 12 months was substantially lower, 50%, ranging between 20 and 66%. No similar pre-post lottery

Table 3. Studies of Juvenile Gambling in Canada (1988–2001)

Investigator(s)	Ladouceur & Mireault (N=1,612)	Omnifacts Research Ltd. (N=300)	Insight Canada Research (N=400)	Govoni et al. (N=965)	Wynne et al. (N=972)	Gupta & Derevensky (N=817)	Ladouceur et al. (N=3426)	Poulin (N=13,549)	Adlaf & Ialomiteanu (N=2371)	Gupta & Derevensky (N=2156)	Median Level
Year survey completed	1988	1993	1994	1996	1996	1998	1999	2000	2000	2001	
Gambled for money in past 12 months	65%	60%	65%	91%	67%	80%	77%	70%	a	63%	67%
Mean age of onset of gambling	a	13 years	a	12 years	12 years	11 years	a	a	a	a	12 years
Province	Quebec b	Nova Scotia b	Ontario b	Ontario b	Alberta b	Quebec b	Quebec b	Atlantic Provinces b	Ontario b	Ontario b	

[a] not reported
[b] lottery operating at time of survey

comparison was possible in Canada between 1988 and 2001, as a lottery had been operating in each of the provinces long before these surveys were initiated. However, the median level of gambling among Canadian youth (67%) is comparable to that observed in American youth (65%), during the same period in states where lotteries had been operating.

Although no direct *causal* effect can be shown between the lottery and an increase of gambling among juveniles, the circumstantial evidence clearly points in that direction. Few would contest the fact that the introduction and continuing advertising and promotion of a lottery creates the most plentiful and easily accessible outlets for gambling. Moreover, a government-supported and promoted lottery fosters a more affirmative and socially acceptable community attitude towards wagering. The impact of this general climate of "it's O.K. to play" does not escape the attention of juveniles who, though legally underage, find easy accessibility to lottery tickets; this behavior is seldom discouraged by vendors and is often aided and abetted by their parents and older relatives (Felsher, Derevensky & Gupta, 2004; Jacobs 1989a; Ladouceur & Mireault, 1988; Westphal, Rush, Stevens & Johnson, 1998; Winters, Stinchfield & Fulkerson, 1990). Westphal et al. (1998), in their state-wide study of juvenile gambling in Louisiana, recommended strict enforcement of existing age restrictions on lottery sales. They found that 65% of their sample had played "scratch off" lottery tickets, as well as other lottery games. Their data revealed that lottery play exceeded all other forms of licensed and social gambling. Volberg and Moore's (1999) replication study of juvenile gambling in Washington found a significant increase in juvenile lottery play between 1993 and 1999. This was found to be directly correlated with increased participation and expenditures by these youth in other types of gambling. Similarly, in Canadian studies the lottery clearly prevailed as the favorite form of wager among juvenile gamblers, including children in grades four through six (Felsher et al., 2004; Gupta & Derevensky, 1996; Ladouceur, Dubé & Bujold, 1994).

These findings support Jacobs' (1994) recommendations for restricting the extent and the seductive content of lottery advertising, rigorous enforcement of laws prohibiting minors from gambling, and holding elected officials and appointed lottery commissioners directly accountable for contributing, however inadvertently, to juvenile gambling in general, and to gambling-related problems. The use of lotteries and other forms of gambling by governments as a major revenue-producing stream needs to be aggressively challenged.

Gender Differences Among Juvenile Players

Like adults, male juveniles tend to gamble earlier, gamble on more games, gamble more often, spend more time and money, and experience more gambling-related problems than females. The preferred games on which male juveniles gamble tend to differ from those of females. Along a skill/knowledge to pure luck continuum, boys tend to cluster at the skill/knowledge end with card and board games, games of personal skill, and sports betting being most popular among them. Girls have been drawn more to games of pure chance (e.g. raffles, bingo, lotteries and pull tabs) (where available). However, where horse and dog tracks and electronic machine games (e.g., video lottery terminals and slot machines) are locally accessible, juvenile participation tends to be similar between boys and girls.

Age of Onset for Gambling Among Juveniles

Studies in this review revealed that children reported their first gambling experience at a surprisingly early age, with median ages ranging between 11 and 13. In fact, by the time children in North America are 12 years old, the majority of these youth have already gambled for money. It is notable that early involvement among juveniles in gambling now precedes the expected onset for their use of cigarettes, hard liquor and marijuana (Gupta & Derevensky, 1998b; Jacobs, 1989a; Westphal et al., 1998).

In general, the earliest gambling experiences among children occur under a set of circumstances where (a) opportunities to wager even small amounts of money are readily accessible; (b) where the social climate of the home and local environment is not only conducive to, but accepting of, such behavior, and (c) where the rules of the games to be played are within the child's capacity to understand. Children simply become involved in social and recreational activities (including gambling) that already have been going on around them, and to which they are welcomed as new players by family members, other adults, and by more sophisticated peers in their home community.

As has long been the case with juvenile drinking, adults appear to overlook their role as an "accessory before the fact," concluding that their children somehow found gambling on their own, rather than having learned it from them (Milgram, 1982). When questioned, the overwhelming majority of youth who gamble reply that they were introduced to this "recreational diversion" by their parents and older relatives. Work by Gupta and Derevensky (1996) revealed that by the age of 12 less than 10% of children fear getting caught gambling. An early study by Ladouceur and Mireault (1988) of high school students in Quebec City found that 66% had placed a bet in the previous year, and 24% said they had gambled at least once a week. Ninety percent of these students reported that their parents knew they gambled and 84% reported their parents did not object. Indeed, 61% of these adolescents said they wagered in the company of their parents and more than 25% reported they had borrowed money from parents or other relatives either to bet, or to repay their gambling debts.

When youth report serious gambling problems being experienced by their parents, age of onset for their own gambling tends to occur much earlier. Jacobs et al. (1989) reported that 75% of high school youth who described one or both of their parents as having a problem with compulsive gambling, had first gambled before age 11, as compared with 34% of their classmates. As is the case with other potentially health threatening behaviors of juveniles (e.g., smoking, alcohol, drug use, and delinquency), an earlier age of onset may result in greater problems later. Winters et al. (1990), concluded that "if early onset is considered grade six or before, there is a definite trend for early gambling onset to decrease as problem severity among youngsters increases" (p. 17). Winters and his colleagues reported that, among a high school sample, early onset (i.e., sixth grade or before) was 40% for the non-problem gamblers group, 52% for at-risk gamblers, and 60% among those described as problem gamblers. They also found that the corollary was true; of those who said they first began gambling when they were in the twelfth grade, 91% were non problem gamblers, 10% were at risk gamblers, and none were problem gamblers. In a similar Canadian study, 48% of problem gamblers, age 12 to 17, had their first gambling experience before age 10, as compared to 34% of at risk gamblers, and 29% of non problem gamblers (Wynne, Smith & Jacobs, 1996).

Two Canadian studies investigated lifetime prevalence rates for gambling among primary school students. Ladouceur, Dubé, and Bujold (1994) found that 81% of fourth graders, 84% of fifth graders, and 92% of sixth graders in Quebec City had gambled sometime in the past. The lottery was by far their favorite wager, followed by cards and sports betting. Similar findings emerged from a second independent Canadian study completed in Montreal (Gupta & Derevensky, 1996). This set of Canadian findings indicates that a substantial majority of primary school children had gambled well before they were eleven years of age. Indeed, evidence is now accumulating that age of onset for gambling among younger juveniles is happening even earlier than once expected.

Prevalence of Serious Gambling-Related Problems Among Juveniles

Dominant Trends of Serious Gambling-Related Problems (SGRP)

From each of the 26 studies the percentage of youth described as either "at-risk" or "potential pathological" gamblers (see Tables 4 & 5) are provided.

Both groups were found to have more gambling-related problems than those of their peers. Individuals classified as "problem," "probable pathological" or "probable compulsive" gamblers were similarly grouped. For purposes of highlighting major trends over the past two decades, a single category of juvenile gamblers described as "serious gambling-related problems" (SGRP) has been produced. Moreover, describing juveniles with SGRP appeared more operational, than to cast children under Volberg and Abbott's (1994) adult designation of "problem gamblers"; primarily since some of the latter group would then be expected to reveal a "chronic and progressive condition" which would be highly unlikely in 12 to 17 year olds.

As seen in Table 4, during the period between 1984–1988, four studies in the United States noted the prevalence of SGRP among juveniles. When taking the sums in rows three and four from each study into consideration, one finds that the median level of SGRP among juveniles during the earliest years of the period under study was 10% (range 9–20%). Table 5 summarizes ten studies completed in the United States during the period 1989–2002. Here one finds that the median level of serious gambling-related problems among juveniles has risen to 12% (range 9–26%). An examination of six studies completed in Canada between 1988 and 2001 reveals the median level of serious gambling-related problems to be 14% (range 7–28%).

The findings reveal that the dominant long term trend has been a progressive increase in the amount of serious gambling-related problems reported by juveniles in the United States and Canada. A parallel trend is revealed which shows a marked increase from the earlier to later years in the proportion of juveniles who reported having gambled in a previous year. These parallel developments now provide an objective basis for concluding that as increasing numbers of juveniles participate in an expanding array of gambling opportunities around them an increasing number of them will experience serious gambling-related problems.

Fellow-Travelers Among Juveniles Reporting Serious Gambling-Related Problems

Studies of *adult* pathological gamblers have reported levels of alcohol and drug abuse as high as 50% among those who present for treatment (Jacobs, 1984a; Lesieur & Blume, 1991; Ramirez, McCormick, Russo & Taber, 1984; Winters & Anderson, 2000). On the other hand, 1701 male adults in treatment for substance abuse in five Veterans hospitals reported levels of probable pathological gambling ranging from 13 to 28% (median 20%) (Elia & Jacobs, 1993; Jacobs, 1992). Findings led this author to coin the term, *fellow-travelers,* who are individuals identified as showing a preferred

Table 4. Serious Gambling-Related Problems among
Juveniles in the United States (1984–1988)

Investigator(s)	Lesieur & Klein	Jacobs et al.	Jacobs et al.	Kuley & Jacobs	Steinberg	Median level of Serious Gambling-Related Problems*
Year study completed	1984	1985	1987	1987	1988	
At-risk/Potential	5%	5%	5%	a	5%	10%
Problem/ Pathological	6%	4%	4%	a	5%	
State	NJ	CA	CA	VA	CT	

a not reported

addictive or potentially addictive pattern of behavior, who use other potentially addictive activities or substances as adjunctive methods for reducing their stress and for escaping their problems (Jacobs, 1990a; 1990b).

Many of the juvenile studies sought to determine the relationship between the presence of SGRP among these youth and their concurrent use of psychoactive substances (e.g., tobacco, alcohol and illicit drugs). It was consistently found that the SGRP groups reported twice the rate of frequent tobacco use, and twice the weekly rate of alcohol use compared to their peers. Alcohol was by far the favorite substance of choice among all juvenile groups, followed at a much lesser level by tobacco use. Use of marijuana and other illicit drugs was less often reported, but when they were the SGRP groups showed patterns of usage that were 2–4 times greater than peers. An important related finding is that participation in gambling has risen to equal alcohol use, thereby making gambling one of the two most popular choices for "recreational diversion" among North American middle and high school age youth.

Another fellow-traveler noted in the history of adult pathological gamblers has been the presence of excessive parental gambling (Custer & Custer, 1978; Jacobs, 1984b; Jacobs, Marston & Singer, 1985b; Taber and McCormick, 1987). When this relationship was explored, the SGRP groups reported consistently higher levels of both parental gambling and excessive parental gambling, compared to their non-problem peers by ratios of 3:2. Still another fellow-traveler noted among adult pathological gamblers is a very high level of illegal activity, which co-occur in 60 to 80% of individuals, resulting in judicial problems (Custer & Milt, 1985; Jacobs, 1984b, 1988b; Lesieur, 1987). Findings from several studies revealed that, while

Table 5. Serious Gambling-Related Problems among Juveniles in the United States (1989–2002)

Investigator(s)	Kuley & Jacobs	Winters et al.	Wallisch	Volberg	Shaffer et al.	Wallisch	Volberg	Westphal et al.	Proimos et al.	Volberg & Moore	Volberg	Median level of Serious Gambling-Related Problems*
Year study completed	1989	1990	1993	1993	1994	1995	1996	1998	1998	1999	2002	
At-risk/ Potential	a	20%	12%	9%	14%	10%	9%	10%	7%	8%	10%	12%
Problem/ Pathological	a	6%	5%	1%	9%	2%	2%	6%	a	1%	2%	
State	VA	MN	TX	WA	MA	TX	GA	LA	VT	WA	NV	

a not reported

* Serious Gambling-Related Problem (SGRP) terminology is based on the sum of the "At-risk/Potential" and "Problem/Pathological" findings in each column.

approximately 10% of youth reported recent involvements in illegal activities and/or problems with the police, the SGRP groups were at least twice as likely to admit being involved. The SGRP groups also emerged as more likely to report poor school performance, truancy, higher levels of unhappiness, anxiety and depression.

A Composite Profile of Juveniles Reporting
Serious Gambling-Related Problems

What follows is a composite profile, drawn from frequently reported demographic, behavioral, and psychological features that have characterized the SGRP groups described in the 26 studies included in this review.

Demographic Features

AGE OF ONSET. Current age differences among 12 to 17 year olds no longer differentiate juveniles with very few gambling problems from those with many. However, an earlier age of onset, well before age 12, consistently distinguishes the SGRP groups from the No Problem groups.

GENDER DIFFERENCES. Boys dominate the ranks of juveniles with SGRP by ratios ranging from 3:1, to extremes as large as 5:1 over girls.

PARENTAL GAMBLING. Growing up in a home where parents gamble, especially when one or both are perceived by the child as gambling excessively, is a situational factor found much more often among the SGRP groups. The same trend is true for reports of gambling problems among other relatives or close friends.

REGIONAL DIFFERENCES. Youth with SGRP are more likely to live in a metropolitan area, than in an outlying suburban or rural area. The exception is for Native Americans, living on reservations.

ETHNIC GROUP MEMBERSHIP. For a number of reasons, the sampling procedures did not include appreciable numbers of ethnic minority youth. However, one is impressed by reports that note an unusually high prevalence of gambling-related problems among Native American youth in both the United States and Canada (Nechi Institute, 1995; Zitzow, 1993, 1996).

Although not a part of the studies selected for this review, but offering further evidence of the special vulnerability of ethnic minority groups, is the very large scale study of gambling behaviors among Minnesota youth by Stinchfield, Cassuto, Winters and Latimer (1997). They found that Latin American, African American and American Indian students in grades nine and twelve had gambled more frequently than their Caucasian and Asian American classmates. Similarly, Wallisch (1993, 1995), reported Hispanic youth in Texas were more frequent weekly gamblers than their peers, and also experienced higher rates of problems with gambling. Clearly, there is an urgent need for additional studies of ethnic minority juveniles to determine reasons for differences in gambling behavior.

Behavioral Features

GAMES PLAYED. Juveniles reporting SGRP are distinguished by their preference for rapid, continuous and interactive games on which to wager. These include video arcade games, card games, games of personal skill, sports betting and machine games (in and out of casinos). These youth are much more likely to have gambled on multiple games, spent more time gambling, and bet larger amounts of money.

SOURCES OF MONEY FOR GAMBLING. The SGRP groups reported greater use of lunch money, selling personal belongings, "borrowing" someone else's property to sell (without their knowledge), utilizing bank or credit cards, as well as stealing or other illegal means to obtain money to gamble, or to repay gambling debts. They also are more likely to work, and to work longer hours in part time jobs.

FELLOW-TRAVELERS. The SGRP groups are more extensively involved in frequent and heavy use of alcohol and psychoactive drugs. They also report more illegal activities and problems with the law, poorer school performance, and more truancy. They are more likely to seek help for alcohol or drug problems, however, very few acknowledge or seek help for their gambling-related problems. This underscores the importance of incorporating a gambling screen in the routine initial assessment of juveniles who present with substance abuse or delinquency problems.

Psychosocial Features

REASONS GIVEN FOR GAMBLING. Researchers have observed a number of psychosocial factors that are more often reported by SGRP youth. These motives and psychological states may predispose juveniles to become gamblers, trigger returns to gambling, or otherwise maintain gambling involvement by reinforcing gratifications obtained by a gambling activity (Jacobs, 1982, 1989b; Winters & Stinchfield, 1993). Statements indicating reasons for more prevalent gambling among SGRP groups included seeking excitement, for entertainment, to win money, because I'm good at it, to escape, as a distraction from daily problems, to relieve boredom, because I'm alone, to diminish sadness or depression, to feel more powerful, to be in control of social situations, to feel less shy, and to make friends.

ATTITUDES ABOUT GAMBLING.   The SGRP groups are far more positive in their attitudes and expectations regarding gambling. They tend to agree with statements such as: gambling should be legal for teenagers; teenagers should be able to gamble; lotteries are a good idea; winning a big lottery jackpot is not very rare; luck or fate plays a big part in my life; gambling is a harmless pastime; there are tricks to gambling; betting for money is not harmful; I can make a lot of money playing games of chance.

DISSOCIATIVE REACTIONS WHILE GAMBLING.   Studies by Jacobs (1982, 1988a, 1989b; Jacobs et al., 1985b) and by Kuley and Jacobs (1988) were the first to identify extremely high rates of dissociative reactions, while gambling, that significantly differentiated adult pathological gamblers from adult social gamblers, and from normative controls of adults and adolescents who gamble. More recent studies have shown strikingly similar results. Much more frequent and pervasive dissociative reactions were noted among juveniles reporting SGRP (Gupta & Derevensky, 1998a, 1998b, 2001; Insight Canada Research, 1994; Wynne et al., 1996).

Findings of high rates of dissociation while gambling are consistent with Jacobs' (1986, 1998, 2000) *General Theory of Addictions*. They offer strong support for the position that all addictive patterns of behavior, including pathological gambling, basically represent a person's deliberately chosen vehicle that is used (a) to escape from highly stressful internal and external reality conditions, and (b) to experience an altered, much more pleasant, state of consciousness while indulging. Support for this direct problem-solving paradigm is further found in the sampling of reasons provided for gambling by youth who report serious gambling-related problems. Consequently, future gambling screens for both juveniles and adults must go beyond the more obvious phenotypic behavioral indices, and also tap into the deeper motives and the psychosocial rewards anticipated by those who find gambling so rewarding that they doggedly persist and accelerate their involvement in this activity, despite increasingly punishing consequences for themselves and others.

Future Prospects

Prospects Regarding Prevalence Rates

Between the years 1984 to 2002 the median prevalence rates for juvenile gambling (past year) rose from 45–66%. This same period saw progressive increases in both the activities and the accessibility of gambling venues and opportunities. The empirical data suggests that the extent and nature of juvenile involvement in any given jurisdiction tends to vary directly with the length of time that legalized forms of gambling have been available and readily accessible to juveniles.

Table 6. Potential Effects of Gambling on
Personality among Ontario Adolescents

Personality Effects SOGS[1] Score	% No Problems (0) (N=252)	% Some Problems (1–2) (N=92)	% Some Problems (3–4) (N=40)	% Probable Pathological (5+) (N=16)
Lost track of time while gambling	12%	36%	55%	65%
Felt like you were a different person	3%	10%	26%	53%
Felt like you were outside of yourself, watching yourself gamble	2%	8%	9%	29%
Felt like you were in a trance	0%	8%	7%	24%
Experienced a memory blackout for things that happened, while you were gambling	0%	3%	2%	12%

Compiled by D. F. Jacobs, Ph.D.
* Reprinted with permission of Insight Canada Research (1994).
[1] Lesieur & Blume (1987)

Table 7. Dissociative Responses and Gambling
Severity among Alberta Adolescents

Dissociative State	% Non-Problem Gamblers (N=430)	% At-Risk Gamblers (N=148)	% Problem Gamblers (N=77)
Lost track of time while gambling	24	56	75
Felt like you were a different person	7	23	29
Felt like you were outside yourself, watching yourself gamble	2	7	26
Felt like you were in a trance	1	12	27
Experienced a memory blackout for things that happened, while you were gambling	1	6	20

* Classification of gambler categories is based on SOGS scores.
** Reprinted with permission of Wynne Resources, Ltd. (1996).

North America has not yet reached its saturation point for per capita expenditures on gambling. Consequently, during the next five years one can expect that the numbers and variety of readily accessible gambling outlets will continue to increase, as will the numbers of adult and juvenile players and the revenues from gambling. Throughout North America, casino-style operations will continue to appear and to expand on state, provincial, and on native lands. They will continue to be breached by under-age players. Expanding opportunities for gambling on the Internet and on home television sets is certain to attract more juvenile players, who will seek and find ingenious ways to join the fun.

Unfortunately, there is little of substance on the immediate horizon that promises any large-scale interventions by government, the private gaming industry or school-based prevention programs that will dramati-cally reduce underage gambling. Therefore, it is more than a safe bet that juvenile gambling will continue to increase over the next five years such that by the year 2009 the median prevalence rates for juvenile gambling can be expected to approach 80% throughout North America.

Prospects for Changes in Favored Games

Strongly influencing the types of games played by juveniles in the future will be the ever expanding menu of offerings by state and provincial lot-teries. Future prospects are for bigger payouts at closer intervals, plus more interactive and more continuous, rapid outcome machine games (e.g., Scratch Offs, Keno and Video Lottery Terminals). The new interactive lottery games also can be expected to produce increased participation and expenditures by juvenile players of both sexes.

Non-lottery fast action machine games will compete for preferential status with games of personal skill for boys, and with bingo for girls. Among boys, one can anticipate increased sports betting with fellow students in middle and high school settings, as well as with the off-campus bookmaker. It is thought that boys will supplement sports betting with high stakes poker games in home settings. Juvenile involvement in both these latter kinds of gambling will continue to increase, so long as parents and educators remain unaware of the potential severity of gambling problems among youth.

Prospects for Increased Gambling by Girls

Gambling as a traditionally male-dominated activity shows early signs of moving towards a unisex recreational and diversionary pursuit. Studies over the past two decades note an increasing proportion of girls in the ranks of juvenile gamblers. This reflects the rapidly disappearing moral-social-economic constraints against participation. Paralleling and enhancing the effects of the changing social climate, is the increasing accessibility of lot-tery, high stakes bingo, pull tabs, slots and VLTs games that appeal more to the female player.

Prospects for Changes in Age of Onset

In past studies of representative adult populations the first gambling experience reported by older adults, aged 46–70, ordinarily did not occur until their early to late twenties. Average age of onset reported by 30–45 year old groups typically occurred during high school years (i.e., 14–18 years of age). Among the 20 juvenile studies reviewed, the reported age of onset for first gambling ranged from 11–13 years of age with an overall median of age 12 (i.e., seventh graders). These dramatically differing *cohort effects*, observed across older to progressively younger age groups, are particularly concerning.

Today's juveniles are the first generation to grow up in a society where an ever increasing number of socially acceptable and readily accessible forms of legalized gambling exist all around them. Therefore, it is not surprising that the current age of onset is much younger than previous generations. The median age of onset for gambling will likely continue to decrease among juveniles over the next five years. First and foremost, this is because increasing numbers of their parents and relatives will be gambling. These adults are the principal channel, facilitators, and role models through which children are introduced to gambling. Secondly, increasingly permissive social attitudes towards gambling by parents, other family members and society at large will result in progressively younger participation in gambling opportunities.

The growing body of evidence in the field of adolescent gambling challenges any a priori expectation that juvenile gamblers who already show serious gambling-related problems will somehow "mature out" in short order—particularly in environments where ever expanding gambling continues to be socially acceptable, actively promoted by governments, and readily accessible. Only a series of prospective research studies will provide definitive answers regarding at what adult age today's cohort of juvenile gamblers will peak and then decline in terms of gambling problems. Meanwhile, as a society, one cannot wait to see the outcome. The emphasis must be on early identification and prompt assistance to those middle and high school age youth first beginning to experience serious gambling-related problems, coupled with prevention programs for all juveniles.

To further stimulate our efforts we need only to recall that the prevalence rates for serious gambling-related problems among juveniles consistently are found to be 2–4 times those found for adults in the same communities (Jacobs, 1989a; Shaffer, Hall & Bilt, 1997). There simply is no alternative to strict enforcement of existing laws, meant to prevent gambling by minors. Such efforts could easily and inexpensively be incorporated into ongoing campaigns, including "sting" operations, to prevent sale of tobacco and alcohol products to underage youth.

Prospects about Gambling Screens

A major shortcoming of current gambling screens is that the anonymity accorded both juveniles and adults precludes any form of feedback to them, regarding the possible clinical significance of their responses. All too familiar is the paradox of an individual obtaining high SOGS scores in company with a denial that a problem with gambling had ever existed (Wynne et al., 1996). This highlights the desirability and ethical correctness of providing some form of direct feedback to individuals scoring within the parameters of serious gambling-related problems. Feedback for moderate to high scorers could be programmed to follow immediately upon completion of the telephone interview. Adolescents, who initially had agreed to receive such feedback, could be informed of potential risks suggested by their responses, along with directions for obtaining more detailed information or assistance.

Another method would be to cast a given gambling screen in a *self-test* format. Upon completion of this kind of questionnaire in school settings, adolescents would be directed to an accompanying self-scoring section, wherein they could discover how they placed in the range of scores denoting increasing levels of risk for problems associated with their gambling (Jacobs, 1995). The opportunity to receive such feedback without risk of embarrassment or loss of anonymity might even encourage more candid responses. The prospects for improved and more socially responsive gambling screens by the year 2009 are very exciting. It is expected that future screens will build in a *self-awareness feedback* feature of one kind or another.

Prospects Regarding Public, Governmental, and Gaming Industry Reactions to Juvenile Gambling

In his first review of teen-age gambling Jacobs (1989a) noted:

> Indeed, teenage gambling was not yet conceptualized as an issue fifteen years ago, even though teenage involvement with potentially addictive substances such as alcohol and illicit drugs were matters of serious concern, and have remained the subject of systematic nationwide evaluation since 1975 (Johnston et al., 1979). Potentially harmful effects of teen-age gambling simply had not been a matter of professional, scientific, governmental, or lay scrutiny, as attested to by the virtually silent literature on this topic before 1980 (p.263).

The matter of government-promoted gambling requires consideration. Among the thirty-six states and the District of Columbia that in 1995 enjoyed revenues of over $32 billion from lotteries alone (Keating, 1996), only a limited number provided any measure of financial support for education, treatment, prevention or research to assist those who already were experiencing, or who were at risk for developing, serious gambling-related problems. To date, helping responses by state governments have been modest at best.

The National Survey of Problem Gambling Programs completed by the National Council on Problem Gambling (1999) with the assistance of the American Gaming Association (1996, 1998) and the North American Association of State and Provincial Lotteries revealed that, during 1998, only half of the 37 states with ongoing lotteries received any funding for the above stated purposes from their respective lottery commissions. During 1998, apart from funding that may have been provided by their respective lottery commissions, only one third of the 47 state governments that enjoyed revenues from legalized gambling provided financial support for such programs. Past experience has shown that the lottery, and other sources of state funding for gambling programs, have been subject to the vagaries of subsequent legislative priorities that often have reduced the original appropriations. Prospects over the next five years are less than certain that states will appreciably increase funding for the range of educational, prevention and research initiatives necessary.

At the federal level in the U.S. nothing has been done to assist juveniles with serious gambling-related problems. Indeed, diagnosed pathological gamblers of any age were specifically excluded from consideration under the 1990 Americans With Disabilities Act, although protection was assured for recovering alcoholics and drug addicts (Pertzoff, 1990). A recent inquiry found that even the Justice Department's Office of Juvenile Justice and Delinquency Prevention had no efforts focused on teenage gambling.

Governmental reactions to juvenile gambling in Canada have been considerably more forthcoming, compared to U.S. responses. Several Canadian provinces have set aside substantial funding from lottery and other gaming revenues to address problem gambling. Since 1993, four provinces have financed prevalence studies of juvenile gambling. Substance abuse agencies in several provinces have expanded their ongoing adult drug and alcohol programs to include increased public awareness, treatment, and prevention activities for juvenile gamblers. Still, within the next five years much more remains to be done in Canada, before the needs of its youth are adequately addressed.

Summary

There is no consensus on how children should be prepared for growing up in a society where most everyone gambles. Indeed, today's juveniles are the first generation to be raised in an environment where legalized gambling is so pervasive, readily accessible, and socially acceptable. The surprisingly early age of onset for gambling makes it imperative that cautionary educational programs be introduced by grade six, or earlier, and continued throughout high school. In each of these settings children and pre-adolescents should be taught age appropriate social skills, communication skills, stress management, and a range of coping and problem-solving strategies (including the laws of probability), that will anticipate, and place them in better stead to deal with the physical, psychological, social, and occupational stresses that characterize passage through the adolescent years. Meanwhile, adequate funding and prompt availability of counseling and treatment must be organized for those juveniles throughout North America who report serious gambling-related problems. Such resources could rather quickly and economically be integrated into existing adolescent substance use programs, currently functioning in schools, residential and drop-in centers, and out-patient settings.

Long past due are additional state-, provincial-, and federally-funded social impact studies to track the extent to which current and subsequent forms of legalized gambling contribute to rates of problem gambling among potentially vulnerable groups, including juveniles. The scientific literature consistently indicates that those under eighteen years of age are most at risk for developing addictive patterns of behavior, including pathological gambling. Therefore, the already high rates of gambling problems among middle and high school students accentuate the urgent need for increased public awareness, early screening, determined outreach efforts, and enhanced educational, counseling and preventive interventions. The early years of the twenty first century will mark the historic hey-day for legalized gambling throughout North America and the world at large. How the United States and Canada prepare to address this eventuality will determine the extent to which the present and future generations of their children will be placed at risk.

References

Adlaf, E. M. & Ialomiteanu, A. (2000). Prevalence of problems gambling in adolescents: Findings from the 1999 Ontario Students Drug Use Survey. *Canadian Journal of Psychiatry, 45,* 752–755.

American Gaming Association. (1996, 1998). *Responsible Gaming Resource Guide.* Washington, D.C.: American Gaming Association,

Custer, R. L., & Custer, L. F. (1978). *Characteristics of the recovering compulsive gambler: A survey of 150 members of Gamblers Anonymous.* Paper presented at the Fourth National Conference on Gambling, Reno, NV.

Custer, R. L., & Milt, H. (1985). *When luck runs out.* New York: Facts on File Publications.

Elia, C., & Jacobs, D. F. (1993). The incidence of pathological gambling among Native Americans treated for alcohol dependence. *The International Journal of the Addictions, 28,* 659–666.

Felsher, J.R., Derevensky, J.L. & Gupta, R. (in press) Lottery playing amongst youth: Implications for prevention and social policy, *Journal of Gambling Studies, 20*, 127–153.

Govoni, R., Rupcich, N., & Frisch, G. R. (1996). Gambling behavior of adolescent gamblers. *Journal of Gambling Studies, 12*, 305–317.

Gupta, R., & Derevensky, J. L. (1996). The relationship between gambling and videogame playing behavior in children and adolescents. *Journal of Gambling Studies, 12*, 375–394.

Gupta, R., & Derevensky, J. L. (1998a). An empirical examination of Jacobs' General Theory of Addictions: Do adolescent gamblers fit the theory? *Journal of Gambling Studies, 14*, 17–49.

Gupta, R., & Derevensky, J. L. (1998b). Adolescent gambling behavior: A prevalence study and examination of the correlates associated with problem gambling. *Journal of Gambling Studies, 14*, 319–345.

Gupta, R. & Derevensky, J. L. (2001). *An Evaluation of the different coping styles of adolescents with gambling problems.* Report prepared for the Ontario Ministry of Health and Long Term Care, Toronto, Ontario.

Insight Canada Research. (1994, December). *An exploration of the prevalence of pathological gambling behaviour among adolescents in Ontario.* Report prepared for the Canadian Foundation on Compulsive Gambling. Toronto, Ontario: Author.

Jacobs, D. F. (1982). The addictive personality syndrome: A new theoretical model for understanding and treating addictions. In W. R. Eadington (Ed.) *The gambling papers, Vol. 2: Pathological gambling, theory and practice* (pp. 1–55). Reno, NV: University of Nevada Press.

Jacobs, D. F. (1984a). Factors alleged as predisposing to compulsive gambling. In *Sharing recovery through Gamblers Anonymous* (pp. 227–233). Los Angeles, CA: Gamblers Anonymous Publishing Inc.

Jacobs, D. F. (1984b). Study of traits leading to compulsive gambling. In *Sharing recovery through Gamblers Anonymous* (pp. 120–123). Los Angeles, CA: Gamblers Anonymous Publishing, Inc.

Jacobs, D. F. (1986). A General Theory of Addictions: A new theoretical model. *Journal of Gambling Behavior, 2*, 15–31.

Jacobs, D. F. (1988a). Evidence for a common dissociative reaction among addicts. *Journal of Gambling Behavior, 4*, 27–37.

Jacobs, D. F. (1988b). Problem gamblers and white collar crime. In W. R. Eadington (Ed.) *Gambling research: Gamblers and gambler behavior* (pp. 272–278). Reno, NV: University of Nevada Press.

Jacobs, D. F. (1989a). Illegal and undocumented: A review of teenage gambling and the plight of children of problem gamblers in America. In H. J. Shaffer, S. Stein, B. Gambino, & T. Cummings (Eds.), *Compulsive gambling: Theory, research and practice* (pp. 249–292). Lexington, MA: Lexington Books.

Jacobs, D. F. (1989b). A General Theory of Addictions: Rationale for and evidence supporting a new approach for understanding and treating addictive behaviors. In H. J. Shaffer, S. Stein, B. Gambino, & T. Cummings (Eds.), *Compulsive gambling: Theory, research and practice* (pp. 35–64). Lexington, MA: Lexington Books.

Jacobs, D. F. (1990a). Focus on teenage gamblers. *Behavior Today, 21*, 1–4.

Jacobs, D. F. (1990b). Gambling behaviors of high school students: Implications for government-supported gambling. In C. S. Campbell & J. Lowman (Eds.), *Gambling in Canada: Golden Goose or Trojan Horse?* Burnaby, BC: Simon Fraser University.

Jacobs, D. F. (1992). *Prevalence of problem gambling among hospitalized adult male substance abusers.* Paper presented at the Sixth National Conference on Gambling Behavior, Cleveland, OH.

Jacobs, D. F. (1994). *Evidence supporting the "Pied Piper Effect" of lottery promotion and sales on juvenile gambling.* Paper presented at the Eighth National Conference on Gambling Behavior, Seattle, WA.

Jacobs, D. F., (1995). A 14 year old plays cards for cash: Is it more than fun and games? *The Brown University Child and Adolescent Behavior Letter, 4,* 1–3.

Jacobs, D. F. (1998, September). *An overarching theory of addictions: A new paradigm for understanding and treating addictive behaviors.* Paper presented at the National Academy of Sciences, Washington, D.C.

Jacobs, D. F. (2000). Juvenile gambling in North America: An analysis of long-term trends and future prospects. *Journal of Gambling Studies, 16,* 119–152.

Jacobs, D. F., Marston, A. R., & Singer, R. D. (1985a*). Study of gambling and other health-threatening behaviors among high school students.* Unpublished manuscript. Loma Linda, CA: Jerry L. Pettis Memorial Veterans Hospital.

Jacobs, D. F., Marston, A. R., & Singer, R. D. (1985b). Testing a General Theory of Addictions: Similarities and differences between alcoholics, pathological gamblers and compulsive overeaters. In J. J. Sanchez-Soza (Ed.), *Health and clinical psychology* (pp. 265–310). Amsterdam, Holland: Elcevier Publishers.

Jacobs, D. F., Marston, A. R., & Singer, R. D. (1987). *A post-lottery study of gambling behaviors among high school students.* Unpublished manuscript, Loma Linda, CA: Jerry L. Pettis Memorial Veterans Hospital.

Jacobs, D. F., Marston, A. R., Singer, R. D., Widaman, K., Little, T., & Veizades, J. (1989). Children of problem gamblers. *Journal of Gambling Behavior, 5,* 261–268.

Johnston, L., Bachman, J., & O'Malley, P. (1979). *1979 Highlights: Drugs and the nation's high school students: Five year national trends.* Rockville, MD: National Institute of Drug Abuse.

Kallick, M., Suits, D., Dielman, T., & Hybels, J. (1976). *Survey of American gambling attitudes and behavior.* Washington, DC: U.S. Government Printing Office.

Keating, P. (1996, May). Lotto fever: We all lose! *Money,* 142–149.

Kuley, N., & Jacobs, D. F. (1987). *A pre-lottery benchmark study of teenage gambling in Virginia.* Unpublished manuscript. Loma Linda, CA: Loma Linda University Department of Psychiatry.

Kuley, N., & Jacobs, D. F. (1988). The relationship between dissociative-like experiences and sensation seeking among social and problem gamblers. *Journal of Gambling Behavior, 4,* 197–207.

Kuley, N., & Jacobs, D. F. (1989). *A post-lottery impact study of effects on teenage gambling behaviors.* Unpublished manuscript. Loma Linda, CA: Loma Linda University Department of Psychiatry.

Ladouceur, R., Dubé, D., & Bujold, D. (1994). Gambling among primary school students. *Journal of Gambling Studies, 10,* 363–370.

Ladouceur, R., & Mireault, C. (1988). Gambling behaviors among high school students in the Québec area. *Journal of Gambling Behavior, 4,* 3–12.

Ladouceur, R., Boudreault, N., Jacques, C., & Viatro, F. (1999). Pathological gambling and related problems among adolescents. *Journal of Child and Adolescent Substance Abuse, 8,* 55–68.

Lesieur, H. R. (1987). Gambling, pathological gambling and crime. In T. Galski (Ed.), *The handbook of pathological gambling* (pp. 89–110). Springfield, IL: Charles C. Thomas.

Lesieur, H. R. & Blume, S. B. (1987). The South Oaks Gambling Screen (SOGS): A new instrument for the identification of pathological gamblers. *American Journal of Psychiatry, 144,* 1184–1188.

Lesieur, H. R., & Blume, S. B. (1991). Evaluation of patients treated for pathological gambling in a combined alcohol, substance abuse and pathological gambling treatment unit using the Addiction Severity Index. *British Journal of Addictions, 86,* 1017–1028.

Lesieur, H. R., & Klein, R. (1984). *Gambling among high school students in New Jersey.* Unpublished manuscript, John Jay College, New York. .

Milgram, G. G. (1982). Youthful drinking: Past and present. *Journal of Drug Education, 12,* 289–308.

National Council on Problem Gambling. (1999). *National survey of problem gambling programs.* Washington, DC: Author

Nechi Training, Research and Health Promotion Institute. (1995). *Firewatch on aboriginal adolescent gambling.* Edmonton, Canada.

Omnifacts Research Limited. (1993). *An examination of the prevalence of gambling in Nova Scotia.* Research Report Number 93090 for the Nova Scotia Department of Health, Drug Dependency Services. Halifax, Nova Scotia: Author.

Pertzoff, L. (1990). *Americans with Disabilities Act: Compulsive gamblers not covered.* Delaware Council on Gambling Problems Newsletter #6.

Poulin, C. (2000). Problem gambling among adolescent students in the Atlantic provinces of Canada, and the role of age and deception about legal age status as potential risk factors for problem gambling. *Journal of Gambling Studies, 16,* 53–78.

Proimos, J., DuRant, R.H., Pierce, J. D., & Goodman, N. E. (1998). Gambling and other risk behaviors among 8th to 12th grade students. *Pediatrics, 102,* 1–6.

Ramirez, L. F., McCormick, R. A., Russo, A. M., & Taber, J. I. (1984). Patterns of substance abuse in pathological gamblers undergoing treatment: *Addictive Behaviors, 8,* 425–428.

Shaffer, H. J., Hall, M. N., & Bilt, J. V. (1997). *Estimating the prevalence of disordered gambling behavior in the United States and Canada: A meta-analysis.* National Center for Responsible Gambling. Kansas City, MO.

Shaffer, H. J., LaBrie, R., Scanlan, K. M., & Cummings, T. N. (1994). Pathological gambling among adolescents: Massachusetts Adolescent Gambling Screen (MAGS). *Journal of Gambling Studies, 10,* 339–362.

Steinberg, M. (1988). *Gambling behavior among high school students in Connecticut.* Paper presented at the Third National Conference on Gambling. New London, CT.

Stinchfield, R., Cassuto, N., Winters, K., & Latimer, W. (1997). Prevalence of gambling among Minnesota public school students in 1992 and 1995. *Journal of Gambling Studies, 13,* 25–48.

Taber, J. I., & McCormick, R. A. (1987). The pathological gambler in treatment. In T. Galski (Ed.), *The handbook of pathological gambling* (pp. 137–168). Springfield, IL: Charles C. Thomas.

Volberg, R. A. (1993). *Gambling and problem gambling in Washington state.* Report to the Washington State Lottery. Albany, NY: Gemini Research.

Volberg, R. A. (1996). *Gambling and problem gambling in Georgia.* Report to the Georgia Department of Health. Roaring Springs, PA: Gemini Research.

Volberg, R. A. (2002). *Gambling and problem-gambling among adolescents in Nevada.* Report to Nevada Department of Human Resources. Carson City, NV: Nevada Department of Human Resources.

Volberg, R. A., & Abbott, M. W. (1994). Lifetime prevalence estimates of pathological gambling in New Zealand. *International Journal of Epidemiology, 23,* 976–983.

Volberg, R. A., & Moore, W. L. (1999). *Gambling and problem gambling among adolescents in Washington State: A replication study, 1993–1999.* Report to the Washington State Lottery. Albany, NY: Gemini Research.

Wallisch, L. (1993). *Gambling in Texas: The 1992 Texas survey of adolescent gambling behavior.* Austin, TX: Texas Commission on Alcohol and Drug Abuse.

Wallisch, L. (1995). *Gambling in Texas: The 1995 Texas survey of adolescent gambling behavior.* Austin, TX: Texas Commission on Alcohol and Drug Abuse.

Westphal, J. R., Rush, J. A., Stevens, L., & Johnson, L. J. (1998). *Pathological gambling among Louisiana students: Grades six through twelve*. Paper presented at the American Psychiatric Association Annual Meeting, Toronto, Canada.

Winters, K. C., & Anderson, N. (2000). Gambling involvement and drug use among adolescents. *Journal of Gambling Studies, 16,* 175–198.

Winters, K. C., & Stinchfield, R. D. (1993). *Gambling behavior among Minnesota youth: Monitoring change from 1990 to 1991/1992*. Minneapolis, MN: University of Minnesota, Center for Adolescent Substance Abuse.

Winters, K. C., Stinchfield, R., & Fulkerson, J. (1990). *Adolescent survey of gambling behavior in Minnesota: A benchmark*. Report to the Department of Human Services Mental Health Division. Duluth, MN: Center for Addiction Studies, University of Minnesota.

Wynne, H. J., Smith, G. J., & Jacobs, D. F. (1996). *Adolescent gambling and problem gambling in Alberta*. Alberta, Canada: Alberta Alcohol and Drug Abuse Commission.

Zitzow, D. (1993, July). *Incidence and comparative study of compulsive gambling behaviors between Indians and non-Indians within and near a northern plains reservation*. Paper presented at The Third National Conference on Gambling Behavior, New London, CT.

Zitzow, D. (1996). Comparative study of problematic gambling behaviors between American Indians and non-Indian adolescents within and near a northern plains reservation. *American Indian and Alaska Native Mental Health Research, 7,* 14–26.

Part II

Chapter 2

Demographic, Psychosocial, and Behavioral Factors Associated with Youth Gambling and Problem Gambling

Randy Stinchfield, Ph.D.

With the rapid expansion of the gambling industry into mainstream society has come concerns about the risks of underage gambling (National Research Council, 1999). The expansion of gambling over the past two decades has resulted in almost daily exposure to gambling and its promotion. This is a dramatic shift in our culture and undoubtedly has an effect upon youth. The degree to which it has affected youth is still an empirical question as we are in the process of examining the early effects of gambling on the first generation of youth to be exposed to widespread legalized gambling and its advertising. It is well established that youth participate in gambling to varying degrees, from no gambling at one end of the continuum to excessive and problem gambling at the other end (see Jacobs, this volume). Recent reviews of youth gambling research have concluded that the majority of youth have gambled, but do so infrequently and do not suffer any severe consequences. However, a minority of youth appear to be overinvolved in gambling and are experiencing significant gambling-related problems (Gupta & Derevensky, 2000; Jacobs, 1993; 2000; Shaffer & Hall, 1996; Stinchfield 2002; Stinchfield & Winters, 1998). Estimates are that between 4–8% of youth have a very serious gambling problem; with a greater percentage amongst male adolescents (Jacobs, 1993, 2000; National Research Council, 1999; Shaffer & Hall, 1996).

At this point in time little is known about the antecedents of youth problem gambling. How and why do youth move from social/recreational gambling to problem gambling? Which youth are most likely to become problem gamblers? What variables maintain problem youth gambling? It is critical for researchers to examine variables associated with youth gambling that may be considered risk and protective factors of youth problem gambling.

There are a number of important reasons to identify and study correlates of youth gambling and problem gambling. Correlates can tell us what characteristics young problem gamblers are likely to exhibit and this information can elucidate the nature of youth problem gambling. Second, correlates can help identify problem gamblers by providing warning signs and help guide prevention initiatives. Parents, teachers and youth workers often want to know what warning signs to look for if they are concerned about problem gambling. Warning signs are very important for what has been described as an "invisible" addiction. Youth, like adults, attempt to conceal their gambling problems and therefore warning signs are important indicators for the identification of the problem. Third, correlates identify variables that may be risk factors for the development of problem gambling. Risk factors are those variables that are associated with the likely genesis of the disorder, and increase the severity and duration of the disorder. Some correlates may also provide insight into protective factors that prevent the development of problem gambling. For example, if school failure is associated with problem gambling, school success may serve as a protective factor. Protective factors enhance the individual's ability to overcome the resulting consequences of the disorder. Prevention efforts have been defined as an effort to avoid the onset of a particular problem behavior and to promote positive behavioral outcomes (Luthar, Cicchetti, & Becker, 2000). Considerable research has shown that risk and protective factors and their interaction are helpful in understanding the psychopathology of addictive behaviors (Latimer, Newcomb, Winters, & Stinchfield, 2000). Fourth, correlates can directly assist in developing empirically-based prevention programs and public awareness messages. It will be important to identify specific risk factors that can be minimized and protective factors that can be enhanced. If we can identify those youth most likely to become problem gamblers, we can then tailor prevention efforts to specific types of youth. For example, some youth may need information about gambling, such as knowledge of probabilities, how games of chance work, etc. Other youth may require guidelines on how to gamble without placing themselves at risk of losing more money than they can afford, while other youth who are already exhibiting problem gambling behaviors will require more extensive services.

Investigators are just beginning to examine those variables associated with youth problem gambling. These studies form a foundation from which to further explore these variables and to identify additional variables that are associated with youth gambling that may play a role in the development and/or maintenance of problem gambling. Most of the studies that have identified correlates of problem gambling have been survey research of either youth in the general population (e.g., Wallisch, 1993) or school-based samples (e.g., Gupta & Derevensky, 1998b). Some studies have focused on youth gambling (e.g., Stinchfield, Cassuto, Winters, & Latimer, 1997) while others have focussed on youth problem gambling (e.g., Wynne, Smith, & Jacobs, 1996).

In 1990, Winters, Stinchfield and Fulkerson (1993) conducted a telephone survey of gambling among 702 general population Minnesota youth. Besides measuring the prevalence rate of youth problem gambling, they examined the relationship of a number of demographic and psychosocial variables to problem gambling severity. Those youth with greater gambling involvement were more likely to be male, regular drug users, have parents who gamble, have a history of delinquency, and have poor academic grades. In two consecutive telephone surveys of Texas youth in 1992 and 1995, Wallisch (1993; 1996) reported problem gamblers were more likely to be male, younger, from a minority racial/ethnic group, work 10 or more hours per week, have a weekly income of $10 or more, have favourable attitudes towards gambling, expect to make money at gambling, and have parents who gamble. Volberg (1993), in a telephone survey of 1,054 Washington State adolescents, reported that tobacco, alcohol, and drug use were associated with gambling frequency and problem gambling.

Stinchfield and colleagues (1997, 2000, 2001) have monitored gambling among Minnesota public school students beginning in 1992 with subsequent surveys collected in 1995 and 1998. The Minnesota Student Survey (MSS) is an alcohol and drug use risk survey that has items covering domains of alcohol/drug use, school problems, acting out behavior, and has seven items focused on gambling behavior. Five items measure frequency of play on different types of gambling activities and two items are drawn from the SOGS-RA addressing problem gambling behavior. The MSS is administered every three years to almost the entire population of Minnesota public students in the 9th and 12th grades. The 1992 sample size included 77,072 students and the 1995 sample included 75,900 students. Variables that were positively correlated ($r > .25$) with gambling on a bivariate level included gender, alcohol use, tobacco use, illicit drug use, antisocial behavior, consequences of alcohol and drug use, attitude toward alcohol/drug use, and sexual behavior. While all of these variables were associated with gambling frequency, it was important to control for covariance among variables by using a multivariate analysis and a forward stepwise multiple regression was computed to empirically select correlates from a larger pool of variables. In both the 1992 and 1995 MSS, it was found that antisocial behavior, being male, and alcohol use, in that order, were the primary variables associated with frequent gambling, with these three variables accounting for more than one-quarter of the variance in gambling frequency. Antisocial behavior was found to be the strongest correlate of gambling frequency and was measured by four items that inquired about vandalism, physical fights, stealing, and getting a kick out of doing dangerous activities. These results suggested that frequent gambling may be part of a larger constellation of deviant behaviors, particularly among a subset of boys, that includes physical violence, vandalism, shoplifting, and alcohol use.

Stinchfield (2000) analyzing the 1998 MSS data, computed a forward stepwise multiple regression. However, this analysis was different in that it computed separate regression analyses for the total sample, and for boys, and girls separately. Furthermore, this analysis included two SOGS-RA gambling problem items. Again, variables were included in the multiple regression that obtained a bivariate correlation with gambling frequency of $r > .25$ including gender, age, grade point average, antisocial behavior, tobacco use, alcohol use, marijuana use, felt bad about the amount bet, a desire to stop gambling, sexual behavior, and consequences of alcohol and drug use. These variables were included in the multiple regression for the total sample and the strongest correlates included antisocial behavior, being male, felt bad about gambling, alcohol use, chewing tobacco use, age, and a desire to stop gambling but did not think they could. These seven variables accounted for 41% of the variance in gambling frequency. For boys, the set of correlates included antisocial behavior, alcohol use, felt bad about gambling, would like to stop gambling, age, chewing tobacco use, and number of female sexual partners. These seven variables accounted for 34% of the variance in gambling frequency. For girls, the set of correlates included alcohol use, felt bad about gambling, antisocial behavior, and age, with these four variables accounting for 23% of the variance in gambling frequency.

These results suggest that there are some similarities while differences between correlates of gambling for boys and girls also exist. The four variables associated with gambling frequency for girls were also true for boys, but the order of inclusion in the regression and the magnitude of the correlations were different with boys having additional correlates including a desire to stop gambling, chewing tobacco use, and number of female sexual partners. Again, these results suggest that gambling may be part of a larger constellation of deviant and risk-taking behaviors and that girls who gamble frequently also use alcohol and exhibit antisocial behavior. It should be noted that some of these correlates in the multiple regression made small contributions to the overall regression, such as tobacco use, age, and sexual behavior. Nevertheless, these correlates were associated with gambling frequency and not necessarily gambling severity.

Wynne, Smith and Jacobs (1996) conducted a telephone survey of youth in Alberta. They found that youth with a gambling problem were more likely to (a) be in trouble with the police; (b) feel that they could not confide in parents, teachers, school counsellors, and ministers; (c) feel ignored or rejected by their family; (d) report negative school experience; (e) have started gambling early, often before age 10; (f) report familial gambling; (g) wager large amounts of money; (h) borrow money for gambling; (i) steal or sell personal property; (j) report feeling anxious, worried, upset or depressed; and (k) smoke cigarettes, frequently drink alcohol and use illicit drugs. Adolescent problem gamblers began gambling early in life, gambling was part of their family norm, they had little academic success, they perceived themselves to be alienated from their family and community, they frequently use tobacco, alcohol and other drugs, they have a negative affect, and they engage in antisocial behaviors. Thus, youth problem gamblers exhibit considerable problems and excessive gambling is part of a larger constellation of psychological distress, family dysfunction, acting out, and deviance (Wynne et al., 1996).

Gupta and Derevensky (1998a) in testing a Jacobs' (1986) General Addictions Theory administered an assessment battery of instruments that measured variables believed to be related to problem gambling. Using a sample of 817 youth in grades 7, 9, and 11, with an age range of 12–17, they reported that problem and pathological gamblers were found to have abnormal physiological resting states, reported greater levels of dissociation, and reported higher rates of other addictive behaviors (including tobacco, alcohol, and drug use). There were some gender differences as well, with male problem gamblers being more excitable and female problem gamblers being more depressed. Gupta and Derevensky (1998a) suggested that males were found to fit Jacobs General Addictions Theory better than females.

This same research team (Gupta & Derevensky, 1998b) further found that males were more likely to be regular gamblers and pathological gamblers than females. The investigators reported that adolescent pathological gamblers were more likely to exhibit regular drug, alcohol, and cigarette use and were also more likely to report stealing and borrowing money to finance their gambling than non-pathological gamblers. They also reported that problem and pathological gamblers gambled for the excitement, to make money, escape problems, and alleviate depression. As such, problem and pathological gamblers tended to use gambling as a form of escape from daily problems and stress.

Vitaro, Ferland, Jacques, and Ladouceur (1998) analyzed data from a longitudinal study of 765 adolescent boys in Montreal. They reported that substance abuse was significantly related to gambling problems and that impulsivity was related to both gambling and substance abuse. Vitaro and his colleagues suggested that comorbid gambling and substance abuse problems may originate from impulse control deficits exhibited in childhood and early adolescence.

Vitaro, Brendgen, Ladouceur, and Tremblay (2001) further examined the Montreal longitudinal study database, this time examining gambling, substance use, and delinquency to determine the association between problem behaviors and to assess whether impulsivity, parental supervision, and deviant friends were predictive of the development of problem behaviors. Their results suggest that gambling frequency at age 16 was predictive of gambling problems one year later, and alcohol and drug at age 16 was modestly predictive of gambling frequency and gambling problems one year later. Delinquency at age 16 was not predictive of gambling frequency or problems one year later. Impulsivity and deviant friends in early adolescence were modestly predictive of gambling frequency, gambling problems, delinquency, and substance use. Parental supervision was negatively correlated with delinquency and substance use and showed no relation to gambling. The authors caution the reader that the explained variance was quite low with only 3% of the variance explaining gambling frequency and 5% explaining gambling problems. Gambling did not explain increases in delinquency or substance use from ages 16 to 17, however substance use at age 16 was found to be predictive of gambling at age 17. The authors tentatively interpreted their results as possibly indicating that substance use increased gambling through disinhibition and/or substance users needed money to acquire substances and used gambling for this purpose. Neither of these interpretations is particularly convincing in that the first interpretation assumes the adolescent was inebriated or high at the time they gambled, which is unknown, and the second interpretation assumes the person won more money than they lost, an unlikely scenario. The lack of a relationship between parental supervision and gambling was thought to indicate that gambling is an acceptable adolescent activity to many parents and therefore does not require parental intervention. This study yielded only partial support for the hypothesis that problem gambling is part of the same syndrome of problem behavior as delinquency and substance use. Both of these studies are rigorous in that they employed a longitudinal design and used a multivariate model of analysis.

   Although gambling and problem gambling is correlated with other risky behaviors, the question remains as to whether gambling precedes or follows other risky behaviors. Stinchfield and colleagues have reported on Minnesota Student Survey data that suggests that gambling precedes other risky behaviors such as tobacco, alcohol and other drug use. The 1992 Minnesota student survey data measuring gambling and other risky behaviors for 6th, 9th, and 12th grade public school students, are presented in Figures 1 and 2. It is interesting to note that frequent gambling is more prevalent among 6th graders, particularly boys, than frequent tobacco, alcohol or marijuana use, however, as boys age, more of them take up frequent tobacco and alcohol use such that by the time they are 12th graders frequent tobacco and alcohol use are equal to frequent gambling. Gambling appears at an early age in boys and appears to precede frequent tobacco and alcohol use. For a small percent of girls (5%), frequent gambling also appears at an early age, but is superceded by frequent tobacco and alcohol use by the 9th grade and is only a footnote by the 12th grade, as compared to tobacco use. In the larger scheme of risk behaviors, frequent gambling comes on the scene early for boys and remains a common risky behavior, whereas, a small percent of girls are involved in frequent gambling which is overshadowed by frequent tobacco and alcohol use.

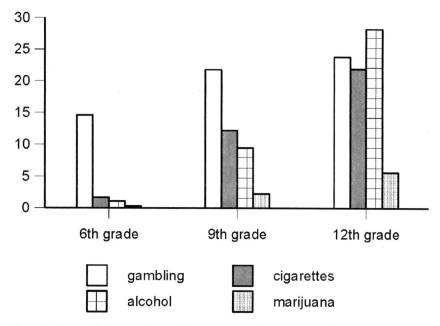

Figure 1. Rates of daily/weekly gambling, cigarette, alcohol, and marijuana use among 6th, 9th, and 12th grade boys. 1992 Minnesota Student Survey (N=122,700).

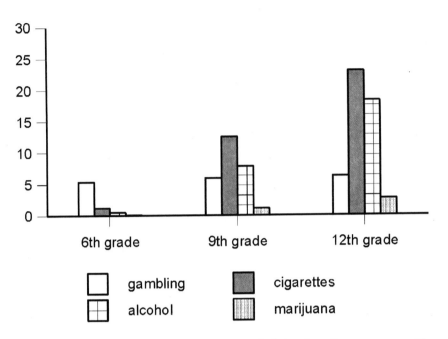

Figure 2. Rates of daily/weekly gambling, cigarette, alcohol, and marijuana use among 6th, 9th, and 12th grade girls. 1992 Minnesota Student Survey (N=122,700).

Winters, Stinchfield, Botzet, and Anderson (2002) followed a sample of 305 youth over an eight year period from adolescents to young adults in one of the few longitudinal studies in this field. They reported that a set of variables observed during adolescence led to problem gambling in young adulthood. Correlates of problem gambling in young adulthood, including early gambling onset, delinquency, gender, school problems, parental gambling history, and substance abuse were identified. These findings corroborate those reported earlier in cross-sectional studies and suggest a causal link between the correlates and problem gambling. This study highlights the importance of identifying risk and protective factors for prevention and the fact that prevention programs need to start early, prior to adolescence.

Derevensky, Gupta, and their colleagues at McGill University have done considerable work in the area of reviewing and organizing correlates of youth problem gambling. In summarizing the existing literature, they have suggested that problem and pathological gambling among adolescents has been shown to be related to delinquency and crime, the disruption of familial relationships and poor academic performance (Gupta & Derevensky, 1998a; Ladouceur & Mireault, 1988; Lesieur & Klein, 1987; Wynne et al, 1996). As well, youth pathological gamblers are reported to have high rates of suicide ideation and suicide attempts (Nower, Gupta, & Derevensky, 2003) and a number of mental health and behavioral problems (Hardoon, Gupta, & Derevensky, 2002). Every study of youth gambling has found that boys are more involved in gambling than girls both in terms of play and problem gambling behaviors (Fisher, 1992; Gupta & Derevensky, 1998a; Ladouceur, Dubé & Bujold, 1994; NORC, 1999; NRC, 1999; Stinchfield, 2000; Stinchfield, Cassuto, Winters & Latimer, 1997; Volberg, 1998; Wynne et al., 1996). Adolescent problem gamblers report that they start gambling at an earlier age (approximately 10 years of age) (Derevensky & Gupta, 2001; Gupta & Derevensky, 1997, 1998b; Wynne et al., 1996), have lower self-esteem (Gupta & Derevensky, 1998b) and report more depressive symptoms compared to social gamblers (Gupta & Derevensky, 1998a, 1998b; Kaufman et al., 2002). Adolescent problem gamblers are also found to score higher on scales measuring dissociation than non-gamblers (Gupta & Derevensky, 1998b), have poorer general coping skills (Nower, Gupta & Derevensky, 2000), and also report more major traumatic life events (Kaufman et al., 2002). A high proportion of youth with gambling problems report poor family connectedness and low perceived social support (Hardoon et al., 2002). Personality traits of adolescent pathological gamblers indicate that they are more excitable, extroverted, anxious, tend to have difficulty conforming to societal norms, and experience difficulties with self-discipline (Hardoon et al., 2002). Adolescents with severe gambling problems also exhibit higher scores on measures of state and trait anxiety (Gupta & Derevensky, 1998b; Ste-Marie, Gupta, & Derevensky, 2002) and are at increased risk for the development of other addictions such as alcohol and drug abuse (Gupta & Derevensky, 1998a, 1998b, 2001; Lesieur & Klein, 1987; Winters & Anderson, 2000).

The McGill group has begun to categorize the above correlates of youth problem gambling by conceptual domains (Hardoon & Derevensky, 2002) and have also attempted to classify which correlates represent risk factors for the development of problem gambling (Derevensky, Gupta, Dickson, Hardoon, & Deguire, 2003; Dickson, Derevensky, & Gupta, 2002; Gupta & Derevensky, 2000). Hardoon and Derevensky (2002) have identified a number of conceptual domains under which correlates can be organized. These conceptual domains include gender differences, physiological factors, personality factors, emotional/mental state, coping skills, problem behavior, gambling behavior, attitudes, familial factors, and accessability/availability. Dickson, Derevensky, and Gupta (2002) have taken the research to date on correlates of problem gambling and adapted it to fit Jessor's (1998) general model of adolescent risk behavior. This is helpful in that it organizes these risk factors into a theoretical framework that can be used to understand youth gambling problems and incorporated into the development of prevention programs. If the risk factors for the development of youth problem gambling are known, we can attempt to ameliorate these factors before problem gambling develops. Furthermore, if the protective factors that prevent youth from developing gambling problems and that lessen the severity of gambling problems are established, we can attempt to bolster these factors.

Conclusions and Future Research Directions

A number of demographic, behavioral, and psychosocial variables associated with youth problem gambling have consistently been reported in the literature. These factors include being male, antisocial behavior, tobacco use, alcohol use, drug use, parental/familial gambling, school failure and school problems, impulsivity, and peer deviance. These correlates associated with gambling may play a role in the development and/or maintenance of gambling behavior and problem gambling. The studies reviewed suggest that problem gambling may be part of a larger constellation of deviant behaviors that are mainly exhibited by males, including frequent alcohol use, tobacco use, drug use and antisocial behavior. It will be important to test the "birds of a feather flock together" hypothesis, that is, the idea that it is the same youth who are involved in multiple risky behaviors, such as cigarette smoking, alcohol use, drug use, etc. For example, Wynne et al. (1996) found that gambling often occurs in groups of youth and that these same youth are involved in other risk behaviors.

There is no one single *type* of youth problem gambler. There are problem gamblers among boys, girls, young, old, etc. It should be noted that the magnitude of these relationships may vary and that many variables obtain only weak correlations with problem gambling. Therefore, these weaker correlates are unlikely to have much practical utility for either predicting problem gambling or for prevention. For example, Vitaro et al. (2001) reported that the predictive variables in their study explained only 5% of the variance in gambling problems; however, these weaker correlates can make contributions to a larger multivariate regression model (Stinchfield, 2000).

Future research needs to focus on the identification of additional risk and protective factors and to confirm the strength of the existing factors to determine if they have practical utility for use in prevention programs. It should also be noted that the set of correlates discovered to date are a function of what investigators were looking for, and there may be other correlates, yet undiscovered, that are equally or more important.

While some variables have been identified as correlates of youth gambling, we do not know if these variables have a causal relationship to gambling or not. Therefore the next step is to conduct longitudinal research to address the question of causality and the order of onset of different problem behaviors as has been done by Vitaro et al. (2001) and Winters et al. (2002) with larger sample sizes using a prospective design.

Dickson, Derevensky, and Gupta's (2002) adaptation of the Jessor general model of adolescent risk behavior is helpful in that it can be used to develop prevention programs, however, the strength of association and practical utility of these variables for prevention still needs to be confirmed. Little is known about what youth problem gambling prevention efforts should be used to reduce youth problem gambling (Stinchfield & Winters, 1998; Winters & Stinchfield, 1999). Few youth problem gambling prevention programs exist and fewer still have been evaluated. Existing prevention programs do not necessarily incorporate empirically-based principles of risk and protective factors. The next steps are to develop an empirically-based youth problem gambling prevention model and evaluate the effectiveness of the program. Prevention programs should not be implemented unless and until they have proven to be effective in reducing or eliminating problem gambling. It is believed that prevention will be effective to the extent that it is based on empirical knowledge of risk and protective factors in youth. Therefore, prevention programs should have a two-pronged approach that includes both the reduction of risk factors and the enhancement of protective factors.

Finally, it is known that youth participate in gambling to varying degrees, from no gambling to excessive problem gambling, and therefore it is likely that youth involved in these different levels of gambling will require different prevention messages and approaches. That is, the prevention approach will need to be targeted to these specific types of youth and providing prevention messages/efforts that are appropriate for the different types of youth gamblers.

This is the first generation of youth to grow up in a society where gambling is a common part of their lives and it is our duty to provide youth with accurate information about gambling so that they may make healthy decisions about their own gambling and avoid excessive gambling. As our knowledge base grows our understanding of adolescent gambling behaviors will help achieve our goal of reducing harm.

References

Derevensky, J. L., & Gupta, R. (2001). Le problème de jeu touché les jeunes. *Psychologie Québec, 18*, 23–27.

Derevensky, J. L., Gupta, R., Dickson, L., Hardoon, K., & Deguire, A. (2003). Understanding youth gambling problems: A conceptual framework. In D. Romer (Ed.), *Reducing adolescent risk: Toward an integrated approach* (pp. 240–246). Beverly Hills, CA: Sage Publications.

Dickson, L. M., Derevensky, J. L., & Gupta, R. (2002). The prevention of gambling problems in youth: A conceptual framework. *Journal of Gambling Studies, 18*, 97–159.

Fisher, S. (1992). Measuring pathological gambling in children: The case of fruit machines in the UK. *Journal of Gambling Studies, 8*, 263–285.

Gupta, R., & Derevensky, J. L. (1997). Familial and social influences on juvenile gambling behavior. *Journal of Gambling Studies, 13*, 179–192.

Gupta, R. & Derevensky, J. L. (1998a). An empirical examination of Jacobs' General Theory of Addictions: Do adolescent gamblers fit the theory? *Journal of Gambling Studies, 14*, 17–49.

Gupta, R. & Derevensky, J. (1998b). Adolescent gambling behavior: A prevalence study and examination of the correlates associated with problem gambling. *Journal of Gambling Studies, 14*, 319–345.

Gupta, R., & Derevensky, J. L. (2000). Adolescents with gambling problems: From research to treatment. *Journal of Gambling Studies, 16*, 315–342.

Hardoon, K. K. & Derevensky, J. L. (2002). Child and adolescent gambling behavior: Current knowledge. *Clinical Child Psychology and Psychiatry, 7*, 263–281.

Hardoon, K. K., Gupta, R. & Derevensky, J. (2002, June). *An examination of the influence of emotional and conduct problems upon adolescent gambling problems.* Paper presented at the annual meeting of the National Council on Problem Gambling, Dallas.

Jacobs, D. F. (1989). Illegal and undocumented: A review of teenage gamblers in America. In H. J. Shaffer, S. A. Stein, B. Gambino, & T. N. Cummings (Eds.), *Compulsive gambling: Theory, research and practice* (pp. 249–292). Lexington, MA: Lexington Books.

Jacobs, D. F. (1993). A review of juvenile gambling in the United States. In W. R. Eadington and J. A. Cornelius (Eds.) *Gambling behavior and problem gambling* (pp. 431–441). Reno, NV: University of Nevada Press.

Jacobs, D. F. (2000). Juvenile gambling in North America: An analysis of long term trends and future prospects. *Journal of Gambling Studies, 16*, 119–152.

Jessor, R. (1998). New perspectives on adolescent risk behavior. In R. Jessor (Ed.), *New perspectives on adolescent risk behavior.* Cambridge, UK: Cambridge University Press.

Kaufman, F., Derevensky, J., & Gupta, R. (2002, June). The relationship between life stresses, coping styles and gambling behavior among adolescents. Poster presented at the annual meeting of the National Council on Problem Gambling, Dallas TX.

Ladouceur, R., Dubé, D., & Bujold, A. (1994). Gambling among primary school students. *Journal of Gambling Studies, 10*, 363–370.

Ladouceur, R. & Mireault, C. (1988). Gambling behaviors among high school students in the Quebec area. *Journal of Gambling Behavior, 4*, 3–12.

Latimer, W. W., Newcomb, M., Winters, K. C., & Stinchfield, R. D. (2000). Adolescent substance abuse treatment outcome: The role of substance abuse problem severity, psychosocial, and treatment factors. *Journal of Consulting and Clinical Psychology, 68*, 684–696.

Lesieur, H. R. & Klein, R. (1987). Pathological gambling among high school students. *Addictive Behaviors, 12*, 129–135.

Luthar, S. S., Cicchetti, D., & Becker, B. (2000). The construct of resilience: A critical evaluation and guidelines for future work. *Child Development, 71*, 543–562.

National Opinion Research Center. (1999). *Gambling impact and behavior study: Report to the National Gambling Impact Study Commission.* Chicago, IL: National Opinion Research Center at the University of Chicago.

National Research Council (1999). *Pathological gambling: A critical review.* National Academy Press, Washington, D.C.

Nower, L., Gupta, R., & Derevensky, J. (2000, June). *Taking risks: A comparison of impulsivity and sensation seeking among youth gamblers.* Paper presented at the 11th International Conference on Gambling and Risk-Taking, Las Vegas, NV.

Nower, L., Gupta, R., & Derevensky, J. (2003, June). *Depression and suicidality among youth gamblers: An examination of comparative data.* Paper presented at the annual meeting of the National Council on Problem Gambling, Louisville, KY.

Shaffer, H. J., & Hall, M. N. (1996). Estimating the prevalence of adolescent gambling disorders: A quantitative synthesis and guide toward standard gambling nomenclature. *Journal of Gambling Studies, 12,* 193–214.

Ste-Marie, C., Gupta, R. & Derevensky, J. (2002). Anxiety and social stress related to adolescent gambling behavior. *International Journal of Gambling Studies, 2,* 123–141.

Stinchfield, R. (2000). Gambling and correlates of gambling among Minnesota public school students. *Journal of Gambling Studies, 16,* 153–173.

Stinchfield, R. (2001). A Comparison of Gambling among Minnesota Public School Students in 1992, 1995 and 1998. *Journal of Gambling Studies, 17,* 273–296.

Stinchfield, R. (2002). Youth Gambling: How Big a Problem? *Psychiatric Annals, 32,* 197–202.

Stinchfield, R., Cassuto, N., Winters, K., & Latimer, W. (1997). Prevalence of Gambling among Minnesota Public School Students in 1992 and 1995. *Journal of Gambling Studies, 13,* 25–48.

Stinchfield, R. & Winters, K. C. (1998). Gambling and problem gambling among youth. *Annals of the American Academy of Political and Social Science, 556,* 172–185.

Vitaro, F., Brendgen, M., Ladouceur, R., & Tremblay, R. E. (2001). Gambling, delinquency, and drug use during adolescence: Mutual influences and common risk factors. *Journal of Gambling Studies, 17,* 171–190.

Vitaro, F., Ferland, F., Jacques, C., & Ladouceur, R. (1998). Gambling, substance use, and impulsivity during adolescence. *Psychology of Addictive Behaviors, 12,* 185–194.

Volberg, R. (1993). *Gambling and problem gambling among adolescents in Washington State.* Albany, NY: Gemini Research.

Volberg, R. A. (1998). *Gambling and problem gambling among adolescents in New York.* Report to the New York Council on Problem Gambling. Albany, NY: New York Council on Problem Gambling.

Wallisch, L. (1993). *Gambling in Texas: 1992 Texas survey of adolescent gambling behavior.* Austin, TX: Texas Commission on Alcohol and Drug Abuse.

Wallisch, L. (1996). *Gambling in Texas: 1995 Surveys of adult and adolescent gambling behavior.* Austin TX: Texas Commission on Alcohol and Drug Abuse.

Winters, K. C., & Anderson, N. (2000). Gambling involvement and drug use among adolescents. *Journal of Gambling Studies, 16,* 175–198.

Winters, K. C., & Stinchfield, R. (1999). Adolescent gambling in Minnesota. *The Prevention Researcher, 6,* 5–8.

Winters, K. C., Stinchfield, R. D., Botzet, A., & Anderson, N. (2002). A prospective study of youth gambling behaviors. *Psychology of Addictive Behaviors, 16,* 3–9.

Winters, K. C., Stinchfield, R., & Fulkerson, J. (1993). Patterns and characteristics of adolescent gambling. *Journal of Gambling Studies, 9,* 371–386.

Wynne, H., Smith, G., & Jacobs, D. (1996). *Adolescent gambling and problem gambling in Alberta.* Edmonton, Alberta: Alberta Alcohol and Drug Abuse Commission.

Chapter 3

Gambling, Depression, and Suicidality in Adolescents

Jennifer Langhinrichsen-Rohling, Ph.D.

Over the past twenty years, prevalence studies have repeatedly shown that many adolescents gamble and that the occurrence of pathological gambling disorders in this age group is considerable (Shaffer & Hall, 1996, Stinchfield & Winters, 1998). More recently, researchers have focused on developing theories to explain why some youth manage to gamble without experiencing negative consequences or dependency, while others develop serious gambling problems (Gupta & Derevensky, 1998; Moore & Ohtsuka, 1997). Some of the central theories of pathological gambling have been adapted from the addictions field under the premise that excessive gambling can best be understood as another type of addictive behavior (Jacobs, 1989). According to Winters and Anderson (2000) three distinct models have been proposed, each of which assumes some commonality between gambling and addiction. In one model, gambling and substance use disorders emerge from the same risk factors. In a second model, gambling evolves out of substance use disorders. In a third model, gambling and substance use disorders both evolve out of conduct disorders. Evidence cited to support the commonality of pathological gambling with other addictions includes studies of the physiological correlates of gambling, data on withdrawal symptoms experienced by gamblers, and the plethora of investigations that have documented comorbidity between gambling disorders and other drug and alcohol dependencies (Gupta & Derevensky, 1998; Winters & Anderson, 2000).

41

The purpose of the current chapter is to consider the associations between gambling and depression as predicted from the theories of addiction, to summarize the findings of empirical studies examining associations between gambling and depression in adolescents, to consider empirical evidence associating depression with suicidality, to present the empirical evidence and theories suggesting a relationship between gambling and suicidality, and to derive an integrative summary of the relations among gambling, depression, and suicidality in adolescents. Directions for future work are also presented.

Addiction Theories Associating Gambling and Depression

In the latter part of the 1980s, Jacobs proposed a *General Theory of Addictions*, which is predicated on a common process for the addictions framework (Jacobs, 1986; 1989). According to Jacobs (1989), all addictions are a "dependent state acquired over time by a predisposed person in an attempt to relieve a chronic stress condition" (p. 35). Jacobs identified two factors as predispositions. The first factor is an under-active or over-active physiological resting state that leaves the individual chronically under- or over-aroused. For the under-aroused individual, it is suggested that gambling is a stimulating activity that provides relief from an underlying boredom and/or possible depression. In contrast, the over-aroused individual is more likely to develop an addiction to alcohol or marijuana, rather than gambling, because these two substances have depressant effects and serve to calm the anxious individual.

The second predisposing factor includes psychological characteristics of the individual such as low self-esteem and/or feelings of inferiority. Jacobs (1989) hypothesized that both sets of predisposing factors had to be present and exerting their effects in a conducive environment in order for the individual to generate and maintain an addiction. For example, an individual who has feelings of inferiority but a normal arousal level would not be expected to become an addict, nor would the over-aroused individual with an adequate self-esteem. Thus, according to his theory, both the presence of an addiction and the choice of addictive substance should be predictable by the number and type of predisposing factors exhibited by the individual.

Jacobs' (1989) assertion that gambling addiction is most likely to occur in depressed, bored, under-aroused individuals with low self-esteem is of key importance. According to this model, depression exists prior to the onset of the gambling disorder. Gambling may even be viewed as a strategy for coping with depression or a way to minimize these symptoms (Beaudoin & Cox, 1999). This stands in contrast to other theories about the relationship between gambling and depression and/or suicidality. For example, Winters and Anderson (2000) raise the issue of whether depression and suicidality can be considered consequences of pathological gambling, or risk factors for the development of a gambling problem. Blaszczynski and Farrell (1998) also argue that pathological gamblers are more likely to experience depression and suicidal behavior as a result of the psychosocial stressors they experience in conjunction with their excessive gambling rather than viewing depression and suicidality as risk factors for the pathological gambling.

Empirical Evidence for the Association Between Gambling and Depression in Adolescents

To date, the majority of research assessing the associations between gambling and depression has focused on adults and has used cross-sectional methodology. Use of cross-sectional methodology makes it much more difficult to answer the question of whether depression is typically a risk factor for, or a consequence of, pathological gambling. However, since longitudinal investigations are often difficult to undertake and more costly to implement than cross-sectional designs, researchers have recently argued that structured clinical interviews with time courses, could be used to further our understanding of the temporal relationship between depression and gambling (Beaudoin & Cox, 1999).

Nonetheless, the existing empirical research findings generally support the notion that there is a significant association, or comorbidity, between depression and gambling in adults. For example, an early study reported that 78% of pathological gamblers who were inpatients received a diagnosis of Major Depressive Disorder (McCormick, Russo, Rameriz, & Taber, 1984). Several other studies published in the late 1980s and early 1990s reported similar findings (e.g., Blaszczynski, McConaghy, & Frankova, 1990; Linden, Pope, & Jonas, 1986; Torne & Konstanty, 1992). More recently, as reported in Table 1, increased reports of depressive symptoms were found in 30 Gamblers Anonymous (GA) adults when compared to 30 controls from the community (Getty, Watson, & Frisch, 2000). Similarly, Beaudoin and Cox (1999) reported the majority of adults seeking treatment for gambling ($n = 57$) indicated that they gambled to relieve dysphoria.

However, more recently published research has also found the association between gambling and depression to be less robust than initially proposed. For example, Cunningham-Williams, Cottler, Compton, Spitznagel, and Ben-Abdallah (2000) recruited 990 adults from drug treatment settings and a community sample. They reported non-significant associations between

Table 1. Summary of recent empirical studies of the association between gambling and depression in adults and adolescents

		Adults		
Sample	Sample Characteristics	Measures	Findings	Authors
Adults seeking treatment for gambling	$N = 57$	Self-report measure	Majority reported that they gambled to relieve dysphoria	Beaudoin & Cox (1999)
Adult Community Recruits	$N = 990$ adults Recruited from drug treatment settings and community	DIS—Diagnostic Interview Schedule	Nonsignificant associations gambling and depression, 59% of the cases pathological gambling preceded the depression, 18% concurrent, 23% gambling problem after MDD	Cunningham-Williams, Cottler, Compton, Spitznagel, & Ben-Abdallah (2000)
Adult GA members and matched controls	GA adults ($N = 30$; 20 males) Matched controls ($N = 30$)	Beck Depression Inventory SOGS	GA members reported significantly more depression	Getty, Watson, & Frisch (2000)
Community older adults and Gambling patrons	Community sample ($N = 224$) Gambling patrons ($N = 91$) Mail-in Form	Geriatric Depression Scale Short Form SOGS-R	No significant between group differences in depression	McNeilly & Burke (2000)
Male undergraduates in fraternities	$N = 93$	SOGS CES-D	Gambling and depression were positively correlated	Murtha (2001)
Pathological gamblers and matched controls in Italy	$N = 48$ male and female gamblers $N = 48$ matched controls	SOGS Symptom Rating Scale	Higher depression scores in pathological gamblers than in controls	Savron, Pitti, DeLuca, & Guerreschi (2001)
Convenience sample of adults playing video poker in Victoria, BC	$N = 163$ women	ICOG WCCL-R coping	Loss of control over gambling associated with emotion focused	Scannell, Quirk, Smith, Maddern, & Dickerson (2000)

Sample	Sample Characteristics	Measures	Findings	Authors
American Indian adults living on or near a reservation	$N = 119$ American Indians $N = 102$ Non-Indian controls	Self-report measures DSM-III-R pathological gambling section	Depression related to pathological and problematic gambling in American Indian adults	Zitzow (1996)
Adolescents				
Sample	Sample Characteristics	Measures	Findings	Authors
Female children, adolescents and adults from Spain	$N = 308$	SOGS-RA BDI or CDI	54.6% of participants at-risk for gambling problems; 37.5% of probable pathological gamblers had moderate or severe depression	Arbinaga (2000b)
Adolescents whose parents belonged to Parents of Young Gamblers	$N = 19$	Self-report	11/19 young gamblers reported feeling fed-up /sad /depressed before gambling	Griffiths (1993)
High School students	$N = 817$	Self-report DSM-IV-J	Pathological gamblers were significantly more likely to report that they gambled to relieve depression or to escape problems	Gupta & Derevensky (1997)
High School students	$N = 817$	RADS DSM-IV-J	Pathological gamblers had higher rates of depression	Gupta & Derevensky (1998)
High School students from three states	$N = 1846$	CES-D self-report SOGS-RA	Pathological gamblers reported more depression than all other adolescents, $F = 7.54, p = .0001$	Langhinrichsen-Rohling, Rohling, Rohde, & Seeley (2004)
Telephone survey of older adolescents	$N = 702$	SOGS-RA Self-report	Gambling groups not differentiated on question about personal satisfaction	Winters, Stinchfield, & Fulkerson (1993)

diagnoses of pathological gambling and major depressive disorder. Of interest, however, is their finding that the majority of individuals with both a gambling and DSM-III-R depression diagnosis indicated through self-report data that their gambling problem occurred prior to the development of the depressive diagnosis. These findings were obtained through structured clinical interviews and are in contrast to Jacobs' (1986) contention that depressive symptoms function primarily as a risk factor for pathological gambling. McNeilly and Burke (2000) also failed to find significant associations between gambling and depressive disorders in their study of elderly gambling patrons who were matched to community controls. Thus, it appears that the strength of the association between depressed mood and gambling in adults may be partially a function of sample characteristics, methodology, operational definitions of depression and dysphoria, and measurement instruments used to assess gambling severity.

The extent to which there is an association between depression and pathological gambling has only recently been investigated in adolescents. Much of this work is summarized in Table 1. In one important test of the model, Gupta and Derevensky (1998) collected cross-sectional data from 817 adolescents specifically to test Jacobs' (1986) model. Consistent with their expectation, they found that problem and pathological gamblers reported significantly more depressive symptoms than individuals in their other three groups (non-gamblers, occasional gamblers, and regular gamblers). Specifically, the rate of clinical depression (using a cut score of 77 or greater on the Reynolds Adolescent Depression Scale) was 23% for the problem gambling group, compared to rates of about 10% for the other three groups (Gupta & Derevensky, 1998). This is especially noteworthy given that the majority of pathological gamblers were male and that males generally tend to have lower depression scores than females during adolescence. However, Gupta and Derevensky (1998) indicated that only 13.2% of the pathological adolescent gamblers reported that they gambled to alleviate dysphoria. One possible interpretation of this finding might be that, for most problematic adolescent gamblers, the gambling disorder preceded the depressive symptoms rather than developed as a coping mechanism. However, it might be that pathological adolescent gamblers have multiple factors underlying their addiction (including, but not limited to depression) as these data do not fully support the notion that gambling is an antidepressant for youth. It is also plausible that there are different subtypes of problem gamblers and that differences among predisposing factors may be an important way of differentiating among subtypes (see Nower & Blaszczynski, in this volume).

Another recent test of the association between adolescent gambling and depression used a sample of 1,846 high school students from three states (Langhinrichsen-Rohling, Rohde, Seeley, & Rohling, 2004). Similar to Gupta and Derevensky's (1998) results, adolescents with pathological gambling problems reported more symptoms of depressed mood on the Center for Epidemiology Scale for Depression (CES-D) than other adolescents (from non gamblers to at-risk gamblers). Whether the depressive symptoms occurred before or after the gambling problems was not ascertained in their cross-sectional design (Langhinrichsen-Rohling et al., 2004). Clearly, the need for more longitudinal studies of adolescent gambling and the impact of depression remains.

Theories Associating Depression and Suicidality

Research documenting an association between depression and suicidality is widespread. For example, according to the DSM-IV-TR (American Psychiatric Association, 2000), up to 15% of individuals with severe and recurrent Major Depressive Disorder eventually complete suicide. Conversely, researchers estimate that about half of those who die as a result of suicide do so during the recovery phase of a depressive episode (Isacsson & Rich, 1997). Common biological mechanisms have been considered as an explanation for these findings. For example, low serotonin levels have been shown to increase the risk of depression, as well as enhance the probability of engaging in impulsive and/or violent behavior, including suicide (Arango & Underwood, 1997). In a separate line of research, other researchers have reported that the cognitive state of hopelessness is another strong predictor of suicidal behavior (Beck, 1986). Specifically, the NIMH Collaborative Depression study proposed three affective disorder symptom clusters as important influences on the increased rate of suicide found in individuals with affective disorders. They include impulsivity/aggression, hopelessness, and agitation/panic (Fawcett, Busch, Jacobs, Kravitz, & Fogg, 1997).

Suicide has also been associated with other mood disorders besides major depression as 10–15% of individuals with bipolar disorders also die by suicide (American Psychiatric Association, 2000). Furthermore, diagnoses of schizophrenia, anxiety, and/or certain personality disorders also enhance the risk of suicidal behavior (Tanney, 2000). Of particular importance is evidence that the co-occurrence of addictive behaviors (e.g., alcohol and drug abuse) and depression significantly enhance the risk of suicidal behavior (Cornelius et al., 1995; Driessen & Veltrup, 1998). Certainly, any theory of the association between gambling and suicidality should account for these additional psychological, biological, and cognitive correlates of suicidal behavior.

Empirical Evidence for the Association
Between Gambling and Suicidal Behavior

The majority of empirical work considering whether gambling is related to suicidal behavior has occurred with adults. Samples have included problem gamblers seeking treatment, those attending Gamblers Anonymous, general adult volunteers, and comparison groups of suicide attempters and completers. For example, Blaszczynski and Farrell (1998) conducted psychological autopsies of 44 individuals who had a well-established connection between suicide and gambling. These individuals were also found to have high rates of comorbid depression, relationship problems, and substantial gambling-related debt. Recent empirical studies of the co-occurrence between gambling disorders and suicidality are presented in Table 2. When suicidal data are obtained from adults with heavy gambling problems or from epidemiological studies of communities with increased gambling, significant associations between gambling and suicidality are often obtained (e.g., Campbell, Simmons, & Lester, 1998; Frank, Lester, & Wexler, 1991; Phillips, Welty, & Smith, 1997).

However, it is also important to note that nonsignificant associations between gambling and suicidality have been obtained in several recently obtained community samples (Cunningham-Williams et al., 2000) and when comparing the prevalence of gambling problems in individuals identified as suicide completers, suicide attempters, or non-psychiatric controls (Holmes, Mateczun, Lall, & Wilcove, 1998). One interpretation of these mixed results is that suicidal ideation and behavior is not purely a function of increased gambling. Rather, it may be a consequence of multiple variables associated with pathological gambling in more severely disordered samples (e.g., being in treatment, relationship difficulties, significant financial debt, comorbid depression).

Only a few studies have focused on whether gambling is associated with suicidal behavior in adolescents with the majority of this research being relatively recent. As shown in Table 2, the typical research strategy has been to assess gambling and suicidal behavior concurrently in large samples of school age children. Using this strategy allows only three types of suicidal behavior to be assessed: suicide proneness, suicidal ideation, and suicide attempts. Suicide proneness has been defined as a person's propensity at a given point in time to engage in suicidal behavior (Rohde, Seeley, Langhinrichsen-Rohling, & Rohling, 2003). This construct has been measured in adolescents with the Life Attitudes Schedule–Short Form (LAS-SF; Rohde, Lewinsohn, Seeley, & Langhinrichsen-Rohling, 1996). LAS-SF scores have been shown to be associated with a history of past suicide attempts (Rohde et al., 2003). Generally, with the exception of Canadian

Table 2. Summary of recent empirical studies of the association between gambling and suicidality in adults (1995–present) and adolescents

Sample	Sample Characteristics	Measures	Findings	Authors
		Adults		
Adults seeking treatment for gambling	$N = 57$	Self-report measure	50% reported suicide ideation 16% reported suicide attempts	Beaudoin & Cox (1999)
Collected Data on Adult Gambling in Parishes from State Department	$N = 64$ Louisiana Parishes	State collected Data	Increases in suicide rate associated with increases in money spent on lottery	Campbell, Simmons, & Lester (1998)
Adult community recruits	$N = 990$ adults	DIS	Nonsignificant associations gambling and thoughts of death or suicidality	Cunningham-Williams, Cottler, Compton, Spitznagel, & Ben-Abdallah (2000)
Suicide attempters, completers, and a non-psychiatric control group of active-duty U.S. Marines	$N = 172$ attempters $N = 22$ completers $N = 384$ non-psychiatric	Self-report and a review of military records	Discriminant function analysis indicated that no history of gambling behavior significantly predicted increased suicide risk	Holmes, Mateczun, Lall, & Wilcove (1998)
Analyzed suicide rate changes in three U.S. geographic regions	Las Vegas, Reno, and Atlantic City	Used computerized mortality data from the US National Center for Health Statistics (1969–1991)	Gambling venue cities have increased suicide rates for both residents and visitors	Phillips, Welty, & Smith (1997)

Table 2. Summary of recent empirical studies of the association between gambling and suicidality in adults (1995–present) and adolescents (*continued*)

Adolescents

Sample	Sample Characteristics	Measures	Findings	Authors
Spanish children and adolescents	N = 130 aged 8 to 17	Self-report of suicidal thoughts	42.9% of pathological gamblers have considered suicide	Arbinaga (2000a)
Dutch Secondary School Children	N = 6084 adolescents aged 16–19	Self-report of suicide attempt	Gamblers odds of a suicide attempt were significantly elevated (1.9)	Garnefski & deWilde (1998)
High School Students	N = 817 aged 12–17	Self-report of suicide ideation	Significant differences in suicide ideation across groups, increasing by level of gambling involvement	Gupta & Derevensky (1998)
Canadian youth in Jr. and Sr. High School	N = 3,426 12–18 year olds	Self-report of suicide ideation and attempts	Significant differences in suicide ideation and suicide attempts across groups. 25% of pathological gamblers attempted suicide versus 7.8% of nonproblem gamblers	Ladouceur, Boudreault, Jacques, &Vitaro (1999)
High School students from three states	N = 1846	Life Attitudes Schedule Self-report of suicide attempt	Gambling increases related to increases in suicidal behavior (F = 33.35, p = .000). Gambling increases also related to increases in suicide attempts (F = 4.36, p = .002)	Langhinrichsen-Rohling, Rohling, Rohde, & Seeley (2004)
Canadian youth attending CEGEP's	N = 1,339 youth aged 17–21	Self-report of suicide ideation and attempts	No significant differences in rates of suicide ideation or attempts across gambling groups	Nower, Gupta, Blaszczynski, & Derevensky (in press)

youth, the studies summarized in Table 2 reveal that the rates of suicide attempts (Garnefski & deWilde, 1998; Langhinrichsen-Rohling et al., 2004), suicide ideation (Arbinaga, 2000a; Gupta & Derevensky, 1998), and suicide proneness as defined by the LAS-SF (Langhinrichsen-Rohling et al., 2001) are higher in adolescent pathological gamblers than in other groups of adolescents. These results are noteworthy for their gender paradox. While pathological gambling is primarily a male phenomenon, these males are showing higher rates of depression, suicide ideation, and suicide attempts; typical patterns which have been associated with females.

An Integrated Model of the Associations Between Gambling and Depression and Suicidal Behavior in Adolescents

In contrast to some models of adult behavior, which suggests that men and women may engage in a variety of risky or addictive behaviors in order to ameliorate negative experiences including depression and loneliness, some researchers have argued that youth engage in risk behaviors primarily because of their perceived benefits (e.g., pleasure, peer approval, and/or relaxation) (Moore & Ohtsuka, 1997). Accordingly, adolescents often deny or fail to consider the health-diminishing aspects or potential costs of their risk behavior. Extending this line of reasoning, it is possible that different models may be required for adolescents to explain the associations among depression, suicidal behavior, and gambling. Alternative models may be required because adolescents may be less likely to consider the potential negative outcomes to their risk behavior than adults. Furthermore, as previously noted, in youth, depression, dysphoric affect and suicidality may be more likely to be consequences of excessive gambling than a risk factor for it.

One plausible model that integrates findings on the associations among gambling, depression, and suicidal behavior in adolescents is presented in Figure 1. As proposed, this model may be more applicable for males. Further research on the pathways among depression, suicidality, and pathological gambling in females is needed.

According to this model, adolescent males who are impulsive and integrated into a deviant peer group are more likely to experiment with gambling. Early experimentation for these youth is likely to be centered around card playing and betting on sports or games of skill. Only a subset of these individuals will become problematic or pathological gamblers. According to this model, those individuals are more likely to have experienced an early "big win" to have a relatively large amount of discretionary money accessible, and live in a family where gambling is acceptable, parents abuse

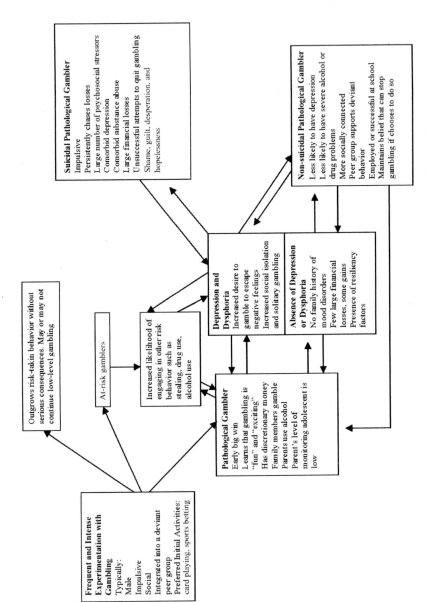

Figure 1. An Integrated Model of the Associations Among Gambling, Depression, and Suicidality in Adolescents.

alcohol, and the level of parental monitoring of adolescent social activities is relatively low. Problematic and pathological adolescent gamblers also have an increased probability of becoming involved in other risky activities. In fact, for some individuals, excessive gambling in early adolescence may be a gateway to other dangerous and deviant behaviors.

In addition, the model proposes that continued pathological gambling, with its associated psychosocial stressors, is likely to increase the probability of the onset of depression and/or increased dysphoric affect. It is likely that further gambling would be undertaken by the individual in an effort to escape their dysphoric mood state. This would be expected to be particularly likely for individuals who experience dissociation while gambling and for individuals who have access to solitary gambling pursuits (i.e., slot machines, lottery, electronic gambling machines).

Finally, in keeping with Blaszczynski and Farrell's (1998) assertions that gambling is likely to be related to suicide, the model also proposes that only a subset of pathological adolescent gamblers will engage in suicidal behavior. Most pathological gamblers who become suicidal will also be experiencing dysphoric affect and/or a clinical diagnosis of depression. They are likely to be highly impulsive. Furthermore, according to the model, pathological gamblers who persistently chase their losses are most likely to become suicidal. This eventually occurs because they expose themselves repeatedly to riskier situations and the probability of greater financial problems as chasing their losses results in greater debt. This, subsequently, will increase the number of psychosocial stressors faced by the gambler (e.g., shame at potential discovery, familial, financial, and relationship stress, and potential absenteeism or reduced performance at work or school). Mounting psychosocial stressors should lead to increased dysphoria, desperation, shame, and hopelessness, which all should, in turn, increase the likelihood of suicidal behavior. A full test of this model, however, awaits future research.

Directions for Future Research

Overall, several directions for future research are proposed:

1. There is a need for prospective, longitudinal studies of the development of gambling disorders, depression, and suicidal behavior in adolescents. Understanding the co-occurrence and time course of these behaviors in their developmental context will be essential for prevention and intervention efforts.
2. The same processes may not explain the occurrence of addiction in adolescents and the elderly, in males and in females, or in the affluent versus those living in poverty. Models of the associations

among gambling, depression, and suicidality may also need to be age, culture, and gender-specific. Future work will be needed to determine the consistency of the proposed model across different subgroups.

3. Dysphoric affect is not the same as depression. Negative affect and dysphoria may be mood states that are likely to precipitate the act of gambling for some individuals. However, it is argued that clinical depression typically occurs primarily as a consequence of pathological gambling and its related psychosocial stressors, rather than a risk factor for excessive gambling in youth, which may not be the case for dysphoric affect.

4. Furthermore, adolescents may gamble initially because of the perceived benefits of gambling, whereas, adults may experiment with gambling to ameliorate their negative mood states. Researchers should consider both the positive and negative motivations for engaging in gambling behavior, across the life cycle and amongst different cultural groups.

5. There is still a need to specify the negative consequences that are directly associated with gambling problems and those attributable to other co-occurring addictive behaviors or psychopathology (Winters & Anderson, 2000). Furthermore, since evidence suggests that the probability of suicide attempt increases as the number of risky behaviors engaged in increases (Garnefski & deWilde, 1998), it is important to study a variety of risky behaviors across time. Use of a multi-modal, multi-risk factor, multi-informant, multi-subgroup research design is likely to enhance our understanding of the interrelationships among gambling, depression, and suicidality in youth. Consistent with this reasoning, Jessor (1993, 1998) articulates a conceptual framework for adolescent risk behaviors that includes risk and protective factors, risk behaviors, and risk outcomes. It is likely that continued use of complex, conceptual, and multi-model research strategies will best inform both prevention and intervention efforts, while providing multiple targets by which to ascertain the success of clinical efforts.

References

American Psychiatric Association. (2000). *Diagnostic and statistical manual of mental disorders, Fourth Edition, Text Revision.* Washington, D.C., American Psychiatric Association.

Arango, V., & Underwood, M. D. (1997). Serotonin chemistry in the brain of suicide victims. In R. W. Maris, M. M. Silverman, & S. S. Canetton (Eds.), *Review of suicidology.* New York: Guilford.

Arbinaga, F. (2000a). Descriptive study of pathological gambling in underage students: Sociodemographic characteristics, use of drugs, and depression. *Adicciones, 12,* 493–505.

Arbinaga, F. (2000b). Sociodemographic characteristics, use of drugs, depression, and pathological gambling in a group of women from Punta Umbria: A descriptive study. *Anales de Psicologia, 16,* 123–132.

Beaudoin, C. M., & Cox, B. J. (1999). Characteristics of problem gambling in a Canadian context: A preliminary study using a DSM-IV based questionnaire. *Canadian Journal of Psychiatry, 44,* 483–487.

Beck, A. T. (1986). Hopelessness as a predictor of eventual suicide. *Annals of the New York Academy of Sciences, 487,* 90–96.

Blaszczynski, A. P., & Farrell, E. (1998). A case series of 44 completed gambling related suicides. *Journal of Gambling Studies, 14,* 93–109.

Blaszczynski, A. P., McConaghy, N., & Frankova, A. (1990). Boredom proneness in pathological gambling. *Psychological Reports, 67,* 35–42.

Campbell, F., Simmons, C., & Lester, D. (1998–99). The impact of gambling on suicidal behavior in Louisiana. *Omega, 38,* 235–239.

Cornelius, J. R., Salloum, I. M., Mezzich, J., Cornelius, Jr., M.D., Fabrega, H., Ehler, J. G., Ulrich, R. F., Thase, M. E., & Mann, J. J. (1995). Disproportionate suicidality in patients with comorbid major depression and alcoholism. *American Journal of Psychiatry, 152,* 358–364.

Cunningham-Williams, R. M., Cottler, L. B., Compton, W. M., Spitznagel, E. L., & Ben-Abdallah, A. (2000). Problem gambling and comorbid psychiatric and substance use disorders among drug users recruited from drug treatment and community settings. *Journal of Gambling Studies, 16,* 347–376.

Driessen, M., & Veltrup, C. (1998). Psychiatric co-morbidity, suicidal behavior, and suicidal ideation in alcoholics seeking treatment. *Addiction, 93,* 889–896.

Fawcett, J., Busch, K., Jacobs, D., Kravitz, H., & Fogg, L. F. (1997). Suicide: A four-pathway clinical biochemical model. In D. Stoff & J. J. Mann (Eds.), *The Neurology of suicide–From the bench to the clinic* (pp. 288–301). New York: New York Academy of Sciences.

Frank, M., Lester, D., & Wexler, A. (1991). Suicidal behavior among members of Gamblers Anonymous. *Journal of Gambling Studies, 7,* 249–254.

Garnefski, N., & deWilde, E. J. (1998). Addiction-risk behaviors and suicide attempts in adolescents. *Journal of Adolescence, 21,* 135–142.

Getty, H. A., Watson, J., & Frisch, G. R. (2000). A comparison of depression and styles of coping in male and female GA members and controls. *Journal of Gambling Studies, 16,* 377–391.

Gupta, R., & Derevensky, J. L. (1997). Adolescent gambling behavior: A prevalence study and examination of the correlates associated with problem gambling. *Journal of Gambling Studies, 14,* 319–345.

Gupta, R., & Derevensky, J. L. (1998). An empirical examination of Jacobs' General Theory of Addictions: Do adolescent gamblers fit the theory? *Journal of Gambling Studies, 14,* 17–49.

Griffiths, M.D. (1993). Factors in problem adolescent fruit machine gambling. *Journal of Gambling Studies, 9,* 31–45.

Holmes, E. K., Mateczun, J. M., Lall, R., & Wilcove, G. L. (1998). *Psychological Reports, 83,* 3–11.

Isacsson, G., & Rich, C. L. (1997). Depression, antidepressants, and suicide: Pharmacoepidemiological evidence for suicide prevention. In R. W. Maris, M. M. Silverman, & S. S. Canetton (Eds.). *Review of suicidology.* New York: Guilford.

Jacobs, D. F. (1986). A general theory of addictions: A new theoretical model. *Journal of Gambling Behavior, 2,* 15–31.

Jacobs, D. F. (1989). A general theory of addiction: Rationale for and the evidence supporting a new approach for understanding and treating addictive behaviors. In H. J. Shaffer, S. A. Stein, & B. Gambino (Eds.), *Compulsive gambling: Theory, research, and practice.* Toronto: Lexington Books.

Jessor, R. (1993). Successful adolescent development among youth in high-risk settings. *American Psychologist, 48,* 117–126.

Jessor, R. (1998). *New perspectives on adolescent risk behavior.* New York: Cambridge University Press.

Ladouceur, R., Boudreault, N., Jacques, C., & Vitaro, F. (1999). Pathological gambling and related problems among adolescents. *Journal of Child and Adolescent Substance Abuse, 8,* 55–68.

Langhinrichsen-Rohling, J., Rohde, P., Seeley, J. R., & Rohling, M. L. (2004). Individual, family, and peer correlates of adolescent gambling. *Journal of Gambling Studies, 20,* 23–46.

Linden, R., D., Pope, H. G., & Jonas, J. M. (1986). Pathological gambling and major affective disorder: Preliminary findings. *Journal of Clinical Psychiatry, 47,* 201–203.

McCormick, R. A., Russo, A. M., Rameriz, L. F., & Taber, J. (1984). Affective disorders among pathological gamblers seeking treatment. *American Journal of Psychiatry, 141,* 215–218.

McNeilly, D. P., & Burke, W. J. (2000). Late life gambling: The attitudes and behaviors of older adults. *Journal of Gambling Studies, 16,* 393–415.

Moore, S. M., & Ohtsuka, K. (1997). Gambling activities of young Australians: Developing a model of behavior. *Journal of Gambling Studies, 13,* 207–236.

Murtha, F. (2001). Gambling behavior, depression, and cognitive errors in undergraduate fraternities. *Dissertation Abstracts International: Section B: The Sciences and Engineering, 61,* 6715.

Nower, J. D., Gupta, R., Blaszczynski, A., & Derevensky, J. (in press). Suicidal ideation among youth problem gamblers. *International Gambling Studies.*

Phillips, D. P., Welty, W. R., & Smith, M. M. (1997). Evaluated suicide levels associated with legalized gambling. *Suicide and Life-Threatening Behavior, 27,* 373–378.

Rohde, P., Lewinsohn, P. M., Seeley, J. R., & Langhinrichsen-Rohling, J. (1996). *The Life Attitudes Schedule Short Form:* An abbreviated measure of life-enhancing and life-threatening behaviors in adolescents. *Suicide and Life-Threatening Behavior, 26,* 272–282.

Rohde, P., Seeley, J. R., Langhinrichsen-Rohling, J., & Rohling, M. (2003). The Life Attitudes Schedule-Short Form: Psychometric properties and correlates of adolescent suicide proneness. *Suicide and Life-Threatening Behavior, 33,* 249–260.

Savron, G., Pitti, P., DeLuca, R., & Guerreschi, C. (2001). Psychopathology and gambling: A preliminary study in a sample of pathological gamblers. *Rivista di Psichiatria, 36,* 14–21.

Scannell, E. D., Quirk, M. M., Smith, K., Maddern, R., & Dickerson, M. (2000). Females' coping styles and control over poker machine gambling. *Journal of Gambling Studies, 16,* 417–432.

Shaffer, H. J., & Hall, M. N. (1996). Estimating the prevalence of adolescent gambling disorders: A quantitative synthesis and guide toward standard gambling nomenclature. *Journal of Gambling Studies, 12,* 193–214.

Stinchfield, R. D., & Winters, K. C. (1998). Adolescent gambling: A review of the prevalence, risk factors and health implications. *Annuals of American Academy of Political and Social Science, 556,* 172–185.

Tanney, B. L. (2000). Psychiatric diagnoses and suicidal acts. In R. W. Maris, A. L. Berman, & M. M. Silverman (Eds.), *Comprehensive textbook of suicidology* (pp. 311–341). New York: Guilford Press.

Torne, I. V., & Konstanty, R. (1992). Gambling behavior and psychological disorders of gamblers on German-style slot machines. *Journal of Gambling Studies, 8,* 39–59.

Winters, K. C., & Anderson, N. (2000). Gambling involvement and drug use among adolescents. *Journal of Gambling Studies, 16,* 175–198.

Winters, K. C., Stinchfield, R., & Fulkerson, J. (1993). Patterns and characteristics of adolescent gambling. *Journal of Gambling Studies, 9,* 371–386.

Zitzow, D. (1996). Comparative study of problematic gambling behaviors between American Indian and non-Indian adults in a northern plains reservation. *American Indian and Alaska Native Mental Health Research, 7,* 27–41.

Chapter 4

Gambling and Drug Abuse in Adolescence[1]

Ken C. Winters, Ph.D., Nikki Arthur, M.A.,
Willa Leitten, M.Ed. and Andria Botzet, M.A.

In recent literature, adolescent gambling has become a hot topic of discussion. There are several reasons for this phenomenon. During the past decade, legalized gambling, such as lotteries, high-stakes casinos, and video lottery terminals have expanded rapidly. In the developmental course, adolescents are susceptible to the engagement of health risk behaviors and frequently disregard their possible negative consequences (Clayton, 1992). With regard to gambling, the predominant belief is that it is a mode of entertainment and it has very few, if any, negative consequences. It is partly due to this perception that implementing programs to treat adolescents with gambling problems have not been widely accepted or developed in the past. It is known that some adolescent problem behaviors are connected with morbidity and mortality (e.g., automobile accidents resulting from drinking and driving) (Chassin & DeLucia, 1996).

The prevalence data on adolescent gambling behaviors are provocative. Among young people, gambling involvement is common, with some gambling occurring among most American adolescents (Jacobs, 1989a, 2000, in this volume; Stinchfield & Winters, 1998). The estimates of problem or

1. Support for this chapter was partially provided by a grant from the National Center for Responsible Gaming.

pathological gambling rates among youth, while not excessive, range from 1–9% past year (median = 6%), while pathological gambling rates are two to four times higher than that of adult populations (Gupta & Derevensky, 1998a; Jacobs, 2000; National Research Council, 1999; Shaffer, Hall & Vander-Bilt, 1997). Youth who are in psychiatric hospitals, chemical dependency programs and juvenile detention centers display gambling rates that are approximately double that of adolescents from school or community samples (Stinchfield & Winters, 1998). The young person who is considered to have a gambling problem or who is a compulsive gambler has been connected to a rise in criminal activities and delinquency, familial difficulties, and poor academic performance (Fisher, 1993; Gupta & Derevensky, 1997). It is therefore safe to assume that gambling behaviors can lead to delinquency and that delinquent behaviors can lead to gambling among youth (Gupta & Derevensky, 1998a). In retrospective reports of adult pathological gamblers, a higher percentage of these individuals have indicated that they began their gambling during adolescence (National Research Council, 1999). Discussions about the origins and course of adolescent gambling often point to the apparent connection between adolescent gambling and drug use.[2] Researchers have noted that the prevalence rates of general gambling involvement and drug use are in most cases are comparable, and that many behavioral and social consequences of each domain are similar. Researchers have also recognized that several psychosocial factors linked to adolescent drug behaviors have emerged as correlates of gambling behaviors as well (Lesieur, Blume & Zoppa, 1986; Stinchfield, in this volume; Stinchfield & Winters, 1998).[3]

This chapter explores the extent to which insights about adolescent gambling behaviors can be enhanced by studying the relationship between gambling and drug use behaviors. Clearly, we are a distance from knowledge parity with respect to these two behavioral domains. Relatively little is known about the origins, course, and responsivity of the treatment of gambling compared to that of drug involvement. In this chapter, we will focus on five issues pertaining to the relationship of gambling and drug use: definitions and measurement, prevalence of the two domains including their co-occurrence, psychosocial factors that may mediate and moderate these behavioral domains, and prevention and treatment implications.

---

2. The terms drugs and substances are used throughout this chapter to refer to alcohol and other drug use.
3. Many points of overlap between adult pathological gambling and substance use disorders have been noted in the literature as well (see National Research Council, 1999).

Definitions and Measurement

At an elemental level, there is not a great deal of controversy in defining *general* drug and gambling involvement for adolescents. Conventional definitions of gambling behavior (playing games of chance for money) and drug use (self-administration of a psychoactive substance) are appropriate when applied to young people. However, there is a greater controversy and more uncertainty as to how we define, classify and measure the varying levels of involvement in these two behavior domains. The specific classification system that is typically chosen, the definitions and criteria subsumed under that system, and the instruments to measure the phenomena are fundamental to how we conceptualize a behavior disorder (Kendell, 1975). A discussion of substance abuse disorders is useful in the discovery of the connection between drug abuse and gambling problems.

Recent literature has given attention to the validity of formal diagnostic criteria for substance use disorders among adolescents. The DSM-IV's (American Psychiatric Association, 1994) two-category system of substance *abuse* and *dependence* are presumed to be indirectly appropriate for youth given that youth-specific criterion are not offered. It is therefore presumed that the validity data cited for substance abuse disorders in the DSM-IV are relevant across age groups. This research is generally supportive with regard to the usefulness of abuse and dependence diagnostic criteria when applied to adolescents. As an example, studies by Stewart and Brown (1995) and Martin and colleagues (Martin, Kaczynski, Maisto, Bukstein, & Moss, 1995) have indicated that youth who are multiple or chronic drug users frequently report abuse and dependence symptoms. Winters and colleagues (Winters, Latimer & Stinchfield, 1999) reported external validity that supported the DSM-IV distinctions of abuse and dependence for both alcohol and cannabis. Those who met the dependence criteria consistently scored higher on independent ratings of problem severity by clinicians compared to those meeting abuse criteria.

Regardless of this milieu of validity evidence, there are rising concerns that the adult-based criteria for substance use disorders are less than ideal when applied to youth. Martin and Winters (1998) have discussed several failings of the DSM-IV criteria for alcohol use disorders in adolescents. Examples of these weaknesses include weaknesses that are not typically experienced by adolescent problem drinkers (e.g. withdrawl and alcohol-related medical problems); some criteria have limited value because they tend to only occur in particular subgroups of youth (e.g. hazardous use of alcohol while driving is essentially limited to youth old enough to drive); and one symptom that is tolerance, has a questionable specificity for adolescents given that its rate is roughly equivalent in both non-problem drinking and problem drinking groups.

When applied to gambling problems, several terms and classification systems have been proposed to describe the levels of adolescent gambling. However, very little validity data has been reported to date. Some investigators have utilized the South Oaks Gambling Screen (SOGS) in adolescent surveys. In these cases, the problem severity groups have naturally been delineated with accordance to the SOGS criteria (e.g., a score of 5 or higher identifies a probable pathological gambler). Because the SOGS is based on American Psychiatric Association's definition of pathological gamblers, using these categories demonstrates the opinion that severe-end gamblers might suffer from a chronic and progressive failure to resist the temptation to gamble, and they indicate negative personal consequences in the face of continued gambling. Investigators have been faced with making subjective classification decisions when SOGS-adapted measures have been used in surveys. Winters and colleagues (Winters, Stinchfield & Fulkerson, 1993a) provided a good example of this difficulty by defining their "problem" gamblers as those who had a higher score on the SOGS-RA *or* those who reported daily gambling, regardless of the SOGS-RA score. The use of the term problem gambler was meant to consider a broadly defined group at the extreme end of the distribution of scores. In other instances, researchers have used the problem gambler label to reflect a sub-pathological group, who are, nonetheless, more disordered in their behavior than the occasional or recreational gambler (National Research Council, 1999; Shaffer et al., 1997). The second example offers the problem gambling category as a similar function as the abuse category provides in the classification of substance use disorders.

Shaffer and Hall (1996) have proposed a five-level classification system for groups of adolescent gamblers (see Table 1). Levels 0 (no gambling history) to 3 (pathological or compulsive gambling based on formal guidelines) indicate an increased involvement and produce signs of impairment due to gambling. Level 4 is assigned to the individuals who meet Level 3 guidelines but are prepared to undertake treatment for their problem. This system is enticing due to the fact that it offers two levels of gambling that are sub-threshold in nature. Level 1 shows recreational gambling while Level 2 distinguishes the "in-transition" or "problem" gambler who is exhibiting signs of over-involvement and may progress toward the more impaired level of pathological gambling. Shaffer and Hall (1996) appropriately noted the proposed five-level classification system has use for advancing communication among researchers and policy makers. However, important research work is necessary to prove the system's validity.

Instrumentation for assessing gambling problems has yet to fully evolve. The increasing and rather abundant assessment literature for the adolescent drug abuse field has been summarized elsewhere (Leccese & Waldron, 1994; Martin & Winters, 1998; SAMHSA, 1999). Countless screening and

Table 1. Shaffer and Hall's (1996) Proposed Classification
System for Levels of Adolescent Gambling

Levels of Gambling Involvement and Experience	Operational Definition
Level 0: No Gambling History	Individual has never gambled.
Level 1: Non-Problem Gambling	Individual has gambled recreationally and does not experience any signs or symptoms of gambling-related disorder.
Level 2: In-Transition or Problem Gambling	Individual experiences symptoms or displays signs of problems related to gambling activity; may be progressing either toward more serious or intense symptoms (i.e., progression) or away from these symptoms (i.e., during recovery).
Level 3: Gambling-Related Disorder with Impairment, such as Pathological or Compulsive Gambling	Individual meets diagnostic criteria (e.g., DSM-IV, MAGS, SOGS) for biologic, sociologic, or psychologic impairment.
Level 4: Pathological/Compulsive Gambler Who Displays Willingness to Enter Treatment	Individual satisfies Level 3 requirements and, in addition displays interest in entering the health care domain (with or without existing obstacles).

all-inclusive questionnaires and interviews exist for researchers and clinicians, with a few including effective psychometric properties (SAMHSA, 1999). Contrary to this is the fact that only a limited number of instruments in the literature pertain to adolescent problem/pathological gambling, and none can be thought of as multi-dimensional, comprehensive tools. Prevalence studies with adolescents have used the SOGS (Lesieur & Blume, 1987) or variations of it (e.g., SOGS-RA; Winters, Stinchfield & Fulkerson, 1993b). Other investigators have created their own instrument (e.g., Massachusetts Gambling Screen; Shaffer, LaBrie, Scanlan & Cummings, 1994) or have assessed youth with the DSM criteria for pathological gambling (e.g., DSM-IV-J; Fisher, 1992). The validity data for these tools are in the early stages of development, and the data indicates a general consistency in terms of discriminant validity. For example, when researchers have compared infrequent gamblers with those who gamble habitually, group differences are consistent with expectations (Derevensky & Gupta, 2000). These studies have found that the SOGS-RA, DSM-IV-J, and Gamblers Anonymous (GA) 20 questions were greatly interrelated (range of inter-correlations .61 to .68), while the DSM-IV-J was the most conventional in the identification of the lowest rate of problem/pathological adolescent gamblers (3% compared to 5% and 6% for the previous two instruments) (see Derevensky & Gupta, in this volume).

Screening tools may error substantially in terms of false positives. This fact has been brought to light by a recent study on the validity of the gambling assessment measures. Ladouceur and colleagues (Ladouceur, Bouchard, Rheaume, Ferland, Leblond & Walker, 2000) examined the speculation that the SOGS-RA (Winters et al., 1993b) overestimates the prevalence of pathological gambling. Followed by an individual interview by a researcher, blind to the subjects' prior responses, children in grade school and adolescents were initially given the SOGS-RA. During the interview phase, the children were asked to clarify the meaning of the items. If the child showed a misunderstanding, the researcher explained the item. Each of these participants then completed the SOGS-RA a second time. The outcome of the collected data confirmed the authors' expectations in that the prevalence rates of the potential pathological gambler (i.e., a score of 3+) was reduced by 65% among grade school children. This reduction was found among adolescents to be more than 47% when the results of the second testing were compared to the first testing data. Furthermore, there were no cases in which a second SOGS-RA score was 3 or higher when the first score was below the 3+ threshold. The study by Ladouceur et al. (2000) is significant for two reasons. First, it puts forth a warning to researchers that screening instruments (e.g. SOGS-RA) may produce an increased prevalence of the estimation of pathological gambling among adolescents. Second, the research presents a hint of the urgent need for further investigation concerning the measurement of gambling behaviors, and in particular, problem and pathological gambling in this field. Nevertheless, it is important to note that in a recent paper by Derevensky, Gupta and Winters (2003) Ladouceur and his colleagues work was methodologically challenged and that a replication study with adults failed to substantiate their assertions (see Derevensky & Gupta in this volume for a more complete discussion).

There are more contrasts than similarities in the separate terminology and classification systems that describe the levels of gambling and drug involvement. The area of adolescent drug abuse is much more cultivated in terms of empirically developing and validating a youth-specific classification system. In addition, the field of adolescent drug abuse has benefited from relatively less contention in regards to the organization of the classification, and from a more highly evolved instrumentation when related to the gambling domain. This is not to say that the conceptions of substance abuse and dependence for adolescents are not without faults; there are still concerns that the DSM-IV criteria for abuse and dependence require a developmental modification (Martin & Winters, 1998). However, investigators and clinicians in the gambling area do not gain from a significant empirical base, resulting in several basic classification and measurement issues that are yet to be determined.

Epidemiology of Youth Gambling
and Drug Use in the United States

More of the epidemiology of youth gambling and drug use studies comes from local surveys which make it problematic to compare one with the other on a national scale. As a result, we do not have the same national viewpoint of gambling behaviors as those available for adolescent drug use. Moreover, it is only recently that adolescent surveys have included both drug and gambling items to permit a more accurate comparative picture of the relative prevalence of the two behavior domains and the boundary of their co-association.

A recent statewide survey in Minnesota of these two behavior sets offers another comparison among gambling involvement and drug use (Stinchfield, Cassuto, Winters & Latimer, 1997). Health behavior statistics were collected in 1995 from nearly all sixth, ninth, and twelfth grade students who attended Minnesota's public schools. A statistical examination was employed for over 18,000 students who were randomly chosen from the full data set. These numbers are significant for the present discussion because they are (a) reasonably up to date, and (b) the survey included comparable items for both prior year frequency of drug use (across six categories) and gambling involvement (for five gambling activities). Table 2 offers a summary of the results of this research for prior year drug use and gambling, with respect to the following data points: *any* involvement and *weekly/daily* involvement.

These two indices were used because they were mutually included in the response options for both sets of survey items and they provided a comparison at two end points along a continuum of involvement. The data indicate that: (a) between ninth and twelfth grade students, at least some participation in drug use and gambling was the rule rather than the exception; (b) rates of any gambling and any drug use were roughly equivalent across grades and gender, with some exceptions (sixth grade girls and ninth grade boys showed higher gambling rates than drug use rates); (c) weekly and daily gambling participation was not reported by the majority of the students who were surveyed, with sixth graders reporting a very low rate at this level, meanwhile older students reported weekly and daily involvement in the range of 20% –25%; (d) there was a partiality for sixth and ninth graders to report higher weekly/daily gambling rates compared to weekly/daily drug use rates, twelfth graders following the opposite trend; and (e) boys were inclined to report gambling and drug use more often when compared to girls, with these reported differences being relatively larger for gambling. A final detail about gender differences is worthy of discussion. In the Minnesota sample, girls were almost equal to boys in terms

Table 2. Comparison Youth Gambling and Drug Use (Prior Year)

| Group | Any Involvement | | Weekly/Daily | |
	Gambling %	Drug Use %	Gambling %	Drug Use %
6th Graders				
Boys (n=4,104)	19.3	24.0	14.8	2.8
Girls (n=4,417)	46.0	21.7	5.4	1.2
9th Graders				
Boys (n=3,759)	77.4	50.5	20.4	14.0
Girls (n=3,714)	49.9	49.5	4.5	9.6
12th Graders				
Boys (n=2,309)	82.7	71.7	22.7	28.7
Girls (n=2,354)	58.7	66.3	5.0	16.4

Data based on *1995 Minnesota Student Survey* (Minnesota Department of Children, Families and Learning, 1995).
Gambling = cards, sports teams, games of skill, scratch tabs and lottery.
Drug Use = alcohol, cannabis, amphetamines, barbiturates, cocaine and inhalants.

of any drug use across the three grades, however, girls tended to have about half of the rate of weekly or daily drug use when compared to that of boys. In contrast, the rate of weekly or daily gambling among boys was about three to four times greater than that of girls, and except for sixth graders, boys also indicated significantly more gambling in general. To summarize, the Minnesota Student Survey data provide indications of considerable topographical overlap between gambling and drug use behaviors. Boys showed more involvement in gambling and drug use when compared to girls. Additionally, while there were many similarities when comparing the two behaviors in terms of general and weekly/daily participation, weekly/daily *gambling* was more widespread in the sixth and ninth grade students in comparison to weekly/daily *drug use,* but the pattern shifted at the twelfth grade when the prevalence rate of weekly/daily *drug use* was higher than that of *gambling.*

The discussion of the comparative rates of drug use and gambling behaviors would not be complete without examining the possible similarities of the *consequences* of the two behavior domains. Several behavioral and social consequences have been noted in the literature with regard to drug involvement (SAMHSA, 1999). Of particular note is that alcohol-related motor vehicle accidents account for nearly half (45.1%) of all traffic fatalities among adolescent drivers (Center for Disease Control and Prevention, 1996). Moreover, when substance use disorders begin at an early age, especially when there is no remission of the disorder, they exact substantially more economic and social costs to society. These costs include a heightened risk for suicide, sexually transmitted diseases, AIDS, and continued criminal activity when compared to those with a later onset of drug use (Children's Defense Fund, 1991).

The empirical picture is uncertain with respect to the consequences linked to adolescent gambling. Even though studies have shown that adolescents who gamble frequently also report elevated rates of poor school performance, legal problems, and loss of interest in normal activities compared to non-gambling peers (Griffiths, 1995; Winters et al., 1993a), it is not clear if these (or other) problems are genuine consequences of gambling involvement. The perceptible difficulty in empirically connecting adolescent gambling to distinguishable consequences may be compounded by several factors, including (a) the possibility that adolescent gambling may hardly ever produce dramatic consequences; (b) the absence in the literature of *clinical studies*, which would possibly draw attention to the presence of severe consequences; and (c) the lack of *prospective studies*, which would help to sort out the temporal relationships between the onset of the disorder and the resulting consequences.

In order to extend our epidemiological examination, we must examine the co-occurrence of the two sets of behaviors. Considerations are given to the extent to which involvement in one behavior domain increases the likelihood of involvement in the other. The literature with regard to adults has indicated that there is a co-association of substance use disorders and pathological gambling. In a review by Crockford and el Guebaly (1998), pathological gamblers were found to have lifetime rates of substance use disorders ranging from 25–63%. Estimates that have been reported by others are comparable (e.g., Lesieur, Blume & Zoppa, 1986; Steinberg, Kosten & Rounsaville, 1992). Studies have additionally discovered that individuals in treatment for alcoholism or drug addition are more likely to report a current or past problem with gambling when compared to those in the general population (National Research Council, 1999). The co-occurrence of gambling and drug use behaviors among youth has been studied on a much smaller scale. The link between adolescent gambling and drug use behaviors has been observed primarily in surveys (Shaffer et al., 1994; Wallisch, 1993; Zitzow, 1996). Conceivably this is also illustrative in the series of Minnesota youth studies that have consistently found an increased link between gambling participation and drug use. For example, a community survey of older adolescents in 1990 found that 62% of problem gamblers reported monthly use of a substance, compared to 28% of the non-problem group (Winters et al., 1993a). Another analysis of statewide data collected in 1992 and 1995 of public school students revealed that lifetime alcohol use was one of the strongest predictors of the highest level of gambling for both cohorts (Stinchfield et al., 1997). In addition, the outcome from a survey of two colleges in Minnesota indicated that weekly or more frequent use of substances increased the odds of being in the probable pathological gambling group (based on the SOGS score) by a factor that ranged from 4.5 (for illicit use) and 2.3 (for licit use) (Winters, Bengston, Dorr & Stinchfield, 1998).

The degree of co-occurrence between gambling and drug use using a large sample available from the 1995 Minnesota student survey was examined further. The authors computed a separate odds ratio for the two end point variables reported in Table 2 (no involvement and weekly/daily involvement). Students were 3.1 times more likely to have never gambled if the individual had never used drugs compared to those who had used drugs. In addition, students were 3.8 times more likely to be a weekly or daily gambler if they were also a weekly or daily drug user compared to those who used drugs less than that (including no use at all). This information provides additional support that gambling involvement is connected to the level of drug use among adolescents.

Due to the methodological problems noted previously, comparisons of gambling and drug use survey data must be interpreted with caution. The data is ambivalent as to which behavior domain is more commonly engaged in by youth, and which "disorder" is more prevalent than the other. Suffice to say that at this point we can conservatively conclude that for adolescents (at least in the United States), (a) some drug use and some gambling is a common developmental experience, (b) a significant but undersized percentage of youth who engage in these behaviors meet the criteria for the respective disorder, and (c) participation in one behavior predisposes the participation in the other, although the direction of the relationship is not clear at this time. As for the comparisons of behavioral and social consequences, the most remarkable observation is the relative scarcity of documentation in the adolescent gambling area compared with the adolescent drug abuse literature.

Exploring the Dual Function of Psychosocial Factors

The nature of the co-association between drug use and gambling involvement is still clearly open for speculation. As a result, it is relevant to further consider this issue by examining the possible intersection of psychosocial factors for these two behavioral domains.

A current perspective on the genetic, inter-personal and intra-personal risk factors for adolescent drug use behaviors, which begin during the childhood years, are influenced by multiple trajectories (e.g., Cadoret, Yates,

Troughton, Woodworth & Stewart, 1995). An individual attribute, situational condition, or environmental context that increases the probability of participating in the target behavior (in this case, drug use and gambling) and possibly leads the individual to continue that involvement can be conceptualized as a risk factor (Clayton, 1992). In contrast, a protective factor decreases the probability of the onset or severity of the target behavior. While a protective factor is the conceptual opposite of a risk factor, for the sake of frugality, we will incorporate protective factors into this discussion by conceptually recasting them as risk factors. An assortment of literature reviews provide a small consensus as to specific adolescent risk factors that fall within these broad genetic and inter- and intra-personal categories (see Clayton, 1992; Hawkins, Catalano & Miller, 1992; Petraitis, Flay & Miller, 1995; Weinberg & Glanz, 1999). While the level of wisdom regarding the vulnerability to problem gambling is still new compared to that of drug abuse vulnerability literature, is has been noted that these two behavioral domains share similar risk factors and thus may share common etiological processes (Jacobs, 1989a).

Findings from the summaries of the adolescent drug abuse risk literature by Stinchfield and Winters (1998) have been compared to the limited literature on the risk factors of adolescent gambling behavior (Derevensky, Gupta & Della-Cioppa, 1996; Dickson, Derevensky & Gupta, 2002; Gupta & Derevensky, 1997, 1998a; Jacobs, 1989a; Stinchfield et al., 1997; Winters et al., 1993a). It is due to this lack of literature that most studies reviewed did not include appropriate measures of both problem gambling and drug abuse, nor included a comprehensive list of candidate risk factors. One has to keep in mind that the following comparison is far less than ideal from an empirical standpoint. For example, it is not known to what end the list of common risk factors capitalizes on methodological and measurement differences across studies. Furthermore, because adolescent gambling studies have typically borrowed psychosocial measures from the drug abuse vulnerability literature, it is reasonable to assume that research has not adequately or fully studied the extent to which the non-convergence of underlying risk factors occurs.

Despite these cautions, the following variables were identified by Stinchfield and Winters (1998) as having a dual status as a risk factor for both drug abuse and problem gambling: low self-esteem, depressive mood or suicidal, being a victim of physical or sexual abuse, poor school performance, history of delinquency (and the related personality trait of disinhibition or poor impulse control), being male, early onset, parental history of the respective problem, and community and family norms that promote accessibility to the respective activity. As a group, these dual-acting variables represent genetic or biological, personality, familial and/or community factors, suggesting that the origins of both of these behaviors are heterogeneous and likely character-ized by various and combined pathways.

The notable extension of tangible psychosocial risk factors with respect to both adolescent problem gambling and drug abuse suggests that the association of the two behavior patterns is not insignificant. The nature of this relationship however is less clear. As shown in Figure 1, several path-ways for risk, substance use disorders and problem gambling are credible.

One direction to consider is that a high-risk status may lead to a devel-opmental disorder (e.g. conduct disorder), which then can influence other disorders such as substance use disorder and problem gambling (path #1). On the other hand, the risk status may increase the vulnerability directly to a substance use disorder and problem gambling independently (path #2). An additional consideration is the plausible interaction between problem gambling and substance use disorders. For example, adolescent problem gambling may be the result of an adolescent substance use dis-order (path #3).

We continue to develop this discussion of common psychosocial inter-actions by contemplating the limit to which hypotheses of early drug use and abuse may generalize to models of vulnerability of gambling involve-ment. Efforts put forth by social scientists to learn why some adolescents experiment and abuse substances have led to the identification of so many constructs and theories integrating these constructs that it has become dif-ficult to clearly understand this phenomenon. Pertraitis, Flay and Miller

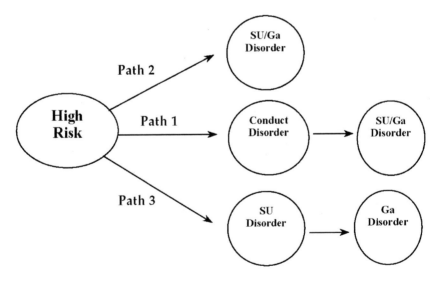

Figure 1. Possible Pathways for Risk and Substance Use (SU) and Gambling (Ga) Disorders

(1995), in their comprehensive review of this research, suggest that "the puzzle of adolescent use is far from complete, and probably few social scientists would argue that existing theories successfully integrate current knowledge about the causes of adolescent substance use, make sense out of seemingly unrelated research findings, lead to accurate predictions regarding adolescent substance use, and form the foundation of effective prevention programs" (p. 67).

How then does one embark on developing reliable theories of adolescent gambling given that this field is in its empirical infancy? While some reliable psychosocial variables have come together as vulnerability factors for adolescent gambling, we are still some distance away from characterizing how all of these concepts are interrelated to form a lucid view of what contributes to the onset and maintenance of gambling behaviors and how to prevent problem gambling among adolescents. As a result, there seems to be evidence of commonalities between adolescent gambling and drug use behaviors. It stands to reason that the familiar theories of adolescent drug abuse may contribute as a foundation from which youth gambling models materialize.

Multivariate theories that exist on adolescent substance use can be structured around four major themes (Lettieri, Sayers, & Pearson, 1980; Moncher, Holden, & Schinke, 1991; Petraitis, Flay, & Miller, 1995; Weinberg & Glantz, 1999). The *cognitive-affective* explanations of drug use are the first group of theories. The primary focus of this hypothesis is how self-perceptions of the costs and benefits of drug involvement are influential with the adolescents' choice to experiment with them. One assumption of this theory is that the individual's expectations and perceptions about a drug's psychological and physiological effects are a primary cause of the decision to use specific drugs. Other influences, such as the individual's personality traits or association with delinquent peers, are mediated through their effects on these drug-specific cognitions (e.g., Fishbein & Ajzen, 1975). A second premise from this literature is based on *social learning theory* (e.g., Bandura, 1982; Krohn, Akers, Radosevich, & Lanza-Kaduce, 1982). The primary factors that endorse drug use, more willingly than cognitive-affective factors are perceived as the interpersonal or social influences. This viewpoint declares that adolescents initially develop delinquent attitudes and behaviors through observation and imitation of role models, especially close friends and siblings (particularly older and same-sex siblings), and in some cases, parents. Social reinforcement for using drugs occurs from encouragement from peers and siblings, which is then followed by expectations of positive social and physiological consequences from drug use in the future. The third theory addresses the role of the *conventional commitment and social attachment.* Within this framework deviant impulses that all people presumably have as a shared trait are often hindered or controlled by firm attachments to social and interpersonal conventions, (i.e. family and religious beliefs). However, some adolescents are deficient in these controlling influences. Consequently, the adolescents with vulnerable conventional bonds are less inclined to follow the typical standards of behavior (Hawkins & Weis, 1985; Jessor, Donovan, & Costa, 1991). The final leading theme discussed in the literature focuses on how *intra-personal characteristics*, some of which may be genetically influenced, interrelate with the adolescents' social settings and community norms and values to either encourage or discourage drug involvement. This group of theories claims that adolescents will vary from each other in their attachment to drug-using peers and their motivation to use drugs by virtue of differences in personality traits, mental health status, affective states, and behavioral skills (Brook, Gordon, Brook & Brook, 1989; Jessor et al., 1991; Kaplan, Martin & Robins, 1984; Kumpfer & Turner, 1990–1991; Rose, 1998). The empirical defense for these various drug abuse theories are inconsistent (Petraitis et al., 1995; Weinberg & Glantz, 1999), an aspect that is important when evaluating the possible utilization of drug use theories to model the development for adolescent gambling. Furthermore, youth gambling models should include factors that are likely to be exceedingly specific to gambling behaviors, such as attributions of luck and skill (Derevensky et al., 1996), outlook concerning money, and the role of gambling on mood enhancement. Moreover, there is a demand for an increase of our understanding concerning the similarities and differences of existing conceptualizations of adolescent gambling, to what extent they can be integrated into prescribed theories of youth gambling, and what empirical tests are required to investigate their validity.

The most unequivocal attempt at bridging the etiological commonalities of gambling and drug involvement is provided by Jacobs' (1989b) *General Theory of Addictions*. Jacobs argues for the etiological connection between drug use and gambling on the basis of the innermost functionality of each of the behaviors in attaining altered states of identity or consciousness for susceptible individuals. Thus, Jacobs' theory seems reliable with the intra-personal characteristic theories described previously. Specifically, Jacobs hypothesizes that such altered states are manifested by dissociative-like reactions when engaging in the addictive behavior (e.g., "I feel like I am in a trance"; "I feel outside of myself"). The empirical defense for Jacobs' theory is provided by findings indicating that problem gamblers and addicts more often report dissociative-like experiences when gambling and drinking when compared to "normals" (Jacobs 1989b). Additional data from youth surveys in which problem gamblers report increased rates of dissociative-like states when compared to non-problem gambling youth (Jacobs, 1989b; Winters, Stinchfield & Fulkerson, 1990) also defined this theory.

Gupta and Derevensky (1998b) tested Jacobs' theory more comprehensively amongst adolescents. Based upon on data from a large school model (N = 817), problem and pathological gamblers demonstrated more abnormal physiological inactive states and self-reported more emotional distress, greater levels of dissociation, and higher rates of frequent substance use compared to non-gamblers and infrequent gamblers.

An important research priority for improving our understanding of the nature of adolescent gambling is the possible dual role of mediating and moderating the risk factors in the onset of gambling involvement and drug behaviors, as well as in the development of resulting gambling and substance use disorders. The existing literature, however limited, proposes that more than a few psychosocial risk factors may significantly overlap, even as the testing of developmental models that incorporate these factors is in the early stages. It is important to take into account that any discussion about dual risk factors should not disregard the possible influence of each behavior domain on the other. Because the two disorders show a high co-occurrence, the inception or desistence of one disorder may impact the status of the other disorder. Unmistakably, comprehensive prospective research is considered necessary to help classify the precise relationship of the two disorders. Nevertheless, it is due to these commonalities that prevention specialists are initiating the examination of the existing treatment methods for substance abuse and how these tools can be developed to treat adolescents with gambling problems.

Prevention and Treatment Issues

When it comes to prevention and treatment research, the knowledge base concerning the connection of gambling and drug involvement is to a certain extent one-sided. Despite the fact that the past 25 years has witnessed a reasonably broad prevention and treatment literature on youth drug abuse emerge (SAMHSA, 1999), there is very little in the sphere of adolescent gambling prevention and treatment. In a literature review by the authors, only one adolescent gambling study regarding treatment was cited. Ladouceur, Boisvert, and Dumont (1994) reported on the efficacy of cognitive-behavioral treatment for four adolescent male pathological gamblers. The post-treatment findings illustrated that all four adolescents were abstinent from gambling at all follow-up periods (one-, four-, and six-months). Not only is gambling treatment minimally discussed in the literature but very few youth gambling treatment services are in existence. The authors found an entry in the literature regarding a Young Gamblers Anonymous program in New Jersey (Ziegler, 1995), and the McGill research group has produced and put into practice a clinical intervention for adolescent and young adult problem gamblers (Gupta & Derevensky, 1999, 2000). The virtual absence of literature on the treatment of youth problem gambling may perhaps be due to several factors, including the deficiency of research funding in this area, being incomplete in the of awareness of adolescent problem gambling by the general public and youth service providers, and low base rates of pathological gambling as a presenting problem in youth clinics (see Gupta & Derevensky, this volume).

The prevention area proposes supplementary organization in the areas that overlap with other disorders. Contemporary knowledge recommends that effective youth gambling prevention must capitalize on the *Best Practices* learned from successful drug and alcohol prevention programs (National Research Council, 1999). This may be reasonable given the numerous commonalities between gambling and drug involvement previously discussed. A current review of the prevention research literature by NIDA (1996) highlights the significance that functional prevention programs should (a) recognize that the target behaviors are diverse, (b) integrate into the program what is known in regard to the behavior's psychosocial determinants, and (c) avoid one-shot, one-dimensional prevention efforts (e.g., school-based only effort limited to one grade level).

There are several models of youth gambling prevention programs that have been created (e.g., McGill University, Minnesota Institute on Public Health) (see Derevensky, Gupta, Dickson & Deguire, 2001; this volume for a comprehensive review of programs). One element of prevention efforts presented in the literature emphasizes the mathematical odds of the games and how they significantly disfavor the player. Crites (2003) discusses that if math classes stressed principles of probability and chance, young people may be more prudent when they have opportunities to gambling.

On a limited basis, prevention efforts have been initiated by the gambling industry. The Harrahs' Casino Group developed Project 21 in an effort to prohibit underage youth from gambling in their casinos (Satre, 2003). It was hoped that this project would impact adolescents who live near casinos as well as providing a deterrent to underage gambling in general. The program involves several components, including the training of casino staff to identify and report underage gamblers, collaborating with the media to produce public service announcements, and posting signs within the casino regarding underage gambling. Project 21 also offers scholarships to students who write exemplary articles or develop clever posters about the dangers of underage gambling. Over $70,000 in scholarships have been awarded.

The implementation of a prevention treatment for gambling should include information from the most basic and applicable research to a more multidimensional approach. By covering all aspects of the researched methods in other areas, one must ensure that the prevention process is developmentally acceptable and appropriate for gambling issues.

Risk and Protective Factors

One area that has received a great deal of attention in the past few years is the examination of individual risk and protective factors. Alcohol and drug abuse interventions often focus on risk and protective factors and how each of these has led to the path of use or abuse. The field of resilience has helped to increase these prevention efforts by expanding the range of their efforts to include the promotion of protective factors and the reduction of risk factors. The expectation of this research is that they will discover ways to increase the resilience among the participants. Research has suggested that protective factors act as a defense against the exposure of risk factors so that the modified course is more positive than it would have been without these added protections (Masten, Best & Garmezy, 1990). Risk and protective factors interact with one another so that the protective factor helps to lessen the intensity of the stressor. Jacobs (1989b) believes that all addictive behaviors satisfy a desire to break away from these stressors. Therefore it becomes necessary to study the connection, among the various addictions, by examining their risk and protective factors as well as the coping techniques that are currently employed.

According to current research, adolescent problem gambling has a quite a few distinctive risk factors. Some of these include a father who experiences pathological gambling, ease of access to gambling facilities, anxiety and depression, inadequate coping skills, poor impulse control and depleted conventionality, continuous risky behaviors and an early inception of gambling experiences (Dickson, Derevensky & Gupta 2002).

Specific protective factors related to the field of adolescent problem gambling have yet to be identified. However it is reasonable to include protective factors such as a "connectedness to one's family and school" as they have been validated in other youth prevention efforts.

There have been numerous studies that focus on the risk and protective factors associated with substance abuse (see Coie et al., 1993; Hawkins, Catalano & Miller, 1992; Rossi, 1994). Oftentimes these studies highlight adolescents who sustain a specific risk factor, for example, a substance-abusing parent. The likelihood that the adolescents will develop a problem with other at-risk behaviors (e.g., gambling) is higher than that for other adolescents who do not possess this risk (Hawkins et al., 1992). As the risk factors increase in number, so does the probability of becoming involved with other risky behaviors (Gupta & Derevensky, 1998b). It is important to note here that specific risk factors are characteristically unrelated to specific disorders. Risk factors are consistently changing and their effect and importance fluctuates over time. The exposure to multiple risk factors however, appear to have a collective effect on an individual (Coie, Watt, West, Hawkins, Asarnow, Markman, Ramey, Shure & Long, 1993). A few studies have addressed the identifying risk factors for adolescents who have gambling problems (see Derevensky & Gupta, 2000; Griffiths & Wood, 2000). None have examined the protective factors for these individuals. It is noteworthy to examine the connection of both of these issues in a prevention program designed to treat adolescents with gambling problems.

While it makes theoretical sense that gambling interventions take advantage of the lessons learned in the drug abuse field, more research is needed in this area. However, one should be aware of Dr. Robert Cluster's remark that while gambling and drug abuse may be 90% similar, the 10% differences must be effectively concentrated upon when developing helpful prevention programs (Vander-Bilt & Franklin, 2003).

Harm Reduction as a Prevention Tool

In the recent past, harm reduction has been used as a tool with prevention efforts towards drug use in school-based educational programs. On a wider scale, harm reduction has been utilized, for example, to exchange needles or to check the potency and reliability of the drug that an individual was planning to ingest (e.g. ecstasy). Any behavior change that reduces harm is a positive result. By implementing this more accommodating method, it allows help for the adolescent who initially is resistant to change. Harm reduction goals can include changing the means of administration of a substance, reducing opportunities to drive under the influence, providing safe alternative to substances, and a reduction in the frequency and/or intensity of the usage. The harm reduction approach uses the information reported by the adolescent as a tool to effectively target his or her own specific objectives. The theory of a harm reduction approach is to prevent the misuse or abuse of using substances and/or reduce the participation in risky behaviors such as problem gambling. By using individualized goals and personalized feedback, the treatment can be more directly focused for each adolescent's specific needs.

The goals of harm reduction can be reached by using a variety of techniques. One example may include questioning the adolescent about their substance use and helping them to recognize the consequences of this behavior. The harm reduction method helps the individual recognize the symptoms of abuse themselves and provides guidance towards change. This newly gained knowledge is then used as a platform to expand the awareness when it comes to peers and family members. In a sense, we are teaching these young people to become more critical with their choice to participate in risky behaviors. An examination into the personal risk-taking behaviors and objectives helps to dismiss stereotypes and provide information on how to control and limit the harm of their involvement. The idea is to be non-judgmental, non-labeling, and non-confrontational. The therapist's job is to act as a guide to help the adolescent through the stages of change. The enhancement and support of self-management and coping skills are important aspects of this treatment method.

The difficulty with the harm reduction approach and gambling prevention is that gambling is often viewed as a harmless mode of entertainment and it has very few, if any, visible negative consequences. In addition, gambling does not have the same costs and health risks as other risky behaviors (e.g. smoking). It is due to these issues that preventative pathological gambling requires it's own specific prevention policies that are validated with active research models.

The Stages of Change Model is beneficial in illustrating the level at which young people stand in terms of their degree of involvement and motivation to change. Prochaska and DiClemente (1982) have provided a "stages of change" continuum for the purpose of treating substance abuse. These stages help to explain how changes in one's behavior transpire when applied to the area of substance abuse (Center for Substance Abuse Treatment, 1999). Based on this research, the continuum has been developed into a five-stage model. The U.S. Department of Health and Human Services has provided a clear-cut description of this model (Center for Substance Abuse Treatment, 1999). The stages begin at pre-contemplation where the individual has no intention to change regardless of the possible consequences. The next stage is called contemplation. In this stage the individual has experienced some consequences but is still not committed to change. Preparation comes after contemplation where the person starts to make the preparations for change. Action is next. The person is now putting forth effort to continue the plan to change and is still struggling. The final stage is maintenance. This stage is where the individual begins to learn new behaviors and the long-term objectives are in the process of becoming a permanent part of the individual's behavior.

Much like substance use, gambling involvement can be conceptualized within stage of change theory and incorporated into intervention programs for youthful problem gamblers (Di Clemente, Delahanty & Schlundt, in this volume). Analogous to the field of substance abuse, the harm reduction method may be highly relevant to young people who are in the early stages of the participation in gambling (e.g., Level 2). While the harm reduction method is not without controversy (Des Jarlais & Friedman, 1993; Kalant, 1999; Mugford, 1999; Newcombe, 1992), this approach may be a viable prevention tool (see Dickson, Derevensky & Gupta, 2004 for a comprehensive discussion).

Concluding Thoughts

Gambling and drug use, not unlike other acting-out or risk-taking behaviors, can equally be viewed as characteristics of the experimentation phase of adolescence. However, some youth (few in terms of absolute percentages) engage heavily in these activities. Additionally, some of these adolescents can evolve to the extent of being identified by formal diagnostic criteria or related operational criteria of pathological gambling and drug use disorders. These youth may be on the path towards adulthood plagued by over-indulgence and disorder.

The sizeable overlap of the psychosocial risk factors for adolescent problem gambling and drug abuse shows that these two behaviors share common characteristics. Additional research is necessary to shed light on how these common factors can lead to the co-existence of drug use and gambling in some adolescents and not in others, to what degree these specific risk factors can be recognized, and if prevention strategies directed at these common factors have favorable results with both behavioral domains.

Adolescent gambling as a field has a considerable lack of documentation in terms of the association with negative conduct and social harm. This is a major barrier towards financial support and credit of prevention methods in this area. Even so, it would be wise for communities to focus on the trends in adolescent gambling and for health clinics serving adolescents to increase the detection of those who are demonstrating problematic gambling involvement. At bare minimum, the political practices that have approved gambling should consider assigning similar attention towards policies and programs that promote rational prevention and intervention strategies.

References

American Psychiatric Association (1994). *Diagnostic and Statistical Manual—Fourth Edition.* Washington, D.C.: Author.

Bandura, A. (1982). Self-efficacy mechanism in human agency. *American Psychologist, 37,* 122–147.

Brook, J.S., Gordon, A.S., Brook, A., & Brook, D. (1989). The consequences of marijuana use on intra personal and interpersonal functioning in Black and White adolescents. *Genetic, Social, and General Psychology Monographs, 115*, 349–369.

Cadoret, R.J., Yates, W.R., Troughton, E., Woodworth, G., & Stewart, M.A. (1995). Adoption study demonstrating two genetic pathways to drug abuse. *Archives of General Psychiatry, 42*, 161-167.

Center for Disease Control and Prevention. (1996). Youth risk behavior surveillance in the United States, 1995. *Morbidity and Mortality Weekly Report, 45*, 1–86.

Center for Substance Abuse Treatment, (1999). *Brief interventions and brief therapies for substance abuse* (Treatment Improvement Protocol–34). Substance Abuse and Mental Health Administration: Rockville, MD.

Chassin, L., & Delucia, C. (1996). Drinking during adolescence. *Life-Stage Issues, 20*, 32-44.

Children's Defense Fund. (1991). *The adolescent and young adult fact book.* Washington, D.C.: Author.

Clayton, R. (1992). Transitions in drug use: Risk and protective factors. In M. Glantz & R. Pickens (Eds.), *Vulnerability to drug abuse* (pp.15–52). Washington, D.C.: American Psychological Association.

Coie, J. Watt, N., West, S., Hawkins, J., Asarnow, J., Markman, H., Ramey, S., Shure, M., & Long, B. (1993). The science of prevention. *American Psychologist, 48*, 1013–1022.

Crites, T. W. (2003). What are my chances? Using probability and number sense to educate teens about the mathematical risks of gambling. In H. J. Shaffer, M. N. Hall, J.V. Vander-Bilt, & E. M. George (Eds.), *Futures at stake: Youth, gambling and society* (pp. 63–83). Reno, Nevada: University of Nevada Press.

Crockford, D.N., & el-Guebaly, N. (1998). Psychiatric co-morbidity in pathological gambling: A critical review. *Canadian Journal of Psychiatry, 43*, 43-50.

Derevensky, J.L., & Gupta, R. (2000). Prevalence estimates of adolescent gambling: A comparison of the SOGS-RA, DSM-IV-J and the G.A. 20 Questions. *Journal of Gambling Studies, 16*, 227–252.

Derevensky, J.L., & Gupta, R., & Della Cioppa, G. (1996). A developmental perspective of gambling behavior in children and adolescents. *Journal of Gambling Studies, 12*, 49–66.

Derevensky, J.L., Gupta, R., Dickson, L. & Deguire, A-E. (2001). *Prevention efforts toward minimizing gambling problems.* Paper prepared for the National Council for Problem Gambling, Center for Mental Health Services (CMS) and the Substance Abuse Mental Health Services Administration (SAMHSA), Washington, D.C., 104 pp.

Derevensky, J.L., Gupta, R., & Winters, K. (2003). Prevalence rates of youth gambling problems: Are the current rates inflated? *Journal of Gambling Studies, 19*, 405–425.

Des Jarlais, D.C. & Friedman, S.R. (1993). Aids, injecting drug use and harm reduction. In N. Healther, A. Wodak, E. Nadelmann & P. O'Hare, (Eds.), *Psychoactive drugs and harm reduction: From faith to science.* London: Whurr Publishers, Ltd.

Dickson, L.M., Derevensky J.L. & Gupta, R. (2002). The prevention of gambling problems in youth: A conceptual framework. *Journal of Gambling Studies, 18*, 97–159.

Dickson, L. Derevensky, J.L, & Gupta, R. (2004). Harm reduction for the prevention of youth gambling problems: Lessons learned from adolescent high-risk prevention programs. *Journal of Adolescent Research, 19*, 233–236.

Fishbein, M., & Ajzen, I. (1975). *Belief, attitude, intention and behavior: An introduction to theory and research.* Reading, MA: Addison-Wesley.

Fisher, S. E. (1992). Measuring pathological gambling in children: The case of fruit machines in the U.K. *Journal of Gambling Studies, 8*, 263-285.

Fisher, S. (1993). Gambling and pathological gambling in adolescents. *Journal of Gambling Studies, 9*, 277–288.

Griffiths, M. (1995). *Adolescent gambling.* London, England: Routledge.

Griffiths, M.D. & Wood, R.T. (2000). Risk factors in adolescence: The case of gambling, video-game playing, and the internet. *Journal of Gambling Studies, 12,* 375–394.

Gupta, R. & Derevensky, J.L. (1997). Familial and social influences on juvenile gambling. *Journal of Gambling Studies, 13,* 179–192.

Gupta, R., & Derevensky, J.L. (1998a). Adolescent gambling behavior: A prevalence study and examination of the correlates associated with excessive gambling. *Journal of Gambling Studies, 14,* 319–345.

Gupta, R., & Derevensky, J.L. (1998b). An empirical examination of Jacobs' General Theory of Addictions: Do adolescent gamblers fit the theory? *Journal of Gambling Studies, 14,* 17–50.

Gupta, R., & Derevensky, J.L. (August, 1999). *Treating adolescent problem gamblers.* Presentation at the 105th annual convention of the American Psychological Association, Boston, MA.

Gupta, R., & Derevensky, J.L. (2000). Adolescents with gambling problems: From research to treatment. *Journal of Gambling Studies, 16,* 315–342.

Hawkins, D., Catalano, R., & Miller, J. (1992). Risk and protective factors for alcohol and other drug problems in adolescence and early adulthood: Implications for substance abuse prevention. *Psychological Bulletin, 112,* 64–105.

Hawkins, D., & Weis, J. (1985). The social development model: An integrated approach to delinquency prevention. *Journal of Primary Prevention, 6,* 73–97.

Jacobs, D.F. (2000). Juvenile gambling in North America: An analysis of long-term trends and future prospects. *Journal of Gambling Studies, 16,* 119–152.

Jacobs, D.F. (1989a). Illegal and undocumented: A review of teenage gamblers in America. In H. Shaffer, S. Stein, B. Gambino, and T. Cummings (Eds.), *Compulsive gambling: Theory, research and practice* (pp. 249–292). Lexington, MA: Lexington Books.

Jacobs, D.F. (1989b). A general theory of addiction: Rationale for and the evidence supporting a new approach for understanding and treating addictive behaviors. In H. Shaffer, S. Stein, B. Gambino, and T. Cummings (Eds.), *Compulsive gambling: Theory, research and practice* (pp. 35–64). Lexington, MA: Lexington Books.

Jessor, R., Donovan, J., & Costa, F. (1991). *Beyond adolescence: Problem behavior and young adult development.* Cambridge, England: Cambridge University Press.

Kalant, H. (1999). Differentiating drugs by harm potential: The rational versus the feasible. *Substance Use and Misuse, 34,* 24–34.

Kaplan, H., Martin, S., & Robbins, C. (1984). Pathways to adolescent drug use: Self-derogation, peer influence, weakening of social controls, and early substance use. *Journal of Health and Social Behavior, 25,* 270–289.

Kendell, R.E. (1975). *The role of diagnosis in psychiatry.* Oxford: Blackwell Scientific Publications.

Krohn, M., Akers, R., Radosevich, M., & Lanza-Kaduce, L. (1982). Norm qualities and adolescent drinking and drug behavior: The effects of norm quality and reference group on using and abusing alcohol and marijuana. *Journal of Drug Issues, 12,* 343–359.

Kumpfer, K., & Turner, C. (1990–1991). The social ecology model of adolescent substance abuse: Implications for prevention. *International Journal of the Addictions, 25,* 435–463.

Ladouceur, R., Boisvert, J.M., & Dumont, J. (1994). Cognitive-behavioral treatment for adolescent pathological gamblers. *Behavior Modification, 16,* 230–242.

Ladouceur, R., Bouchard, C., Rheaume, N., Jacques, C., Ferland, F., Leblond, J., & Walker, M. (2000). Is the SOGS an accurate measure of pathological gambling among children, adolescents and adults? *Journal of Gambling Studies, 16,* 1–24.

Leccese, M., & Waldron, H.B. (1994). Assessing adolescent substance use: A critique of current measurement instruments. *Journal of Substance Abuse Treatment, 11,* 553–563.

Lesieur, H. R., & Blume, S.B. (1987). The South Oaks Gambling Screen (SOGS): A new instrument for the identification of pathological gamblers. *American Journal of Psychiatry, 144,* 1184-1188.

Lesieur, H.R., Blume, S., & Zoppa, R. (1986). Alcoholism, drug abuse and gambling. *Alcoholism: Clinical and Experimental Research, 10,* 33–38.

Lettieri, D., Sayers, M., & Pearson, H. (Eds.). (1980). *Theories on drug abuse: Selected contemporary perspectives* (Research Monograph 30). Rockville, MD: National Institute of Drug Abuse.

Martin, C., Kaczynski, N.A., Maisto, S.A., Bukstein, O.M., & Moss, H.B. (1995). Patterns of DSM-IV alcohol abuse and dependence symptoms in adolescent drinkers. *Journal of Studies on Alcohol, 56,* 672-680.

Martin, C., & Winters, K.C. (1998). Diagnosis and assessment of alcohol use disorders among adolescents. *Alcohol Health and Research World, 22,* 95–106.

Masten, A., Best, K., & Garmezy, N. (1990). Resilience and development: Contributions from the study of children who overcome adversity. *Development and Psychopathology, 2,* 425–444.

Minnesota Department of Children, Families and Learning. (1995). *Perspectives on youth.* St. Paul, MN: Author.

Moncher, M.G., Holden, G., & Schinke, S. (1991). Psychosocial correlates of adolescent substance use: A review of current etiological constructs. *International Journal of the Addictions, 26,* 377–414.

Mugford, S. (1999). Harm reduction: Does it lead where its proponents imagine? In N. Heather, A. Wodak, E. Nadelmann & P. O'Hare (Eds.), *Psychoactive drugs and harm reduction: from faith to science.* London: Whurr Publishers, Ltd.

National Institute on Drug Abuse. (1996). *Preventing drug use among children and adolescents: A research-based guide.* Rockville, MD: National Institute of Health.

National Research Council. (1999). *Pathological gambling: A critical review.* Washington, D.C.: National Academy Press.

Newcombe, R. (1992). The reduction of drug-related harm: A conceptual framework for theory, practice and research. In P. O'Hare, R. Newcombe, A. E. Matthews and C. Buning (Eds.), *The reduction of drug-related harm.* London: Routledge.

Petraitis, J., Flay, B., & Miller, T. (1995). Reviewing theories of adolescent substance use: Organizing pieces in the puzzle. *Psychological Bulletin, 117,* 67–86.

Prochaska, J.O., & DiClemente, C.C. (1982). Transtheoretical therapy: Toward a more integrative model of change. *Psychotherapy: Theory, Research and Practice, 19,* 276–288.

Rose, R.J. (1998). A developmental behavioral-genetic perspective on alcoholism risk. *Alcohol Health and Research World, 22,* 131–143.

Rossi, R.J. (1994). *Schools and students at risk: Context and framework for positive change.* Thousand Oaks: Sage.

Satre, P. (2003) Youth gambling: The casino industry's responsibility. In H.J. Shaffer, M. N. Hall, J.V. Vander-Bilt, & E. George (Eds.), *Futures at stake: Youth, gambling and society.* Reno, Nevada: University of Nevada Press.

Shaffer, H.J., & Hall, M.N. (1996). Estimating the prevalence of adolescent gambling disorders: A quantitative synthesis and guide toward standard gambling nomenclature. *Journal of Gambling Studies, 12,* 193–214.

Shaffer, H.J., Hall, M.N., & Vander-Bilt, J.V. (1997). *Estimating the prevalence of disordered gambling behavior in the United States and Canada: A meta-analysis.* Cambridge: Harvard Medical School Division of Addictions.

Shaffer, H. J., LaBrie, R. S., Scanlan, K. M., & Cummings, T. N. (1994). Pathological gambling among adolescents: Massachusetts Gambling Screen (MAGS). *Journal of Gambling Studies, 10,* 339–362.

Stewart, D.G., & Brown, S.A. (1995). Withdrawal and dependency symptoms among adolescent alcohol and drug abusers. *Addiction, 90,* 627-635.

Steinberg, M., Kosten, T., & Rounsaville, B. (1992). Cocaine abuse and pathological gambling. *American Journal on Addictions, 30,* 929-962.

Stinchfield, R.D., Cassuto, N., Winters, K.C., & Latimer, W. (1997). Prevalence of gambling by Minnesota public school students in 1992 and 1995. *Journal of Gambling Studies, 13,* 25-48.

Stinchfield, R.D., & Winters, K.C. (1998). Adolescent gambling: A review of prevalence, risk factors and health implications. *Annals of American Academy of Political and Social Science, 55,* 172-185.

Substance Abuse Mental Health Service Administration. (1999). Screening and assessing adolescents with substance use disorder. *Treatment Improvement Protocol (TIP) Series No. 31,* Rockville, MD: Center for Substance Abuse Treatment.

Vander-Bilt, J.V., & Franklin, J. (2003). Gambling in a familial context. In H.J. Shaffer, M. N. Hall, J.V. Vander-Bilt, & E. George (Eds.), *Futures at stake: Youth, gambling and society.* Reno, Nevada: University of Nevada Press.

Wallisch, L.S. (1993). *Gambling in Texas: 1992 Texas survey of adolescent gambling behavior.* Austin, TX: Texas Commission on Alcohol and Drug Abuse.

Weinberg, N., & Glantz, M.D. (1999). Child psychopathology risk factors for drug abuse: Overview. *Journal of Clinical and Child Psychology, 28,* 290-297.

Winters, K.C., Bengston, P., Dorr, D., & Stinchfield, R.D. (1998). Prevalence and risk factors of problem gambling among college students. *Psychology of Addictive Behaviors, 12,* 127-135.

Winters, K.C., Latimer, W.W., & Stinchfield, R.D. (1999). DSM-IV criteria for adolescent alcohol and cannabis use disorders. *Journal of Studies on Alcohol, 60,* 337-344.

Winters, K.C., Stinchfield, R.D., & Fulkerson, J. (1990). *Adolescent gambling among Minnesota youths: A benchmark study.* Minnesota Department of Human Services, Compulsive Gambling Treatment Division.

Winters, K.C., Stinchfield, R.D., & Fulkerson, J. (1993a). Toward the development of an adolescent gambling problem severity scale. *Journal of Gambling Studies, 9,* 63–84.

Winters, K.C., Stinchfield, R.D., & Fulkerson, J. (1993b). Patterns and characteristics of adolescent gambling. *Journal of Gambling Studies, 9,* 371–86.

Ziegler, A. (1995, January 11). Critics say adults gamble on the future of their children: Teens may bet on elder's example. The Washington Times, p. A2.

Zitzow, D. (1996). Comparative study of problematic gambling behaviors between American Indian and non-Indian adolescents within and near a Northern Plains reservation. *American Indian and Alaska Native Mental Health Research, 7,* 14–26.

Chapter 5

Adolescent Problem Gambling
Neurodevelopment and Pharmacological Treatment

Jon E. Grant, M.D., J.D., R. Andrew Chambers, M.D., and Marc N. Potenza, M.D., Ph.D.

Problem gambling among adolescents can be conceptualized as belonging to a larger constellation of *developmental addictions*. Data support a relationship between behavioral and drug addictions in both adults and adolescents. For example, high rates of both problem gambling and substance use disorders have been reported during adolescence (Chambers & Potenza, 2003; Wagner & Anthony, 2002), with gambling, substance use, and other risk behaviors frequently co-occuring during this developmental stage (Proimos, DuRant, Pierce & Goodman 1998; Romer, 2003). The co-aggregation of risky behaviors appears particularly strong in adolescent males. Arguably the most consistent and robust finding across youth gambling studies is that boys are more involved in gambling and have higher rates of problem gambling than girls (e.g., Gupta & Derevensky, 1998; Stinchfield, 2001; Wallisch, 1993; Wynne, Smith & Jacobs, 1996). Similarly, adolescent males have a greater likelihood of developing a substance use disorder than adolescent females. Nonetheless, the observation that these age-specific trends are observed in both males and females in epidemiological studies performed during different eras and involving different cultures suggests the existence of factors in the developmental onset of addictive disorders that impact both boys and girls (Chambers, Taylor & Potenza, 2003).

In this chapter, we will review a neurodevelopmental model for motivated behaviors, describe changes that occur during adolescence in brain structure and function in regions thought to underlie motivated behaviors, and describe the implications for the pharmacological treatment of adolescent gambling problems. Given that no studies have directly investigated the safety and efficacy of pharmacological treatments for pathological gambling in adolescents, we will briefly review the literature on effective treatments in adults, describe safety data for the use of these drugs in adolescents, and provide a rationale for future investigative studies on the efficacy and tolerability of pharmacotherapies for pathological gambling in adolescents.

Developmental Biology

A growing body of literature suggests the importance of environmental and genetic influences on brain function that leads to vulnerability to, and the expression of, addictive disorders (Shah, Eisen, Xian & Potenza, in press; Slutske et al., 2000; Tsuang, Bar, Harley & Lyons, 2001). Both environmental and genetic factors are important influences on brain function and thus can contribute to addiction vulnerability in adolescence. As such, it is important to consider general changes in brain structure and function that occur during adolescence that might influence the motivation to engage in risk-taking behaviors like gambling.

Motivational Neural Circuits

A wide range of studies across species implicate multiple brain structures as underlying motivated behaviors. We have proposed a model to explain the increased propensity to engage in risk behaviors like gambling (Figure 1) (Chambers & Potenza, 2003). One central aspect involves the ventral striatum, a brain region that includes the nucleus accumbens. The ventral striatum receives input from the ventral tegmental area and prefrontal cortex and has direct access to, and influence on, motor output structures (Chambers et al., 2003; Kalivas, Churchill & Romanides, 1999). As such, the ventral striatum is well-situated as an important node for controlling motivated behavior that is largely determined through a series of cortical-striatal-thalamic-cortical loops.

Motivated behavior involves integrating a wide array of contextual information, including information regarding a person's internal state (e.g., hunger, sexual desire, pain), environmental factors (e.g., resource or reproductive opportunities, the presence of danger), and personal experiences (e.g., recollections of events deemed similar in nature). Specific brain regions

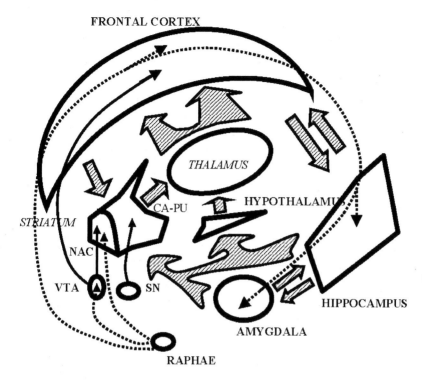

Figure 1. *Major neuroanatomical circuitry involved in motivation and action-oriented decision-making.* Sensory cortices, amygdala, hippocampus, hypothalamus and subcortical autonomic brain centers contribute to highly integrated, multimodal representations in the frontal cortex and striatum of the contextual frame that informs action-oriented decision-making. Frontal/prefrontal cortex (including orbitofrontal, dorsolateral prefrontal, and ventromedial prefrontal cortices), ventral striatum (nucleus accumbens (NAc)), thalamus, and brainstem nuclei (dopaminergic afferents from the ventral tegmental area (VTA); serotonergic afferents from the dorsal raphae) mediate the representation, evaluation and choosing of behavioral response options to this contextual frame. Premotor-motor cortex, dorsal striatum (caudate-putamen (CA-PU)), thalamus, brainstem nuclei (dopaminergic afferents from the substantia nigra (SN)), hypothalamus and cerebellum (not shown) implement and control motor output programs or behavioral responses in execution of the action-decision. Major excitatory glutamatergic projections and important inhibitory GABAergic projections from striatum to thalamus: wide stippled arrows. Dopaminergic afferents: thin dark arrows. Serotonergic afferents: thin stippled arrows (Chambers & Potenza, 2003).

are central in providing the primary motivational system with this information. For example, the hypothalamic and septal nuclei provide information about nutrient ingestion, aggression and reproductive drive, the amygdala about affective information, and the hippocampus about contextual memory data. Although a wide array of neurotransmitters serve to coordinate information processing within this network, including glutamate and gamma-aminobutyric acid (GABA), the neurotransmitters that are arguably the best characterized that influence motivated behavior are dopamine and serotonin.

Dopamine: Promotional Motivation Pathways

Dopamine release into the nucleus accumbens has been implicated in translation of motivated drive into action, serving as a "go" signal. Dopamine release into the nucleus accumbens has also been associated with a wide array of experiences including rewarding and reinforcing, novel and aversive or stressful stimuli (Chambers et al., 2003). Examples of specific stimuli include all drugs with addictive potential, wins and losses in gambling paradigms, and natural rewards such as food or sex. Dopamine release into the nucleus accumbens seems maximal when reward probability is most uncertain, suggesting it plays a central role in guiding behavior during risk-taking situations (Fiorillo, Tobler & Schultz, 2003). Importantly, the structure and function of dopamine neuronal projections to the nucleus accumbens, in conjunction with glutamatergic afferent and intrinsic GABA-ergic activities, change following experiences influencing function of the nucleus accumbens. That is, in reward-related learning, future behavior is determined in part according to past reward-related experiences via neuroplastic changes involving the nucleus accumbens. In this manner, dopamine function within the nucleus accumbens may serve to narrow motivational repertoires over time.

Adolescence, as a developmental period, is a time of profound physical change, and similarly remarkable changes occur in brain structure and function, including within promotivational dopamine systems (Chambers et al., 2003). Developmental changes within primary motivational pathways during adolescence may lead to increased novelty seeking and risk-taking. A number of observations suggest that adolescence represents a state of heightened dopaminergic activity. For example, tic disorders, thought to be driven by a relatively increased dopminergic drive, are most prevalent in childhood and adolescence and tend to remit in adulthood. The pathophysiology of Parkinson's Disease correlates with dopamine neuron loss that occurs with increasing age. Concern has been rising regarding the emergence of gambling problems with pro-dopaminergic agents (Driver-Dunkley, Samantra & Stacy, 2003), suggesting that increased dopamine activity across the lifespan can influence the propensity to engage in risk-taking behaviors. During their period of adolescence, animals show heightened behavioral responses (e.g., increased motoric activity and novelty seeking) following exposure to pro-dopaminergic drugs. Together, the data suggest that vulnerability to addictive behaviors, particularly that observed during adolescence, might be increased by a heightened dopaminergic state.

Serotonin: Inhibitory Motivational Pathways

Diminished inhibitory mechanisms could also underlie risk-taking behaviors like adolescent gambling. Decreased measures of serotonin have been associated with a variety of adult risk-taking behaviors including alcoholism, fire-setting and pathological gambling (Potenza & Hollander, 2002). Although the precise mechanism has not been fully determined, serotonin projections from the raphe nuclei to motivational circuitry, including the ventral tegmental area, nucleus accumbens, prefrontal cortex, amygdala and hippocampus, appear involved (Chambers et al., 2003). For example, blunted serotonergic responses in the ventromedial prefrontal cortex have been observed in individuals with impulsive aggression (New et al., 2002), and this region has been implicated in disadvantageous decision-making as has been observed in adults with gambling or substance use disorders (Bechara, 2003).

Adolescent changes within the prefrontal cortex are profound and are thought to underlie many of the cognitive changes (abstract thinking, complex problem solving) that occur during adolescence (Chambers et al., 2003). For example, during adolescence, substantial increases in myelination and extensive neuronal pruning are observed in the prefrontal cortex, suggesting that adolescence serves as a transition stage for prefrontal cortical functioning. That is, there exists a tradeoff between the capacity to learn new data versus the ability to use and elaborate on previously learned information. Ultimately, the changes in brain structure and function that occur during adolescence are thought to allow in adults for greater computational efficiency in longer cortical-cortical connections rather than more local connections (Lewis, 1997). According to computational models, these differences should allow for the preferential incorporation of information from previously learned experiences into decision-making processes rather than the preferential engagement in more risky, novel or seemingly impulsive behaviors that may represent a corollary of learning during adolescence.

Changes in Secondary Motivational Pathways and Implications for Treatment

Other influences on motivated behaviors likely stem from other neurochemical changes during adolescence. For example, sex steroid changes that occur during adolescence influence activities within the hippocampus and hypothalamus and thus can influence motivated behaviors (Chambers et al., 2003). Together, the data suggest that the adolescent brain is a changing organ and this has several important implications. First, it suggests that treatments for adults might not work in the same manner in adolescents. Second, it suggests that treatments for adolescents might need to differ according to brain maturational stage, and that within individuals the effectiveness of specific treatments might vary over time. Third, treatments during specific developmental epochs in adolescence may have an enduring impact on the presence or manifestation of adult psychiatric syndromes. These points highlight the importance of directly studying the efficacy and tolerability of specific treatments in adolescents.

Assessment of Adolescent Gambling

Adolescents present many diagnostic challenges, and this is no less the case in the area of gambling. As with a disorder such as depression (adolescents with depression often report feeling irritable rather than depressed), adolescents with gambling problems may experience a different pattern of symptoms depending upon their age and developmental stage. At present, there is no evidence of a unique adolescent version of pathological gambling. Accordingly, the diagnostic criteria for pathological gambling in the DSM-IV-TR are identical for adolescents and adults. However, some researchers have questioned whether the diagnostic threshold for pathological gambling should be lowered when assessing adolescents (Fisher, 2000; Winters, Stinchfield & Fulkerson, 1993). Even in the case of adult gamblers, there is debate regarding the most appropriate classification system for defining disordered gambling behaviors and whether there should be distinct diagnostic categories for "problem gambling" and "pathological gambling" (Derevensky, Gupta & Winters, 2003; Potenza, 2002; Stinchfield, 2003).

Given the limited current information and concern regarding symptom classification accuracy in adolescents, and whether there should be a separate diagnostic category for "problem gambling," we have chosen to use the term *pathological gambling* when referring to adolescents and adults who meet diagnostic criteria. An important step in the treatment of pathological gambling in adolescents, therefore, is the requirement for further research into the constituent symptom components of a diagnosis of pathological gambling in adolescent populations, whether additional diagnostic categories such as problem gambling should be entertained, and their concomitant implications for prevention and treatment.

Pharmacotherapy

Given the current prevalence rates of adolescent problem gambling and its impact on affected individuals and their families, effective treatments are important. There are, however, no pharmacological treatments for pathological gambling in children, adolescents or adults that are currently approved by the U.S. Food and Drug Administration (FDA). Thus, it is important for treatment providers, patients, parents and guardians to understand that any use of medications for pathological gambling is off-label, and a review of the benefits and risks of pharmacotherapy and other treatment options is warranted in order to devise an appropriate treatment plan.

Pharmacological treatments have only been examined in adult pathological gamblers, and, therefore, there is no direct evidence of either safety or efficacy of these treatments in adolescents with pathological gambling. Developmental issues are important to consider when prescribing medication for adolescents. It is important to note that because adolescents may metabolize medications more efficiently than adults, that some adolescents may require higher doses relative to body weight compared to adults. Conversely, because adolescents may have less adipose tissue than adults, there may be more bioactive drugs available and therefore a greater likelihood of adverse events or a need for lower doses. Differences in central nervous system functioning and hormonal changes may further influence adolescents' responses to various medications.

Serotonin Reuptake Inhibitors

CLOMIPRAMINE. Serotonin reuptake inhibitors (SRIs), drugs blocking the action of serotonin transporter and thus increasing synaptic availability of serotonin, have been used with varying degrees of success in treating adult pathological gambling. Clomipramine, a relatively non-selective SRI, has demonstrated efficacy in reducing gambling behavior in a double-blind study with one adult subject (Hollander, Frenkel, DeCaria, Trungold & Stein, 1992). At a dose of 125mg/day, the patient showed significant improvement that was later sustained for 28 weeks on a dose of 175mg/day (Hollander et al., 1992).

Clomipramine is currently FDA-approved for the treatment of obsessive-compulsive disorder (OCD) in adolescents. Three separate studies have found the medication safe and effective in treating adolescent OCD. In one double-blind study, a mean dose of 141 mg/day resulted in a significant decrease of OCD symptoms compared to a placebo (Flament et al., 1985). A later study comparing clomipramine to desipramine found that a mean dose of 150mg/day resulted in a significantly greater improvement in OCD symptoms compared to desipramine (Leonard et al., 1989), and a multi-center study of clomipramine further supported the efficacy and safety of clomipramine in the treatment of adolescent OCD (DeVeaugh-Geiss et al., 1992). The most common adverse effects observed in adolescents, including dry mouth, somnolence and dizziness, are comparable to those observed in adults. These studies suggest that while clomipramine may be safe for adolescents with pathological gambling, its effectiveness needs further study.

FLUVOXAMINE. Fluvoxamine, a selective serotonin reuptake inhibitor (SSRI), has demonstrated mixed results in three studies of adult pathological gambling. Two studies, one open-label and one double-blind, support its efficacy at an average end-of-study dose of 195mg/day to 207mg/day (Hollander et al., 1998; Hollander et al., 2000). A longer, six-month double-blind study found that those assigned to fluvoxamine did not demonstrate a statistically significant difference in response rate compared to those taking a placebo, although the high rates of subject drop-out complicate the interpretation of the findings (Blanco, Petkova, Ibanez & Saiz-Ruiz, 2002).

Fluvoxamine was the first SSRI to gain FDA approval for the treatment of adolescent OCD. Both an open-label study (Apter et al., 1994) and a subsequent double-blind study (Riddle et al., 2001) have demonstrated that fluvoxamine, at doses ranging from 50mg to 300mg/day, is effective and safe in the treatment of adolescents with OCD. An independent study in adolescents with anxiety disorders further supports its safety (Walkup et al., 2002).

PAROXETINE. In one double-blind study, the SSRI paroxetine, at doses between 20mg/day and 60mg/day, was found to decrease gambling thoughts and behavior after approximately 6 to 8 weeks of treatment (Kim, Grant, Adson, Shin & Zaninelli, 2002). A multi-center, 16-week, placebo-controlled, double-blind, randomized study using paroxetine (mean end-of-study dose of 50mg/day) also demonstrated improvement for those taking medication, but the proportion of individuals demonstrating improvement on active drug (59%) was not found to be statistically significant different from that receiving a placebo (48%) (Grant et al., 2003).

Although never tested with adolescents having gambling problems, paroxetine has been studied in adolescents suffering from major depressive disorder and OCD. In a double-blind study of adolescent depression, paroxetine was found to be both safe and effective at doses equivalent to those used in adults (20—40mg/day) (Keller et al., 2001). Similarly, in an open-label study of adolescent OCD, paroxetine was effective and well tolerated (Rosenberg, Stewart, Fitzgerald, Tawile & Carroll, 1999). However, a recent study has found paroxetine treatment in adolescents to be associated with an increased risk for suicide (Abbott, 2003). As such, the off-label use of paroxetine in the treatment of adolescent problem gambling should be carefully considered.

CITALOPRAM. Citalopram has been studied in a three-month open-label study of eight adults with pathological gambling in which seven patients responded positively to a mean dose of 37mg/day (Zimmerman, Breen & Posternak, 2002). As in the case of other SSRIs, citalopram has been studied in the treatment of adolescent depression and OCD. In a chart review, citalopram was found to be effective and safe in reducing depressive symptoms in children and adolescents (Baumgartner, Emslie & Crismon, 2002). An open-label study of adolescent OCD suggests that citalopram may also be effective and safe in treating adolescents (Thomsen, 1997). In addition, citalopram was found to reduce adolescent impulsive aggression (mean dose of 27mg/day) and have a low incidence of adverse events (Armenteros & Lewis, 2002).

FLUOXETINE. There has been only a single study using fluoxetine in the treatment of adults with pathological gambling. Fluoxetine (20mg/day) plus monthly supportive psychotherapy was compared against supportive psychotherapy alone in a 6-month study. Those individuals assigned to the combined treatment demonstrated greater improvement in gambling symptoms and greater adherence to treatment than those undergoing supportive therapy alone (De la Gandara, 1999; Potenza & Hollander, 2002).

Although not FDA-approved for adolescent depression, fluoxetine has been examined in one double-blind study. Using a mean dose of fluoxetine of 20mg/day, the adolescents on active medication responded more favorably than those taking placebo. Adverse effects were similar to those reported by adults (Emslie et al., 1997). Fluoxetine has also been tested in two placebo-controlled studies of adolescents with OCD, has demonstrated efficacy in reducing symptoms of adolescent OCD (doses ranging from 20mg/day to 60mg/day), and has been well tolerated (Riddle et al., 1992; Geller et al., 2001). To minimize side effects, lower initial doses are used (for example 2.5mg/day to 5mg/day) depending on the adolescent's age and weight.

5HT$_2$ Receptor Antagonists

NEFAZODONE. Only one non-SRI "antidepressant" has been examined for the treatment of pathological gambling. Nefazodone, a 5-HT$_2$ receptor antagonist, was evaluated in 14 patients in an 8-week open-label trial. Twelve patients responded positively to the medication (Pallanti, Baldini Rossi, Sood & Hollander, 2002a).

Nefazadone has been examined in one open-label pharmacokinetics study of depression in adolescents (Findling et al., 2000) and one open-label treatment study (Goodnick, Jorge, Hunter & Kumar, 2000). Both studies reported that the medication was not only effective in treating depressive symptoms but also well tolerated. Adolescents had low rates of adverse events similar to adults.

Response to SRI and $5HT_2$-receptor-antagonist antidepressants, particularly in the placebo-controlled trials of SSRIs, usually involves decreased thoughts about gambling, reductions in gambling, and improvement in social, educational and/or occupational functioning. Patients may initially report feeling less preoccupied with gambling and feeling less anxious about having thoughts of gambling. As these studies have often excluded individuals with significant depressive or anxious symptoms and changes in gambling behaviors and overall clinical status occur independently from changes in depression or anxiety, the data suggest that modulation of serotonin function in adults with pathological gambling may mediate improvement in symptoms specifically related to gambling.

The evidence of SRI efficacy in the treatment of adult pathological gambling suggests that these medications may be beneficial for adolescents with pathological gambling problems. However, given changes during adolescence in serotonergic neuronal structure and function in such brain regions as the prefrontal cortex, direct investigation of the efficacies and tolerabilities of specific SRIs in adolescents with pathological gambling is warranted. The use of these medications in adolescents suffering from mood disorders or OCD further suggests that many of these medications may be safe in adolescent pathological gamblers. However, without further research, use of these medications for adolescent pathological gambling would necessarily be conducted in an off-label manner and should be carefully considered.

Mood Stabilizers

LITHIUM. Successful response to lithium at 1800mg/day was originally described in an early case report of pathological gambling using three individuals (Moskowitz, 1980). Two larger studies further support these early findings. In a single-blind trial, 14 (60.9%) of 23 pathological gamblers taking lithium and 13 (68.4%) of 19 taking valproate responded positively to treatment (Pallanti, Quercioli, Sood & Hollander, 2002b). A recent double-blind study found sustained-release lithium carbonate superior to a placebo in 29 bipolar-spectrum pathological gamblers (Hollander, Pallanti & Baldini-Rossi, 2002).

Lithium has been FDA-approved for the treatment of bipolar disorder in adolescents. One double-blind study examining lithium in 25 adolescents with co-occurring bipolar disorder and substance use disorders found that after 6 weeks of treatment, those on lithium reported improved functioning and a decrease in the number of positive urine toxicology screens

(Geller et al., 1998). The weekly mean lithium level among responders was 0.9 mEq/L. Common adverse effects of lithium appear similar to those in adults, including nausea, polyuria, tremor and acne.

Given its general safety profile in adolescents and its efficacy in treating adult pathological gambling, lithium may be a potentially useful treatment for adolescent pathological gambling. Nevertheless, studies of lithium in adolescents with pathological gambling are needed.

DIVALPROEX (VALPROIC ACID, VALPROATE). Only one study has examined divalproex in the treatment of adult pathological gambling. In a single-blind study of lithium and valproate, 13 of 19 patients (68.4%) taking divalproex reported improvement in gambling symptoms (Pallanti et al., 2002b). Although only FDA-approved for the treatment of child and adolescent seizure disorders, divalproex has been used in the treatment of adolescent bipolar disorder. Open label studies of divalproex have reported response rates of 53 to 82% for adolescents suffering from acute manic symptoms (Papatheodorou, Kutcher, Katic & Szalai, 1995; Wagner et al., 2002). In general, divalproex is started at 20mg/kg/day in adolescents. As with adults, side effects include weight gain, nausea, sedation and tremor.

CARBAMAZEPINE. Carbamazepine has been described in a case report as effective in the treatment of adult pathological gambling. One patient receiving carbamazepine in a double-blind fashion for 24 weeks experienced complete remission of gambling symptoms while on active medication (Haller & Hinterhuber, 1994). Although only FDA-approved for the treatment of adolescent seizures, carbamazepine has also demonstrated some efficacy in the treatment of adolescent bipolar disorder. An open-label comparison study of lithium, divalproex and carbamazepine in 42 patients, aged 8 to 18 years, suffering from mania or hypomania found positive response rates of 53% (divalproex), 38% (lithium) and 38% (carbamazepine) (Kowatch et al., 2000).

Opioid Antagonists

There is evidence suggesting that naltrexone, a mu-opioid receptor antagonist, is effective in reducing gambling urges and gambling behavior in adult pathological gambling. One case report describes a patient suffering from both pathological gambling and alcohol dependence who responded positively to naltrexone 50mg/day with augmentation by fluoxetine at 20 mg/day (Crockford & el-Guebaly, 1998). An open-label study using naltrexone (mean dose 157mg/day) in adult pathological gambling resulted in a significant decline in the intensity of gambling urges, thoughts and behavior (Kim & Grant, 2001). Additionally, a double-blind, placebo-controlled, randomized 12-week study found naltrexone superior to placebo.

Naltrexone, at a mean end-of-study dose of 188mg/day, resulted in improved control over gambling urges, thoughts, and behavior (Kim, Grant, Adson & Shin, 2001).

Naltrexone has also been used in the treatment of autism and appears to be well tolerated in young patients (Campbell et al., 1993; Kolmen, Feldman, Handen & Janosky, 1995). Although not clearly beneficial for the social deficits of autism, naltrexone has demonstrated efficacy in controlling hyperactivity in autistic children and adolescents (Campbell et al., 1993; Kolmen et al., 1995). Preliminary results in the treatment of alcoholic adolescents support the use of naltrexone on abstinence when combined with a supportive psychotherapy (Lifrak, Alterman, O'Brien & Volpicelli, 1997). A single case report describes the efficacy and safety of naltrexone in the treatment of a 13-year-old female with kleptomania (Grant & Kim, 2002). The medication was well tolerated at 50mg/day with only mild nausea reported at the beginning of the medication trial. Existing data support the efficacy and tolerability of naltrexone in adolescents with a wide array of disorders characterized by impaired impulse control.

Naltrexone has demonstrated some positive results in adolescents with autism, alcohol use disorders, and kleptomania when used at 50mg/day. The findings from studies of adult pathological gamblers suggest that naltrexone may be a promising treatment for adolescents with pathological gambling. The safety of naltrexone at the higher doses used in the adult studies (up to 250 mg/day), however, has not been examined in an adolescent population. Doses of naltrexone greater than 50mg/day have warranted a "black box" warning due to the medication's propensity for hepatotoxicity, particularly at higher doses (Physician's Desk Reference, 2003). Therefore, more research on both the efficacy and safety of naltrexone for adolescent pathological gambling is needed to inform prescribing guidelines.

Atypical Antipsychotics: Serotonin/Dopamine Receptor Antagonists

Atypical antipsychotics, including drugs like risperidone, olanzapine, and ziprasidone, generally share the ability to antagonize serotonin $5HT_2$ and dopamine D_2-like (D_2, D_3, and D_4) receptors (Potenza & McDougle, 1998). These drug have been explored as monotherapies and augmenting agents in the treatment of non-psychotic disorders and behaviors (Potenza & McDougle, 1998), including pathological gambling. One study of olanzapine monotherapy in the treatment of a video poker adult pathological gamblers found similar improvements in individuals treated with active or placebo drug (Potenza, Fiellin, Heninger, Rounsaville & Mazure, 2002; Rugle, 2000). One case report, observed improvement in an adult woman with pathological gambling and co-occurring schizophrenia following initiation of treatment with olanzapine at 10 mg/day (Chambers & Potenza, 2001).

Currently no atypical antipsychotic is FDA-approved for use in adolescents. One open-label study of olanzapine in children and adolescents with bipolar disorder demonstrated an overall response rate of 61% (mean dose was 9.6mg/day). Olanzapine was well tolerated although body weight increased significantly (mean body mass index increased $2.4kg/m^2$ (Frazier et al., 2001). In a double-blind study of a different atypical antipsychotic in the treatment of adolescent bipolar disorder, quetiapine plus divalproex was more effective than divalproex alone in reducing manic symptoms in 15 adolescents (DelBello, Schwiers, Rosenberg & Strakowski, 2002). Although quetiapine and other atypical antipsychotic drugs have been found to be well-tolerated in short-term trials involving adolescents (Stigler, Potenza & McDougle, 2001), increasing concerns have been raised regarding their adverse effect profile, particularly regarding their propensity for impaired glucose control and weight gain in adults and adolescents (Stigler, Potenza, Posey & McDougle, 2004). As such, emerging data regarding the long-term risk-benefit ratio may influence the decision to use these drugs in adolescents. Given the relatively weak support for the use of atypical antipsychotics in treating adults with pathological gambling problems and the potential risks of using these drugs with regard to such adverse effects as weight gain and impaired glucose regulation, their use in adolescents with pathological gambling problems should be cautiously entertained.

Conclusion

Despite the high prevalence rates of pathological gambling in adolescents, research on this disorder is still in its infancy. Our understanding of neurodevelopmental changes that occur during adolescence, and their influence on adolescent behaviors, is still at an early stage. Longitudinal studies involving neuro-imaging, genetics, and behavioral assessments should help advance our understanding of adolescents, and with this understanding should come advances in prevention and treatment strategies for problems frequently experienced by adolescents, including risk behaviors such as pathological gambling.

Available data on pathological gambling in adults suggest several possible pharmacological interventions. At present, the best evidence suggests the use of SRIs, mood stabilizers, and naltrexone in treating pathological gambling in adults (Grant, Kim & Potenza, 2003). However, no data currently exist directly evaluating the efficacy of pharmacological treatments for pathological gambling in adolescents. Pharmacological treatment of other disorders in adolescents suggests that certain medications—SRIs, mood stabilizers, naltrexone—appear safe and effective at certain doses and for certain indications. Although the data suggest potentially promising pharmacological treatments for adolescent pathological gambling, definitive treatment recommendations await completion of controlled treatment studies in this population. As the combination of behavioral and drug therapies has been demonstrated in other addictive disorders to be superior to either treatment alone (Carroll, 1997), future investigations in the treatment of pathological gambling in adolescents and adults should consider empirically validating such combined treatment approaches (Potenza, 2002; Petry, 2003). Such studies offer substantial promise and should contribute to optimizing treatment strategies for pathological gambling.

References

Abbott, A. (2003). British panel bans use of antidepressant to treat children. *Nature, 423*, 792.

Apter, A., Ratzoni, G., King, R. A., Weizman, A., Iancu, I., Binder, M., et al. (1994). Fluvoxamine open-label treatment of adolescent inpatients with obsessive-compulsive disorder or depression. *Journal of the American Academy of Child and Adolescent Psychiatry, 33*, 342–348. Armenteros, J. L. & Lewis, J. E. (2002). Citalopram treatment for impulsive aggression in children and adolescents: an open pilot study. *Journal of the American Academy of Child and Adolescent Psychiatry, 41*, 522–529.

Baumgartner, J. L., Emslie, G. J., & Crismon, M. L. (2002). Citalopram in children and adolescents with depression or anxiety. *Annals of Pharmacotherapy, 36*, 1692–1697.

Bechara, A. (2003). Risky business: Emotion, decision-making, and addiction. *Journal of Gambling Studies, 19*, 23–51.

Blanco, C., Petkova, E., Ibanez, A., & Saiz-Ruiz, J. (2002). A pilot placebo-controlled study of fluvoxamine for pathological gambling. *Annals of Clinical Psychiatry, 14*, 9–15.

Campbell, M., Anderson, L. T., Small, A. M., Adams, P., Gonzalez, N. M., & Ernst, M. (1993). Naltrexone in autistic children: Behavioral symptoms and attentional learning. *Journal of the American Academy of Child and Adolescent Psychiatry, 32*, 1283–1291. Carroll, K. M. (1997) Integrating psychotherapy and pharmacotherapy to improve drug abuse treatment outcome. *Addictive Behaviors, 22*, 233–245.

Chambers, R. A. & Potenza, M. N. (2001). Schizophrenia and pathological gambling [Letter]. *American Journal of Psychiatry, 158*, 497–498.

Chambers, R. A. & Potenza, M. N. (2003). Neurodevelopment, impulsivity, and adolescent gambling. *Journal of Gambling Studies, 19*, 53–84.

Chambers, R. A., Taylor, J. R., & Potenza, M. N. (2003). Developmental neurocircuitry of motivation in adolescence: a critical period of addiction vulnerability. *American Journal of Psychiatry, 160*, 1041–1052.

Crockford, D. N. & el-Guebaly, N. (1998). Naltrexone in the treatment of pathological gambling and alcohol dependence [Letter]. *Canadian Journal of Psychiatry, 43*, 86.

De la Gandara, J. J. (1999). *Fluoxetine: Open-trial in pathological gambling* [Abstract]. Presented at the 152 Annual Meeting of the American Psychiatric Association; May 16–21; Washington, DC.

DelBello, M., Schwiers, M., Rosenberg, H., & Strakowski, S. (2002). Quetiapine as adjunctive treatment for adolescent mania associated with bipolar disorder. *Journal of the American Academy of Child and Adolescent Psychiatry, 41,* 1216–1223.

Derevensky, J. L, Gupta, R., & Winters, K. (2003). Prevalence rates of youth gambling problems: Are the current rates inflated? *Journal of Gambling Studies, 19,* 405–425.

DeVeaugh-Geiss, J., Moroz, G., Biederman, J., Cantwell, D., Fontaine, R., Greist, J. H., et al. (1992). Clomipramine hydrochloride in childhood and adolescent obsessive-compulsive disorder—a multicenter trial. *Journal of the American Academy of Child and Adolescent Psychiatry, 31,* 45–49.

Driver-Dunkley, E., Samantra, J., & Stacy, M. (2003) Pathological gambling associated with dopamine agonist therapy in Parkinson's disease. *Neurology, 61,* 422–423.

Emslie, G. J., Rush, A. J., Weinberg, W. A., Kowatch, R. A., Hughes, C. W., Carmody, T., et al. (1997). A double-blind, randomized, placebo-controlled trial of fluoxetine in children and adolescents with depression. *Archives of General Psychiatry, 54,* 1031–1037.

Findling, R. L., Preskorn, S. H., Marcus, R. N., Magnus, R. D., D'Amico, F., Marathe, P., et al. (2000). Nefazodone pharmacokinetics in depressed children and adolescents. *Journal of the American Academy of Child and Adolescent Psychiatry, 39,* 1008–1016.

Fiorillo, C. D., Tobler, P. N., & Schultz, W. (2003). Discrete coding of reward probability and uncertainty by dopamine neurons. *Science, 299,* 1898–1902.

Fisher, S. (2000). Developing the DSM-IV criteria to identify adolescent problem gambling in non-clinical populations. *Journal of Gambling Studies, 16,* 253–274.

Flament, M. F., Rapoport, J. L., Berg, C.J., Sceery, W., Kilts, C., Mellstrom, B., et al. (1985). Clomipramine treatment of childhood obsessive-compulsive disorder. A double-blind controlled study. *Archives of General Psychiatry, 42,* 977–983.

Frazier, J. A., Biederman, J., Tohen, M., Feldman, P. D., Jacobs, T. G., Toma, V., et al. (2001). A prospective open-label treatment trial of olanzapine monotherapy in children and adolescents with bipolar disorder. *Journal of Child and Adolescent Psychopharmacology, 11,* 239–250.

Geller, B., Cooper, T. B., Sun, K., Zimerman, B., Frazier, J., Williams, M., et al. (1998). Double-blind and placebo-controlled study of lithium for adolescent bipolar disorders with secondary substance dependency. *Journal of the American Academy of Child and Adolescent Psychiatry, 37,* 171–178.

Geller, D. A., Hoog, S. L., Heiligenstein, J. H., Ricardi, R. K., Tamura, R., Kluszynski, S., et al. (2001). Fluoxetine treatment for obsessive-compulsive disorder in children and adolescents: A placebo-controlled clinical trial. *Journal of the American Academy of Child andAdolescent Psychiatry, 40,* 773–779.

Goodnick, P. J., Jorge, C. A., Hunter, T., & Kumar, A. M. (2000). Nefazodone treatment of adolescent depression: An open-label study of response and biochemistry. *Annals of Clinical Psychiatry, 12,* 97–100.

Grant, J. E. & Kim, S. W. (2002). Adolescent kleptomania treated with naltrexone: a case report. *European Child & Adolescent Psychiatry, 11,* 92–95.

Grant, J. E., Kim, S. W., & Potenza, M. N. (2003) Advances in the pharmacotherapy of pathological gambling disorder. *Journal of Gambling Studies, 19,* 85–109.

Grant, J. E., Kim, S. W., Potenza, M. N., Blanco, C., Ibanez, A., Stevens, L. C., et al. (2003). Paroxetine treatment of pathological gambling: a multi-center randomized controlled trial. *International Clinical Psychopharmacology, 18,* 243–249.

Gupta, R. & Derevensky, J. L. (1998). Adolescent gambling behavior: A prevalence study and examination of the correlates associated with problem gambling. *Journal of Gambling Studies, 14,* 319–345.

Haller, R. & Hinterhuber, H. (1994). Treatment of pathological gambling with carbamazepine. *Pharmacopsychiatry, 27,* 129.

Hollander, E., Frenkel, M., DeCaria, C., Trungold, S., & Stein, D. J. (1992). Treatment of pathological gambling with clomipramine [Letter]. *American Journal of Psychiatry, 149,* 710–711.

Hollander, E., DeCaria, C. M., Mari, E., Wong, C. M., Mosovich, S., Grossman, R., et al. (1998). Short-term single-blind fluvoxamine treatment of pathological gambling. *American Journal of Psychiatry, 155,* 1781–1783.

Hollander, E., DeCaria, C. M., Finkell, J. N., Begaz, T., Wong, C. M., & Cartwright, C. (2000). A randomized double-blind fluvoxamine/placebo crossover trial in pathological gambling. *Biological Psychiatry, 47,* 813–817.

Hollander, E., Pallanti, S., & Baldini-Rossi, N. (2002). *Sustained release lithium/placebo treatment response in bipolar spectrum pathological gamblers.* Poster presented at the 42nd Annual New Clinical Drug Evaluation Unit Meeting, Boca Raton, Florida.

Kalivas, P. W., Churchill, L., & Romanides, A. (1999). Involvement of the palladal-thalamocortical circuit in adaptive behavior. *Annals of the New York Academy of Sciences, 877,* 64–70.

Keller, M. B., Ryan, N. D., Strober, M., Klein, R. G., Kutcher, S. P., Birmaher, B., et al. (2001). Efficacy of paroxetine in the treatment of adolescent major depression: a randomized controlled trial. *Journal of the American Academy of Child and Adolescent Psychiatry, 40,* 762–772.

Kim, S. W. & Grant, J. E. (2001). An open naltrexone treatment study of pathological gambling disorder. *International Clinical Psychopharmacology, 16,* 285–289.

Kim, S. W., Grant, J. E., Adson, D. E., & Shin, Y. C. (2001). Double-blind naltrexone and placebo comparison study in the treatment of pathological gambling. *Biological Psychiatry, 49,* 914–921.

Kim, S. W., Grant, J. E., Adson, D. E., Shin, Y. C., & Zaninelli, R. M. (2002). A double-blind placebo-controlled study of the efficacy and safety of paroxetine in the treatment of pathological gambling. *Journal of Clinical Psychiatry, 63,* 501–507.

Kolmen, B. K., Feldman, H. M., Handen, B. L., & Janosky, J. E. (1995). Naltrexone in young autistic children: a double-blind, placebo-controlled crossover study. *Journal of the American Academy of Child and Adolescent Psychiatry, 34,* 223–231.

Kowatch, R. A., Suppes, T., Carmody, T. J., Bucci, J. P., Hume, J. H., Kromelis, M., et al. (2000). Effect size of lithium, divalproex sodium and carbamazepine in children and adolescents with bipolar disorder. *Journal of the American Academy of Child and Adolescent Psychiatry, 39,* 713–720.

Leonard, H. L., Swedo, S. E., Rapoport, J. L., Koby, E. V., Lenane, M. C., Cheslow, D. L., et al. (1989). Treatment of obsessive-compulsive disorder with clomipramine and desipramine in children and adolescents. A double-blind crossover comparison. *Archives of General Psychiatry, 46,* 1088–1092.

Lewis. D. A. (1997). Development of the prefrontal cortex during adolescence: insights into vulnerable neural circuits in schizophrenia. *Neuropsychopharmacology, 16,* 385–398.

Lifrak, P. D., Alterman, A. I., O'Brien, C. P., & Volpicelli, J. R. (1997). Naltrexone for alcoholic adolescents. *American Journal of Psychiatry, 154,* 439–441.

Moskowitz, J. A. (1980). Lithium and lady luck: use of lithium carbonate in compulsive gambling. *New York State Journal of Medicine, 80,* 785–788.

New, A. S., Hazlett, E. A., Buchsbaum, M. S., Goodman, M., Reynolds, D., Mitropoulou, V., et al. (2002). Blunted prefrontal cortical 18fluorodeoxyglucose positron emission tomography response to meta-chlorophenylpiperazine in impulsive aggression. *Archives of General Psychiatry, 59,* 621–629.

Pallanti, S., Baldini Rossi, N., Sood, E., & Hollander, E. (2002a). Nefazodone treatment of pathological gambling: A prospective open-label controlled trial. *Journal of Clinical Psychiatry, 63*, 1034–1039.

Pallanti, S., Quercioli, L., Sood, E., & Hollander, E. (2002b). Lithium and valproate treatment of pathological gambling: a randomized single-blind study. *Journal of Clinical Psychiatry, 63*, 559–564.

Papatheodorou, G., Kutcher, S. P., Katic, M., & Szalai, J. P. (1995). The efficacy and safety of divalproex sodium in the treatment of acute mania in adolescents and young adults: an open clinical trial. *Journal of Clinical Psychopharmacology, 15*, 110–116.

Petry, N. M. (2002). How treatments for pathological gambling can be informed by treatments for substance use disorders. *Experimental and Clinical Psychopharmacology, 10*, 180–192.

Physician's Desk Reference (57th ed.). (2003). Montvale, NJ: Thompson PDR.

Potenza, M. N. (2002). A perspective on future directions in the prevention, treatment and research of pathological gambling. *Psychiatric Annals, 32*, 203–207.

Potenza, M. N., Fiellin, D. A., Heninger, G. R., Rounsaville, B. J., & Mazure, C. M. (2002). Gambling: An addictive behavior with health and primary care implications. *Journal of General Internal Medicine, 17*, 721–732.

Potenza, M. N., & Hollander, E. (2002). Pathological gambling and impulse control disorders. In J. T. Coyle, C. Nemeroff, D. Charney, & K. L. Davis (Eds.), *Neuropsycho-pharmacology: The 5th generation of progress.* (pp. 1725–1741). Baltimore, MD: Lippincott Williams and Wilkins.

Potenza, M. N., & McDougle, C. J. (1998). The potential of atypical antipsychotics in the treatment of non-psychotic disorders. *CNS Drugs, 9*, 213–232.

Proimos, J., DuRant, R. H., Pierce, J. D., & Goodman, E. (1998). Gambling and other risk behaviors among 8th- to 12th-grade students. *Journal of Pediatrics, 102*, e23.

Riddle, M. A., Scahill, L., King, R. A., Hardin, M. T., Anderson, G. M., Ort, S. I., et al. (1992). Double-blind, crossover trial of fluoxetine and placebo in children and adolescents with obsessive-compulsive disorder. *Journal of the American Academy of Child and Adolescent Psychiatry, 31*, 1062–1069.

Riddle, M. A., Reeve, E. A., Yaryura-Tobias, J. A., Yang, H. M., Claghorn, J. L., Gaffney, G., et al. (2001). Fluvoxamine for children and adolescents with obsessive-compulsive disorder: a randomized, controlled, multicenter trial. *Journal of the American Academy of Child and Adolescent Psychiatry, 40*, 222–229.

Romer, D. (2003). *Reducing adolescent risk: Toward an integrated approach.* Sage Publications, Thousand Oaks, CA.

Rosenberg, D. R., Stewart, C. M., Fitzgerald, K. D., Tawile, V., & Carroll, E. (1999). Paroxetine open-label treatment of pediatric outpatients with obsessive-compulsive disorder. *Journal of the American Academy of Child and Adolescent Psychiatry, 38*, 1180–1185.

Rugle, L. (2000). *The use of olanzapine in the treatment of video poker pathological gamblers* [Abstract]. Presented at the conference entitled, "The Comorbidity of Pathological Gambling: A Current Research Synthesis"; December 3–5; Las Vegas, Nevada.

Shah, K. R., Eisen, S. A., Xian, H., & Potenza, M. N. (in press). Genetic studies of pathological gambling: A review of methodology and analyses of data from the Vietnam Era Twin (VET) Registry. *Journal of Gambling Studies.*

Slutske, W. S., Eisen, S., True, W. R., Lyons, M. J., Goldberg, J., & Tsuang, M. (2000). Common genetic vulnerability for pathological gambling and alcohol dependence in men. *Archives of General Psychiatry, 57*, 666–673.

Stigler, K. A., Potenza, M. N., & McDougle, C. J. (2001) Tolerability profile of atypical antipsychotics in children and adolescents. *Pediatric Drugs, 3*, 927–942.

Stigler, K. A., Potenza, M. N., Posey, D., & McDougle, C. J. (2004). Bodyweight gain associated with atypical antipsychotic use in children and adolescents: Epidemiology, clinical relevance and management. *Pediatric Drugs, 6*, 33–44.

Stinchfield, R. (2001). A comparison of gambling among Minnesota public school students in 1992, 1995 and 1998. *Journal of Gambling Studies, 17*, 273–296.

Stinchfield, R. (2003). Reliability, validity, and classification accuracy of a measure of DSM-IV diagnostic criteria for Pathological Gambling. *American Journal of Psychiatry, 160*, 180–182.

Thomsen, P. H. (1997). Child and adolescent obsessive-compulsive disorder treated with citalopram: findings from an open trial of 23 cases. *Journal of Child and Adolescent Psychopharmacology, 7*, 157–166.

Tsuang, M. T., Bar, J. L., Harley, R. M., & Lyons, M. J. (2001). The Harvard twin study of substance abuse: What we have learned. *Harvard Review of Psychiatry, 9*, 267–79.

Wagner, F. A. & Anthony, J. C. (2002). From first drug use to drug dependence: developmental periods of risk for dependence upon marijuana, cocaine, and alcohol. *Neuropsycho-pharmacology, 26*, 479–488.

Wagner, K. D., Weller, E. B., Carlson, G. A., Sachs, G., Biederman, J., Frazier, J. A., et al. (2002). An open-label trial of divalproex in children and adolescents with bipolar disorder. *Journal of the American Academy of Child and Adolescent Psychiatry, 41*, 1224–1230.

Walkup, J., Labellarte, M., Riddle, M. A., Pine, D. S., Greenhill, L., Fairbanks, J., et al. (2002). Treatment of pediatric anxiety disorders: an open-label extension of the research units on pediatric psychopharmacology anxiety study. *Journal of Child and Adolescent Psychopharmacology, 12*, 175–188.

Wallisch, L. (1993). *Gambling in Texas: 1992 Texas survey of adolescent gambling behavior.* Austin, TX: Texas Commission on Alcohol and Drug Abuse.

Winters, K. C., Stinchfield, R., & Fulkerson, J. (1993). Patterns and characteristics of adolescent gambling. *Journal of Gambling Studies, 9*, 371–386.

Wynne, H., Smith, G., & Jacobs, D. (1996). *Adolescent gambling and problem gambling in Alberta.* Edmonton, Alberta: Alberta Alcohol and Drug Abuse Commission.

Zimmerman, M., Breen, R. B., & Posternak, M. A. (2002). An open-label study of citalopram in the treatment of pathological gambling. *Journal of Clinical Psychiatry, 63*, 44–48.

Part III

Chapter 6

Youth and Technology
The Case of Gambling,
Video-Game Playing, and the Internet

Mark Griffiths, Ph.D. and
Richard T. A. Wood, Ph.D.

The field of gambling is certainly not immune to the technological revolution taking place elsewhere in other fields. Technology continues to provide new market opportunities in the shape of advanced slot machines, video-games, Internet gambling, interactive television gambling and telephone/mobile phone gambling. In addition, other established gambling forms are becoming more technologically driven (e.g. bingo, keno); all of which are appealing to adolescents.

The global expansion of gambling coupled with the increased popularity of technology, the Internet, and various digital technologies, has led the gambling industry to invest heavily in Internet gambling. Prospects for new and extended business are potentially large as more people gain access to this technology. Further, it has been alleged that social pathologies are beginning to surface in cyberspace in the form of "technological addictions" (e.g., Griffiths, 1998). The growth of technological forms of gambling raises pertinent questions particularly when it comes to adolescent participation. This chapter provides on overview of three areas of growing interest to adolescents—slot machines, video-games, and Internet gambling.

Adolescent Slot-Machine Gambling

Adolescent gambling is a major problem in society today. Not only is it usually illegal, but it appears to be related to high levels of problem gambling and other delinquent activities such as illicit drug taking and alcohol abuse (e.g., Griffiths & Sutherland, 1998; Gupta & Derevensky, 1998a; Stinchfield, Cassuto, Winters & Latimer, 1997;). Studies in Europe, the U.S., Canada and Australia have noted high levels of gambling among adolescents. In fact, relative to adults, it has been suggested that adolescents may be more susceptible to pathological or problem gambling (Fisher, 1993a; Lesieur & Klein, 1987). Research from Canada, the U.K. and the U.S. has revealed that between 5 and 6% of adolescents under the age of 18 meet criteria for pathological gambling, a figure which is higher than that identified among adults (Fisher, 1993a; Griffiths 1995; Jacobs, this volume; Shaffer, LaBrie, Scanlon & Cummings, 1993).

Evidence suggests that adolescent problem gambling is primarily a male phenomenon (Griffiths 1991a; Stinchfield et al., 1997), and that adults contribute, at least in part, to the development of this phenomenon. For example, studies show that adolescent gambling is strongly associated with parental gambling (e.g., Fisher, 1993a; Griffiths 1995; Gupta & Derevensky, 1997; Wood & Griffiths 1998). According to studies in the U.K. and in Canada, it is not uncommon for parents to purchase lottery tickets or scratchcards for their children (Derevensky & Gupta, 2001; Fisher & Balding, 1998; Wood & Griffiths 1998). This is particularly worrisome given that problem gambling in adulthood is negatively associated with age of onset during adolescence (Fisher, 1993a; Griffiths, 1995; Gupta & Derevensky, 1998a; Winters, Stinchfield & Fulkerson, 1993).

With respect to technological advances in gambling, it is thought that slot machines represent the most pressing problem for adolescents. Worldwide data has clearly shown that electronic gaming machines are potentially addictive (for a comprehensive review see Griffiths, 2002). In the past decade, slot machines and other forms of electronic gaming machines, have been the predominant form of gambling by pathological gamblers treated in self-help groups and professional treatment centres across Europe (Griffiths & Wood, 1999). There are many reasons why this is the case. Slot machines are fast, aurally and visually stimulating and rewarding, require a low initial stake, provide frequent wins, require no special knowledge to play, and may be played alone. Although the excessive play of slot machines is undoubtedly contingent upon biological, psychological, and situational variables, it is clear that the structural characteristics of electronic gaming machines are designed to induce the individual to play and to continue playing. It has been argued that a combination of the technological aspects of the structural characteristics (e.g., event frequencies, near misses, and light and sound effects) may contribute towards habitual and repetitive play in some individuals (Griffiths, 1993a, 1995; Loba, Stewart, Klein & Blackburn, 2001).

Most research on slot-machine gambling in youth has been undertaken in the U.K. where they are legally available to children of any age. For example, Fisher and Balding (1998) found that slot machines were the most popular form of adolescent gambling with 75% of youth (n = 9774) participating. A more thorough examination of the literature (Fisher & Balding, 1998; Griffiths, 1995, 2002; Griffiths & Wood, 2000) suggests that:

- at least two-thirds of adolescents play slot machines at some point during adolescence
- one third of adolescents report having played slot machines in the past month
- 10–20% of adolescents are regular slot machine players (minimum of once a week)
- 0.5–6% of adolescents are probably pathological gamblers and/or have severe gambling-related difficulties.

Why do adolescents play slot machines? This is not easy to answer as there are a host of plausible reasons. However, research indicates that irregular *social* gamblers play for different reasons than the excessive *pathological* gamblers (Griffiths, 1995, 2002). Social gamblers usually play for fun, because their friends or parents play, to win money and/or for excitement and enjoyment. Pathological gamblers appear to play for other reasons such as mood modification and as a means of escape. Young males seem to be particularly susceptible to slot-machine addiction with 6% of adolescents in the U.K. meeting DSM criteria for problematic slot-machine gambling at any given time (Fisher, 1993a; Griffiths, 1995). This does not mean that everyone who plays slot machines will become addicted (in the same way that not everyone who drinks alcohol will become an alcoholic). What it does mean, however, is that in combination biological, social, psychological, situational and structural characteristics lead a proportion of individuals to develop severe gambling-related problems.

Similar to other potentially addictive behaviors, slot-machine addiction is associated with negative behaviors including school truancy (Fisher & Balding, 1998; Griffiths, 1990, 1995), stealing (Fisher & Balding, 1998; Griffiths, 1990; Yeoman & Griffiths, 1996), getting into trouble with teachers and/or parents over machine playing (Griffiths, 1990, 1995), poor schoolwork (Griffiths, 1990, 1995), and in some cases aggressive behavior (Griffiths, 1990, 1995). In addition, slot machine addicts also display signs of addiction including withdrawal effects, tolerance, salience, mood modification, conflict and relapse (Griffiths, 1993b, 1995, 2002). It is also worth noting that the negative consequences associated with slot-machine addiction have also been identified in other more general studies on gambling addiction among youth in the U.S., Canada and Australia (Gupta & Derevensky, 1997; 1998a, 1998b; Lesieur, Cross, Frank, Welch, Rubenstein, Moseley & Mark, 1991; Moore & Ohtsuka, 1997).

Risk Factors in Slot-Machine Gambling

Griffiths (1999) has noted that gambling addictions are not merely measured in terms of simple frequency, but instead encompass a multitude of factors including:

- stake size (including issues around affordability, perceived value for money)
- event frequency (time gap between each gamble)
- amount of money lost in a given time period (important in chasing)
- prize structures (number and values of prizes)
- probability of winning (e.g., 1 in 14 million on the lottery)
- size of jackpot (e.g., over £1 million on the lottery)
- skill and pseudo-skill elements (actual or perceived)
- "near miss" opportunities (number of near winning situations)
- light and colour effects (e.g., use of red lights on slot machines)
- sound effects (e.g., use of buzzers or musical tunes to indicate winning)
- social or asocial nature of the game (individual and/or group activity)
- accessibility (e.g., number of outlets, opening times, membership rules)
- location of gambling establishment (out of town, next to workplace etc.)
- type of gambling establishment (e.g., betting shop, amusement arcade etc.)
- advertising (e.g., television commercials)
- the rules of the game

Although the factors noted above may influence gambling behavior directly, it is generally thought that structural characteristics of the game interact with individual risk factors to promote the development of pathological gambling. As a result of the recent upsurge in research into adolescent gambling behavior, scholars have begun to put together a "risk factor model" of those who might be at the greatest risk of developing gambling-related difficulties. For example, in comprehensive reviews of the literature Griffiths (1991a; 1995) suggests that adolescent problem gamblers are more likely to be male (16–25 years), have begun gambling at an early age (as young as 8 years of age), have had a big win earlier in their gambling careers, consistently chase losses, have begun gambling with their parents or other relatives, be depressed before gambling, be excited and aroused during gambling, be irrational (i.e., have erroneous perceptions) during gambling, have poor school performance, engage in other addictive behaviors (smoking, drinking alcohol, illegal drug use), come from the lower social classes, have parents who have a gambling (or other addiction) problem, have a history of delinquency, steal and/or borrow money to fund their gambling and are truant from school to go gambling.

There is, of course, a problem with the identification of adolescent problem gamblers in that there is no observable sign or symptom like there is with other addictions (e.g., alcoholism, drug addiction, etc.). Although there have been some reports of a personality change in young gamblers (Griffiths, 1995), many parents may attribute the change to those associated with the period of adolescence itself (i.e., evasive behavior, mood swings, etc.). It is often the case that parents do not even realize that their son or daughter has a problem until he or she is in trouble with the police. Research suggests that there are a number of possible warning signs to look for, although taken on their own, many of these signs are commonly attributed to the developmental period of adolescence itself (Griffiths, 1995). However, it is premised that the presence of several of these signs may be indicative of a gambling problem. The signs include:

- a sudden drop in academic performance
- going out each evening and being evasive about where they have been
- personality changes (e.g., sullen, moody, or constantly on the defensive)
- money missing from home
- selling expensive possessions and not being able to account for the money
- loss of interest in activities previously enjoyed
- lack of concentration
- an ambivalent attitude
- lack of concern over their appearance or hygiene

It is important to note that many of these "warning signs" are not necessarily unique to a gambling addiction and can also be indicative of other addictions (e.g., alcohol and drugs).

Video-game Playing in Adolescence

Both video-game machines and slot machines may be considered under the generic label of "amusement machines" (Griffiths, 1991a). The primary difference between video-game machines and slot machines are that video-games are played to accumulate as many points as possible whereas slot machines are played (i.e., gambled upon) to accumulate money. Griffiths (1991a) has suggested that playing a video-game could be considered as a non-financial form of gambling. Both types of machine require insertion of a coin to play, although the playing time on a slot machine is usually much less than on a video-game machine. On video-games the outcome is almost solely due to skill, whereas on slot machines the outcome is more likely to be a product of chance. However, the general playing philosophy of both slot machine players and video-game players is to stay on the machine for as long as possible using the least amount of money (Griffiths, 1990). Griffiths has argued that regular slot machine players play with money rather than for it and that winning money is merely a means to an end, that is, to stay on the machine as long as possible.

Besides the generic labeling, their geographical juxtaposition, and the philosophy for playing, it could be argued that on both a psychological and behavioral level, slot-machine gambling and video-game playing share many similarities (e.g., similar demographic differences such as age and gender in the U.K., similar reinforcement schedules, similar potential for 'near miss' opportunities, similar structural characteristics involving the use of light and sound effects, similarities in skill perception, similarities in the effects of excessive play, etc.). The most probable reason the two forms have rarely been seen as conceptually similar is because video-game playing does not involve the winning of money (or something of financial value) and therefore cannot be classified as a form of gambling.

However, the next generation of slot machines are starting to use video-game graphics and technology. While many of these relate to traditional gambling games (e.g., roulette, poker, blackjack, etc.) there are plans for developing video gambling games in which people would win money based on their game scores (J. Derevensky, personal communication, January 2000). In short, it is becoming increasingly clear that video-games share common ground with slot machines and other gambling mediums; not only in terms of their structural characteristics but also in terms of their potential to create dependency (Fisher & Griffiths, 1995; Griffiths, 1991a; 1997; Gupta & Derevensky, 1996).

Adolescent Gambling and Video-game Playing:
Psychosocial Factors

It has been noted that adolescent video-game playing is also often associated with gambling participation (Gupta & Derevensky, 1996; Wood, Gupta, Derevensky & Griffiths, in press). As such, it is important to consider the psychological features that contribute to why some youth develop gambling-related problems, while others do not. Excessive gambling is derived from a complex interplay between the activity itself (e.g., structural characteristics), the availability of the activity (e.g., situational factors), social factors (e.g., peer influence) and psychological factors (e.g., mood modification). In relation to the latter there are a number of specific factors that have been linked to problem gambling/gaming. It has been noted that problem gamblers often exhibit poor coping skills (Marget, Gupta & Derevensky, 1999; Nower, Gupta & Derevensky, 2000). As such, gambling/gaming may be used as an alternative method of coping that some adolescents use to deal with daily problems. Consequently, when the behavior ceases, the person is faced with the prospect of dealing with underlying problems. The excessive video-game player and/or gambler knows that engaging in these activities provides relief from dealing with daily problems and, consequently, the behavior is likely to be repeated. Wood et al. (in press) found that both excessive video-game playing and excessive gambling were associated with perceived excitement, relaxation, and escape while engaged in the activity. Furthermore, high frequency video-game players and those who reported gambling problems were more likely to report various states of dissociation (e.g., going into a trance-like state, losing track of time etc.) According to Jacobs' *General Theory of Addictions* (1986) activities that have the capacity to be either arousing and/or relaxing, and that allow a person to be distracted from their normal lives, is highly desirable and likely to be participated in excessively by some individuals. Both gambling and video-game playing fall into this category of activity.

Gupta and Derevensky (1996) found that males played video-games significantly more than females, and that high frequency video-game playing males were more likely to gamble at least once per week. Dissociative states while engaging in gambling/gaming also appear to vary significantly between males and females. According to Wood et al. (in press), males find video-games to be significantly more exciting and/or relaxing, and play video-games for much longer periods of time, relative to their female counterparts. The authors also report that compared to low-frequency video-game players, high-frequency players score higher on the Risk-Taking Questionnaire (RTQ), and that as this relationship increased, so too did the probability of being a problem gambler increased. As such, it seems that high-frequency video-game players and problem gamblers tend to be high-risk takers. It is plausible that at-risk adolescents feel under aroused and that engaging in gambling activities, video-game playing, or more general risk-taking behavior is an attempt to increase arousal levels.

Cognitive factors may also contribute to problem gambling/gaming in youth. Wood et al. (in press) reported that those youth who exhibited the most severe gambling-related problems were also those more likely to rate themselves as either excellent or very good video-game players. This may suggest that problem gamblers try to transfer the skills learned as video-game player to gambling situations. This is consistent with holding an illusion of control (Langer, 1975). These players may perceive that gambling skills can be learned and mastered in much the same way as the techniques required to perform well on video-games. Increasingly, many forms of gambling have the appearance of a video-game (e.g., VLTs, CD-ROM, some forms of Internet gambling, etc.) and share many similar structural characteristics (e.g., intermittent rewards, flashing lights, etc.). The convergence of video-games and gambling makes it increasingly difficult to establish what is and what is not a purely chance-based activity. Recently, Loto-Quebec released a series of interactive CD-ROM lottery games. These games have similar structural characteristics to some forms of gambling (e.g., scratchcards, VLTs) combined with graphic animation and the "playability" of a video-game. While these games require no actual skill whatsoever to win and the player can receive help at any stage to solve the problems, the nature of the game contributes to an illusion of control by effectively mimicking the structural characteristics of a video-game (e.g., skill-based problem solving). While this game is currently limited to the format of a CD-ROM, the technology exists to play these types of games over the Internet which ultimately eliminates the need to leave home to purchase these products and allows for continuous play.

Empirical Research on Video-game Addiction

To date, there has been very little research directly investigating video-game addiction, although almost all of it has concentrated on adolescents. Shotton (1989) conducted a study specifically on *computer addiction* using a sample of 127 people, half of whom were adolescents, who reported being "hooked" on home video-games for at least five years. Results showed that computer-dependent individuals were highly intelligent and motivated, but often felt misunderstood. After a five-year follow up, the younger cohort had done well educationally, had gone on to university and achieved high-ranking jobs. However, Shotton's research included people who were familiar with the older generation of video-games, that is, those that were popular in the earlier part of the 1980s. Video-games beginning in the 1990s may in some way be more psychologically rewarding than previous generations of games as they require more complex skills, improved dexterity, and feature socially relevant topics and better graphics. Anecdotal accounts of greater psychological rewards could mean that newer games are more 'addiction inducing'; a conjecture which clearly merits empirical attention.

A more recent study by Griffiths and Hunt (1995, 1998) examined almost 400 adolescents (12–16 years of age) to establish levels of "dependence" using a scale adapted from the DSM-III-R criteria for pathological gambling (American Psychiatric Association, 1987). Questions relating to the DSM-III-R criteria were adapted for computer-game playing and examined a number of components associated with addiction including salience, tolerance, euphoria, chasing, relapse, withdrawal, and conflict. Scores on the adapted DSM-III-R scale indicated that 62 players (19.9%) were dependent on computer games (i.e., scored four or more on the continuous scales). Furthermore, 7% of the sample claimed they played in excess of thirty hours a week. Dependence score correlated with how often individuals played computer games, the mean length of playing session time, and the longest single session playing time. Males were found to be more likely to have high dependence scores.

The above study assumes that computer-game playing overlaps with gambling in terms of the consequences of excessive behavior. Whether excessive computer-game playing should be conceptualized as an addiction or as a preoccupation, it is clear that for some children and adolescents video-games can consume a considerable amount of time. Whether video-games are identified as addictive or not may not be the most salient issue. Rather, the question to ask is what are the longitudinal developmental effects of any activity (not just video-game playing) that can consume up to 30 hours of leisure time a week? It is our contention that children who engage in any activity at excessive frequencies, for long durations (over a number of years), and from a young age, are likely to experience some degree of impairment in psychosocial development.

Excessive Video-game Play: Other Negative Consequences

Back in the early 1980s, rheumatologists described cases of "Pac-Man's Elbow" and "Space Invaders' Revenge" in which players suffered skin, joint and muscle problems from repeated button hitting and joystick pushing on the game machines (Loftus & Loftus, 1983). These researchers found that two-thirds of video-game players examined complained of blisters, calluses, sore tendons, and numbness in the hands as a direct result of excessive play. Among a host of other negative consequences, researchers have also cited photo-sensitive epilepsy (e.g., Millett, Fish & Thompson, 1997), enuresis (Schink, 1991), encoprisis (Corkery, 1990), hand-arm vibration syndrome (Cleary, McKendrick & Sills, 2002), repetitive strain injuries (Mirman & Bonian, 1992), peripheral neuropathy (Friedland & St. John, 1984), increased risk of childhood obesity (e.g., Deheger, Rolland-Cachera & Fontvielle, 1997), decreased participation in educational and sporting pursuits (Egli & Meyers, 1984), and increased social isolation (Zimbardo, 1982) as directly resulting from video-game playing.

Clearly, from case studies, individuals who are excessive users of video-games exhibited some form of negative consequence. From prevalence studies, there is little evidence of serious acute adverse effects on health from moderate play. Adverse effects are likely to be relatively minor, and temporary, resolving spontaneously with decreased frequency of play, or to affect only a small subgroup of players. Although excessive players may be most at-risk for developing health problems, increased research in establishing clearer operational definitions and in shedding light on the prevalence rate of clinically significant problems associated with video-game play is warranted.

Adolescence, Internet Use and Internet Gambling

To a gambling addict, the Internet could potentially be a very dangerous medium. In fact, some observers have argued that Internet gambling provides "a natural fit" for compulsive gamblers (O'Neill, 1998). It would appear that Internet gambling will significantly increase for several reasons. First, it is easy to access and participate in an activity that comes into the home via the computer or television. Second, internet gambling has the potential to offer visually exciting effects similar to slot machines and VLTs (two of the most problematic forms of gambling). Third, the event frequency can be very rapid, particularly if the gambler is subscribed to several sites. Finally, as a result of bigger and better home entertainment systems (e.g., digital television, home cinema systems, and cable and satellite systems) the need and desire to fill leisure time outside the home is greatly reduced (Griffiths & Wood, 2000). It is speculated that in the not-to-distant future, part of this entertainment-seeking pattern may include Internet gambling for many families.

Internet Addiction and Internet Gambling Addiction

Gambling has long been known to be potentially addictive. Coupled with increasing research reports that the Internet, in general, is addictive (e.g., Griffiths, 1998, 2000b; Young, 1996, 1998, 1999), it has been speculated that the risk of problematic Internet gambling is particularly alarming. Technological addictions including, Internet addiction, can be best viewed as a subset of behavioral addictions (see Marks, 1990), which feature the core components of an addiction, namely salience, euphoria, tolerance, withdrawal, conflict and relapse (see Griffiths, 1995). Young (1999) has claimed that an Internet addiction is a broader term that covers a wide variety of behaviors and impulse-control problems, and can be categorized according to five specific subtypes: (a) *Cybersexual addiction:* compulsive use of adult websites for cybersex and cyberporn, (b) *Cyber-relationship addiction:* over-involvement in online relationships, (c) *Net compulsions:* obsessive online gambling, shopping or day-trading, (d) *Information overload:* compulsive web surfing or database searches, and (e) *Computer addiction:* obsessive playing of computer games.

Griffiths (2000b) has argued that many of these excessive users are not *Internet addicts* but rather use the Internet excessively as a medium to fuel other addictions. Put simply, a gambling addict who engages in their chosen behavior online is not addicted to the Internet but rather gambling. However, in contrast, there are case studies of individuals who appear to be addicted to the Internet itself (Griffiths, 2000a; Young, 1996). These are usually people who use Internet chat rooms or play fantasy role playing games—activities that they would not typically engage in except on the Internet itself. Such individuals, to some extent, are engaged in text-based virtual realities and take on other social personas and social identities. In these cases, the Internet may provide an alternative reality to the user and allow them feelings of immersion and anonymity that may subsequently lead to an altered state of consciousness. This in itself may be highly psychologically and/or physiologically rewarding.

The Impact of Technology on Gambling: Salient Factors

To what extent does technology promote excessiveness? There are a number of factors that make online activities potentially seductive and/or addictive. Such factors include accessibility, affordability, anonymity, convenience, escape, dissociation /immersion, disinhibition, event frequency, interactivity/simulation, and asociability. In general, the structural characteristics common to gambling appear to be enhanced through technological innovation.

Some researchers have made attempts to explain the Internet's seductiveness. Cooper (1998) proposed the *Triple A Engine* (Access, Affordability, and Anonymity) which he claimed help to understand the power and attraction of the Internet for sexual pursuits. Young's (1999) *ACE* model (Anonymity, Convenience, Escape) is similar. Neither of these are strictly models as they fail to explain the process of how online use develops. They do, however, provide in acronym form, the primary variables accounting for the acquisition and maintenance of online behaviors. The variables that lead to such activities as virtual adultery (i.e., anonymity, access, convenience, affordability and escape) appear to provide the explanatory building blocks for the development of other online behaviors, including Internet gambling. It would also appear that virtual environments have the potential to provide short-term comfort, excitement and/or distraction.

The Internet's *accessibility* is now commonplace and widespread within homes and the workplace. Given that prevalence of behaviors is strongly correlated with increased accessibility, it is not surprising that the development of regular online use is increasing across the population. Increased accessibility may result in increased problems. Research into other socially acceptable but potentially addictive behaviors (drinking alcohol, gambling etc.) has revealed that increased accessibility leads to increased uptake (regular use) and that this eventually results in increased problems (Griffiths, 1999). In other words, where accessibility of gambling is increased, not only is there an increase in the number of regular gamblers, but also in the number of problem gamblers. While not everyone is susceptible to developing a gambling addiction, it does suggest that on a societal (rather than individual) level, the more gambling opportunities, the greater the number of problems will likely exist.

Given the increase in Internet use and increased competition, the *affordability* of online services has increased. The *anonymity* of the Internet also allows users to privately engage in gambling without the fear of stigma. This anonymity may also provide the user with a greater sense of perceived control over the content, tone, and nature of the online experience (Young, Griffin-Shelley, Cooper, O'Mara & Buchanan, 2000). Anonymity may also increase feelings of comfort since there is a decreased ability to look for, and thus detect, signs of insincerity, disapproval, or judgment in facial expression, as would be typical in face-to-face interactions. For activities such as gambling, this may be a positive benefit particularly when losing as no one will actually see an individual's emotional reactions.

Another relevant factor is *convenience;* interactive online applications such as e-mail, chat rooms, newsgroups, or role-playing games provide convenient mediums to engage in online behaviors. Such behaviors will usually occur in familiar and comfortable environments, thus reducing the feeling of risk and allowing adventurous behaviors which may be potentially addictive. For the gambler, not having to move from one's home or workplace may be perceived to be a significant benefit.

Moreover, feelings of *escape, immersion/dissociation* and *disinhibition* may also promote Internet gambling. For some, the primary reinforcement to engage in Internet gambling is the gratification they experience online. However, the experience of Internet gambling itself, may be reinforced through a subjectively experienced "high." The pursuit of mood-modificating experiences is characteristic of addictions, has the potential to provide an emotional or mental escape, and further serves to reinforce the behavior. Online behavior can provide potential to relieve the stresses and strains of real life, and these activities falling on a continuum from life enhancing to pathological and addictive behaviors (Cooper, Putnam, Planchon & Boies, 1999).

Also promoting gambling behavior is *event frequency.* Defined as the number of opportunities to gamble in a given time period, event frequency is a structural characteristic designed and implemented by the gaming operator. The length of time between each gambling event may be critical in the development of problems with particular types of gambling. Gambling activities that offer intermittent outcomes every few seconds, such as slot machines, will likely result in greater problems than activities with less frequent outcomes, such as weekly lotteries or sports pools. Slot machines' event frequencies, linked to (a) the win/lose outcome of the wager and (b) the actual time until winnings (reinforcements) are received, exploits certain basic psychological principles of learning (Moran, 1987). Rapid event frequency also suggests that the loss period is brief, with little time given to financial considerations, and more importantly, winnings can be rewagered almost immediately. Internet gambling has the potential to offer visually exciting effects similar to slot machines and VLTs.

Finally, *interactivity/stimulation* and *asociability* also contribute to the seductive and/or addictive potential of online gambling. In terms of interactivity/stimulation, studies have shown that one's personal involvement in a gambling activity can increase the illusion of control which, in turn, results in increased gambling (Langer, 1975). With increased time spent interacting online, less time is spent interacting face-to-face in the social world. One of the consequences of technology has been to reduce the fundamentally social nature of gambling to an activity that is essentially asocial. Both Fisher (1993b) and Griffiths (1991b) have carried out observational analyses of slot machine players (particularly adolescents) and have reached similar conclusions. Those who experience problems are more likely to be those playing on their own. Moreover, most problem gamblers report that at the height of their problem gambling, it was a solitary activity (Griffiths, 1995). It is possible that gambling in a social setting provides some kind of "safety net" for over-spenders. One of the primary influences of technology appears to be the shift from social to asocial forms of gambling. It is speculated that as gambling becomes more technological, gambling problems will increase due to its asocial nature.

Other Factors Relating to Internet Gambling

There are many other technological developments that are likely to increase Internet gambling including (a) sophisticated gaming software, (b) integrated e-cash systems (including multi-currency), (c) multi-lingual sites, (d) increased realism (e.g., real gambling via webcams, player and dealer avatars), (e) live remote wagering (for both gambling alone and gambling with others), and (f) improving customer care systems. According to some estimates, $2.3 billion (US) a year is being spent on Internet gaming worldwide, and the market has more than tripled in size since 1997 (Mitka, 2001). One study, which featured details on more than 1,400 gambling sites available worldwide, estimated that the number of Internet gamblers will grow from approximately 4 million in 1999 to 15 million individuals by the year 2004 (Sinclair, 2000).

Recent surveys have revealed that the majority of Internet users are male although the number of female Internet users is rising (Morahan-Martin, 1998). Other studies have begun to examine excessive Internet use among student populations (e.g., Morahan-Martin & Schumacher, 1997). Although unrepresentative of the general public, college students are considered high-risk for Internet problems because of ready access, technological sophistication, ample financial resources and flexible time schedules (Moore, 1995). To date there has been little empirical research into Internet gambling and such studies have not focused on youth.

Griffiths (2001) carried out a UK prevalence survey examining Internet gambling. Of the 2098 people surveyed (918 male and 1180 female) only 495 of them (24%) were Internet users. The results showed that not one person gambled regularly on the Internet (i.e., once a week or more) and that only 1% of the Internet users were occasional Internet gamblers (i.e., less than once a week). Results also revealed that a further 4% had never gambled but would like to do so whereas the remaining 95% had never gambled on the Internet and said they were unlikely to do so. Participants who were between 15 and 19 years old (n=119) were also asked about whether they had ever gambled on the Internet, and if they had whether they had used a parent's credit card. No one in the sample had done so although 4% said they have a desire to do so. Griffiths (2001) argued that the results were not that surprising given the relatively low overall use of the Internet in the UK (i.e., traditionally in the UK most people have to pay by the minute for Internet access which likely inhibits use). Although there has been speculation that Internet gambling will be addictive, there was no evidence from this study. However, it is important that this study be viewed within context in that it was carried out at a time when Internet use was an irregular activity amongst individuals in the UK.

In Canada, Ialomiteanu and Adlaf (2001) reported on the prevalence of Internet gambling among Ontario adults. Their data were collected by a random telephone survey of 1,294 Ontario adults. Overall, 5.3% reported having gambled on the Internet during the past 12 months. Although women were more likely to report gambling on-line than males (6.3% vs. 4.3%), the difference was not statistically significant. There were no dominant age, regional, educational or income differences. Although rates of Internet gambling were not excessive, they argued that the simultaneous expansion and diffusion of both Internet access and gambling requires monitoring.

Higher Internet gambling rates were reported in a study by Ladd and Petry (2002) in the U.S. among 389 patients (seeking free or reduced cost dental care). They found that 8.1% of participants reported Internet gambling, with 3.7% gambling at least weekly. Compared to non-Internet gamblers, Internet gamblers were more likely to be younger, non-Caucasian and to have higher scores on a psychometric gambling measure. Only 22% of the participants without Internet gambling experience were problematic or pathological gamblers, as compared to 74% of those with Internet gambling experience.

Finally, a recent study by Hardoon, Derevensky and Gupta (2002) found that 25% of adolescents with serious gambling problems and 20% of those at-risk for a gambling problem reported playing on-line gambling type games using practice sites (gambling activities where points are won/lost without the use of real money). The use of the Internet may present a special danger for individuals at high-risk for developing a gambling problem (Messerlian, Byrne & Derevensky, 2004).

Conclusions

It is clear that excessive involvement with gambling, video-games and the Internet may result in an increase in adolescent problems. The technologies involved in gambling, video-game playing, and Internet use are growing. Adolescents, already living and interacting in a multi-media world, are discovering that leisure opportunities are becoming more easily accessible and widespread. Although the risk factors involved in youth problem gambling are becoming clearer, more research is needed to identify specific risk models for both excessive video-game playing and excessive Internet use. Jacobs (1997) has suggested that without early and appropriate prevention, intervention and treatment, adolescents are high-risk candidates for developing a variety of dysfunctional behaviors including a range of addictive behavior patterns.

By analyzing situational and structural characteristics in gambling, video-game and Internet activities, it is our contention that situational characteristics impact most on the acquisition of gambling behavior, while structural characteristics impact most on its development and maintenance. Furthermore, the most important of these factors appear to be accessibility of the activity and event frequency (both of which are critical to the success of gambling, video-games and the Internet). It is when these two characteristics combine that the greatest problems likely occur. This is well demonstrated by the worldwide proliferation in electronic gambling machines and the associated problems that accompany them. As Griffiths (1999) points out, it could be that slot machine gambling has more "gambling inducing" structural characteristics (as a result of the inherent technology) than other forms of gambling, and may account for the relatively large minority of gamblers "addicted" to slot machines (many of whom are adolescents) in the UK. With their integrated mix of conditioning effects, rapid event frequency, short pay out intervals and psychological rewards, it is not hard to see how slot machine gambling can become a repetitive habit. It may also provide insight into the possible problems created by the spread of interactive Internet gambling.

At the moment, the laws relating to Internet gambling vary from country to country and are often difficult to apply. For example, if a gaming operator runs an Internet gambling site from the Dominican Republic, then how can another country's laws be applied? The need for effective legislation, although difficult to administer and enforce still needs urgent attention. Some Internet gaming operators appear to be trying to overcome the problem of adolescent and/or problem gamblers by introducing security and monitoring initiatives. For instance, some companies have developed Internet gaming sites which require an account to be set up in advance, have passwords to prohibit minors, and monitor spending levels to discourage excessive gambling. However, it is difficult to define what is "excessive" as this will largely depend on the person's income, and currently there is no control over how many other Internet gambling sites to which a gambler can subscribe. The challenge for researchers is to examine the impact of these systems and devise ways of minimizing their harm.

Finally, it is perhaps worth speculating about the impact that new technologies are having on child development. Technological advances have created an 'instant' culture where everything can be achieved and attained very quickly at the touch of a button. The youth of today expect instantaneous access to almost everything and there is no longitudinal research that provides insight to the longer-term effects of such a culture. Anecdotally, it would appear that in social situations youth seem to expect more stimulation and interaction in all they do, often having a hard time attending to tasks that are not as stimulating. The emergence of these new technologies may be having detrimental effects such as a shortening of attention span, although such an assertion is highly speculative. It is our contention that these emerging technologies support and encourage this trend and that further research is needed to assess their impact.

References

American Psychiatric Association (1987). *Diagnostic and statistical manual of mental disorders* (3rd Edition—Revised). Washington D.C.: Author.

Cleary, A.G., McKendrick, H., & Sills, J.A. (2002). Hand-arm vibration syndrome may be associated with prolonged use of vibrating computer games. *British Medical Journal, 324,* 301.

Cooper, A. (1998). Sexuality and the Internet: Surfing into the new millennium. *CyberPsychology and Behavior, 1,* 181–187.

Cooper, A., Putnam, D.E., Planchon, L.A., & Boies, S.C. (1999). Online sexual compulsivity: Getting tangled in the net. *Sexual Addiction & Compulsivity: The Journal of Treatment and Prevention, 6,* 79–104.

Corkery, J.C. (1990). Nintendo power. *American Journal of Diseases in Children, 144,* 959.

Deheger, M., Rolland-Cachera, M.F., & Fontvielle, A.M. (1997). Physical activity and body composition in 10 year old French children: Linkages with nutritional intake? *International Journal of Obesity, 21,* 372–379.

Derevensky, J., & Gupta, R. (2001). Le problème de jeu touché aussi les jeunes. *Psychologie Québec, 18,* 23–27.

Egli, E.A., & Meyers, L.S. (1984). The role of video game playing in adolescent life: Is there a reason to be concerned? *Bulletin of the Psychonomic Society, 22,* 309–312.

Fisher, S.E. (1993a). Gambling and pathological gambling in adolescence. *Journal of Gambling Studies, 9,* 3, 277–287.

Fisher, S.E. (1993b). The pull of the fruit machine: A sociological typology of young players. *Sociological Review, 41,* 446–474.

Fisher, S.E., & Balding, J. (1998). *Gambling and problem gambling among young people in England and Wales.* London: Office of the National Lottery.

Fisher, S.E., & Griffiths, M.D. (1995). Current trends in slot machine gambling: Research and policy issues. *Journal of Gambling Studies, 11,* 239–247.

Friedland, R.P., & St. John, J.N. (1984). Video-game palsy: Distal ulnar neuropathy in a video game enthusiast. *New England Journal of Medicine, 311,* 58–59.

Griffiths, M.D. (1990). The acquisition, development and maintenance of fruit machine gambling in adolescence. *Journal of Gambling Studies, 6,* 193–204.

Griffiths, M.D. (1991a). Amusement machine playing in childhood and adolescence: A comparative analysis of video games and fruit machines. *Journal of Adolescence, 14,* 53–73.

Griffiths, M.D. (1991b). The observational analysis of adolescent gambling in UK amusement arcades. *Journal of Community and Applied Social Psychology, 1,* 309–320.

Griffiths, M.D. (1993a). Fruit machine gambling: The importance of structural characteristics. *Journal of Gambling Studies, 9,* 101–120.

Griffiths, M.D. (1993b). Tolerance in gambling: An objective measure using the psychophysiological analysis of male fruit machine gamblers. *Addictive Behaviors, 18,* 365–372.

Griffiths, M.D. (1995). *Adolescent Gambling.* London: Routledge.

Griffiths, M.D. (1998). Internet addiction: Does it really exist? In J. Gackenbach (Ed.), *Psychology and the Internet: Intrapersonal, interpersonal and transpersonal applications.* New York: Academic Press.

Griffiths, M.D. (1999). Gambling technologies: Prospects for problem gambling. *Journal of Gambling Studies, 15,* 265–283.

Griffiths, M.D. (2000a). Does internet and computer "addiction" exist? Some case study evidence. *CyberPsychology and Behavior, 3,* 211–218.

Griffiths, M.D. (2000b). Internet addiction—Time to be taken seriously? *Addiction Research, 8,* 413–418.

Griffiths, M.D. (2001). Internet gambling: Preliminary results of the first UK prevalence study. *e-Gambling: Journal of Gambling Issues, 5,* [http://www.camh.net/egambling/issue5/research/griffiths_article.html].

Griffiths, M.D. (2002). *Gambling and gaming addictions in adolescence.* Oxford: British Psychological Society, Blackwells.

Griffiths, M.D., & Hunt, N. (1995). Computer game playing in adolescence: Prevalence and demographic indicators. *Journal of Community and Applied Social Psychology, 5,* 189–194.

Griffiths, M.D., & Hunt, N. (1998). Dependence on computer game playing by adolescents. *Psychological Reports, 82,* 475–480.

Griffiths, M.D., & Sutherland, I. (1998). Adolescent gambling and drug use. *Journal of Community and Applied Social Psychology, 8,* 423–427.

Griffiths, M.D., & Wood, R.T.A. (1999). *Lottery gambling and addiction: An overview of European research.* Lausanne: Association of European Lotteries.

Griffiths, M.D., & Wood, R.T.A. (2000). Risk factors in adolescence: The case of gambling, video-game playing and the internet. *Journal of Gambling Studies, 16,* 199–225.

Gupta, R., & Derevensky, J.L. (1996). The relationship between gambling and video-game playing behavior in children and adolescents. *Journal of Gambling Studies, 12,* 375–394.

Gupta, R. & Derevensky, J.L. (1997). Familial and social influences on juvenile gambling behavior. *Journal of Gambling Studies, 13,* 179–192.

Gupta, R., & Derevensky, J.L. (1998a). Adolescent gambling behavior: A prevalence study and an examination of the correlates associated with problem gambling. *Journal of Gambling Studies, 14,* 319–345.

Gupta, R., & Derevensky, J.L. (1998b). An experimental examination of Jacobs' General Theory of Addictions : Do adolescent gamblers fit the theory? *Journal of Gambling Studies, 14,* 17–49.

Hardoon, K., Derevensky, J., & Gupta, R. (2002). *An examination of the influence of familial, emotional, conduct and cognitive problems, and hyperactivity upon youth risk-taking and adolescent gambling problems.* Guelph, ON, Canada: Ontario Problem Gambling Research Centre.

Ialomiteanu, A., & Adlaf, E. (2001). Internet gambling among Ontario adults. *Electronic Journal of Gambling Issues, 5,* 1–10.

Jacobs, D. F. (1986). A general theory of addictions: A new theoretical model. *Journal of Gambling Behavior, 2,* 15–31.

Jacobs, D.F. (1997, June). *Effects on children of parental excesses in gambling*. Paper presented at the National Conference on Problem Gambling, Orlando, Florida.

Ladd, G.T., & Petry, N.M. (2002). Disordered gambling among university-based medical and dental patients: A focus on Internet gambling. *Psychology of Addictive Behaviors, 16,* 76–79.

Langer, E. J. (1975). The illusion of control. *Journal of Personality and Social Psychology, 32,* 311–328.

Lesieur, H.R., Cross, J., Frank, M., Welch, C., Rubenstein, G., Moseley, K. & Mark, M. (1991). Gambling and pathological gambling among college students. *Addictive Behaviors, 16,* 517–527.

Lesieur, H.R., & Klein, R. (1987). Pathological gambling among high school students. *Addictive Behaviors, 12,* 129–135.

Loba, P., Stewart, S.H., Klein, R.M. & Blackburn, J.R. (2001). Manipulations of the features of standard video lottery terminal (VLT) games: Effects in pathological and non-pathological gamblers. *Journal of Gambling Studies, 17,* 297–320.

Loftus, G.A., & Loftus, E.F. (1983). *Mind at play: The psychology of video games.* New York: Basic Books.

Marget, N., Gupta, R., & Derevensky, J. (1999, August). *The psychosocial factors underlying adolescent problem gambling*. Poster presented at the annual meeting of the American Psychological Association, Boston.

Marks, I. (1990). Non-chemical (behavioural) addictions. *British Journal of Addiction, 85,* 1389–1394.

Messerlian, C., Byrne, A., & Derevensky, J. (2004). Gambling, youth and the Internet: Should we be concerned? *The Canadian Child and Adolescent Psychiatry Review, 13,* 12–15.

Millett, C.J., Fish, D.R. & Thompson, P.J. (1997). A survey of epilepsy-patient perceptions of video-game material/electronic screens and other factors as seizure precipitants. *Seizure, 6,* 457–459.

Mirman, M.J., & Bonian, V.G. (1992). "Mouse elbow": A new repetitive stress injury. *Journal of the American Osteopath Association, 92,* 701.

Mitka, M. (2001). Win or lose, Internet gambling stakes are high. *Journal of the American Medical Association, 285,* 1005.

Moore, D. (1995). *The Emperor's virtual clothes: The naked truth about the Internet culture.* Chapel Hill, NC: Algonquin.

Moore, S.M., & Ohtsuka, K. (1997). Gambling activities of young Australians: Developing a model of behaviour. *Journal of Gambling Studies, 13,* 207–236.

Morahan-Martin, J.M. (1998, March). *Women and girls last: Females and the internet*. Paper presented at the Internet Research and Information for Social Scientist Conference, University of Bristol, UK.

Morahan-Martin, J.M. & Schumacher, P. (1997, August). *Incidence and correlates of pathological internet use*. Paper presented at the 105th Annual Convention of the American Psychological Association, Chicago, Illinois.

Moran, E. (1987). *Gambling among schoolchildren: The impact of the fruit machine.* London: National Council on Gambling.

Nower, L., Gupta, R., & Derevensky, J. (2000, June). *Youth gamblers and substance abusers: A comparison of stress-coping styles and risk-taking behavior of two addicted adolescent populations*. Paper presented at the 11th International Conference on Gambling and Risk-Taking, Las Vegas.

O'Neill, K. (1998, June). *Internet gambling*. Paper presented at the 13th National Council on Problem Gambling Conference, Las Vegas.

Schink, J.C. (1991). Nintendo enuresis. *American Journal of Diseases in Children, 145,* 1094.

Shaffer, H.J., LaBrie, R., Scanlon, K.M., & Cummings, T.N. (1993). *At risk, problem and pathological gambling among adolescents : Massachusetts Adolescent Gambling Screen (MAGS)*. Cambridge, MA: Harvard Medical School.

Shotton, M. (1989). *Computer addiction? A study of computer dependency.* London: Taylor and Francis.

Sinclair, S. (2000). Wagering on the Internet: Final Report [electronic document]. St. Charles, MO: Christiansen Capital Advisors, Inc. and River City Group. Available: http://www.igamingnews.com/Stata Corporation. (1999).

Stinchfield, R., Cassuto, R., Winters, K., & Latimer, W. (1997). Prevalence of gambling among Minnesota public school students in 1992 and 1995. *Journal of Gambling Studies, 12,* 25–48.

Winters, K.C., Stinchfield, R.D. & Fulkerson, J. (1993). Patterns and characteristic of adolescent gambling. *Journal of Gambling Studies, 9,* 371–386.

Wood, R.T.A., Gupta, R., Derevensky, J. L., & Griffiths, M.D. (in press).Video game playing and gambling in adolescents: Common risk factors. *Journal of Child & Adolescent Substance Abuse.*

Wood, R.T.A., & Griffiths, M.D. (1998). The acquisition, development and maintenance of lottery and scratchcard gambling in adolescence. *Journal of Adolescence, 21,* 265–273.

Yeoman, T. & Griffiths, M.D. (1996). Adolescent machine gambling and crime. *Journal of Adolescence, 19,* 183–188.

Young, K. (1996). Psychology of computer use: XL. Addictive use of the internet: A case that breaks the stereotype. *Psychological Reports, 79,* 899–902.

Young, K. (1998). *Caught in the net: How to recognize the signs of Internet addiction and a winning strategy for recovery.* New York: Wiley.

Young K. (1999). Internet addiction: Evaluation and treatment. *Student British Medical Journal, 7,* 351–352.

Young, K., Griffin-Shelley, E., Cooper, A., O'Mara, J., & Buchanan, J. (2000). Online infidelity: A new dimension in couple relationships with implications for evaluation and treatment. In A. Cooper (Ed.), *Cybersex: The dark side of the force.* Philadelphia: Brunner Routledge.

Zimbardo, P. (1982). Understanding psychological man: A state of the science report. *Psychology Today, 16,* 15.

Chapter 7

The Measurement of Youth Gambling Problems
Current Instruments, Methodological Issues, and Future Directions

Jeffrey L. Derevensky, Ph.D. and
Rina Gupta Ph.D.

Large-scale prevalence studies conducted in the United States, Canada, England, Europe, New Zealand and Australia all confirm the high prevalence rates of gambling participation among youth. Shaffer, Hall and Vander-Bilt (1997) in their meta-analysis reported that adolescent lifetime gambling rates ranged from 39 to 92%, the median being 85%. When examining pathological gambling among adolescents, Shaffer and Hall (1996) concluded that between 4.4 and 7.4% of adolescents exhibit seriously adverse patterns of compulsive or pathological gambling, with another 9.9 to 14.2% remaining at-risk for either developing or returning to a serious gambling problem. Based upon the current conceptualization, understanding and measurement of pathological gambling, and acknowledging difficulty in comparing data sets, the National Research Council (1999) reported that the level of adolescent pathological gambling ranged between 1.2 and 11.2%, with a median of 5.0%. Once again, acknowledging difficulties in interpretation of the data, the National Research Council concluded that the proportion of pathological gambling among adolescents in the United States could be more than three times that of adults.

Our basic conceptualization about the nature of pathological gambling has been continuously evolving (Volberg, 1994) with differences between diagnostic criteria established in the DSM-III (American Psychiatric Association, 1980), DSM-III-R (American Psychiatric Association, 1987), and DSM-IV (American Psychiatric Association, 1994) clearly denoting changes in our understanding and conceptualization of adult pathological gambling. Debates about the appropriate inclusion criteria and the concerns for validity and reliability of screens as measures of pathological gambling have been reiterated amongst researchers and clinicians since the establishment of the original criteria. Having established 10 diagnostic criteria for adult pathological gambling, each having an equal weighting, the DSM-IV (APA, 1994) became the gold standard for clinically assessing adult pathological gambling. Individuals exhibiting five or more of the criteria were thought to exhibit persistent and maladaptive gambling behaviors.

As the interest in pathological gambling grew in the 1980s and 1990s the number of instruments for assessing pathological gambling amongst adults also grew. While the original DSM-III classification and subsequent modifications were thought to be truly representative of maladaptive

Table 1. DSM-IV Criteria for Pathological Gambling (APA, 1994)

Behavior	Description
Preoccupation	Is preoccupied with gambling (e.g., preoccupied with reliving past gambling experiences, handicapping or planning the next venture, or thinking of ways to get money with which to gamble)
Tolerance	Needs to gamble with increasing amounts of money in order to achieve the desired excitement
Withdrawal	Is restless or irritable when attempting to cut down or stop gambling
Escape	Gambles as a way of escaping from problems or relieving dysphoric mood (e.g., feelings of helplessness, guilt, anxiety or depression)
Chasing	After losing money gambling, often returns another day in order to get even ("chasing one's losses")
Lying	Lies to family members, therapists or others to conceal the extent of involvement with gambling
Loss of control	Has made repeated unsuccessful efforts to control, cut back or stop gambling
Illegal acts	Has committed illegal acts (e.g., forgery, fraud, theft or embezzlement) in order to finance gambling
Risked significant relationship	Has jeopardized or lost a significant relationship, job or educational or career opportunity because of gambling
Bailout	Has relied on others to provide money to relieve a desperate financial situation caused by gambling

gambling behavior, it did not lend itself well to screening surveys. As a result, a number of screening surveys were developed as a quick tool to assess severity of gambling problems. Shaffer, LaBrie, LaPlante, Nelson and Stanton (2004) have identified over 30 instruments for identifying disordered problem gambling with more in development; the vast majority of the instruments being aimed at adults.

Survey instruments, in general, have received serious criticism (see Ferris, Wynne & Single, 1999; Volberg, 1994; Volberg & Steadman, 1992). Nevertheless, the commonality within existing instruments and measures has focused upon behavioral indicators of problem playing, the emotional and psychological correlates associated with pathological gambling, the adverse consequences of excessive playing, and the economic and sociological aspects directly associated with excessive gambling (see Ferris et al., 1999 and Volberg, 2001 for a review of adult instruments).

The issue of nomenclature concerning disordered gambling (i.e., compulsive, pathological, problem, disordered) and instrumentation has recently received considerable attention. Independent of perspective, there remains considerable concern and interest amongst researchers, clinicians and policy makers toward developing some uniformity in the nomenclature, definition of disordered/pathological gambling, and the development of a new *gold standard;* a standardized instrument with acceptable reliability and validity that would be accepted as the instrument to be used in psychiatric, psychological, and sociological gambling research and treatment with adolescents. An important assumption predicating this discussion is that an acceptable *screening inventory* may not be appropriate as a *diagnostic instrument* and/or may require different scoring criteria. While these instruments may share similar items, their purpose is significantly different.

Instruments Used To Assess Youth Problem Gambling

Despite progress in gambling research and treatment approaches in the last decade, new screening instruments for adolescent problem gambling are still lacking (It should be noted that the Canadian Centre for Substance Abuse and the Ontario Problem Gambling Research Centre are currently working on developing a new adolescent instrument). Due to the growing awareness of gambling problems amongst adolescents, a number of instruments have been adapted for this age group. More specifically, the SOGS-RA (Winters, Stinchfield & Fulkerson, 1993), DSM-IV-J (Fisher, 1992) and its revision the DSM-IV-MR-J (Fisher, 2000), and the MAGS (Shaffer, LaBrie, Scanlan & Cummings, 1994) have been used in a large number of adolescent prevalence studies. Similar to adult instruments (e.g., SOGS, DSM-IV, NODS, GA-20, CPGI), there exist common constructs underlying all the instruments. The notion of deception (lying), stealing money to support gambling, preoccupation, and chasing losses are common amongst these instruments. Similarly, while the number of items and constructs differ, each criterion item has equal weighting, and a cut score is provided identifying pathological gambling for each respective instrument.

South Oaks Gambling Screen-Revised for Adolescents (SOGS-RA)

A revised version of the South Oaks Gambling Screen (SOGS) (Lesieur & Blume, 1987), the SOGS-RA (Winters et al., 1993) was developed as a screening instrument to more accurately assess severity of adolescent gambling problems. This 16-item scale (four items are omitted for scoring) assesses past year gambling behavior and gambling related problems while maintaining a single dimension of problem gambling. Items from the original SOGS were reworded to make it more age appropriate and the scoring scheme was adjusted. The screen emphasizes the frequency of gambling behavior and the behavioral indices often accompanied by problem gambling in contrast to emphasizing money expended. Winters et al. (1993) report satisfactory reliability (.80) and validity measures (adequate construct validity as well as discriminating between regular and non-regular gamblers). However, Ferris et al. (1999) has noted that the instrument has not been adequately tested with adolescent females given the low prevalence rate of female problem gamblers in the original sample (a problem common to many adolescent instruments).

A number of studies based on the SOGS and SOGS-RA have been carried out in high schools in Alberta, Connecticut, Louisiana, New Jersey, New York and Quebec (Ladouceur & Mireault, 1988; Lesieur & Klein, 1987; Steinberg, 1997; Volberg, 1998; Westphal, Rush & Stevens, 1997; Wynne, Smith & Jacobs, 1996). More recently, Ladouceur, Bouchard, Rhéaume, Jacques, Ferland, Leblond, and Walker (2000) questioned the validity of the SOGS-RA as they contend that the high rates of prevalence by youth are a result of individuals misunderstanding the intent of the items.

Diagnostic Statistical Manual-IV-MR-J (Adapted-Multiple Response format for Juveniles) (DSM-IV-MR-J)

A revised version of the DSM-IV criteria, and the DSM-IV-J (Fisher, 1992), the DSM-IV-MR-J (Fisher, 2000) consists of 12 items. The DSM-IV-J and the

Table 2. South Oaks Gambling Screen-Revised for Adolescents

SOGS-RA Items

What is the largest amount of money you have ever gambled in the past 12 months?

$50–$99

$100–$199

$200 and more

Do you think that either of your parents gamble too much?

mother

father

both mother and father

In the past 12 months, how often have you gone back another day to win back the money you lost? (Every time)

In the past 12 months when you were betting, have you ever told others you were winning money when you really weren't winning?

Has your betting, in the past 12 months, ever caused any problems for you such as arguments with family and friends, or problems at school or work?

In the past 12 months, have you ever gambled more than you had planned to?

In the past 12 months, has anyone criticized your betting or told you that you had a gambling problem, regardless of whether you thought it was true or not?

In the past 12 months, have you ever felt bad about the amount you bet, or about what happens when you bet money?

Have you ever felt, in the past 12 months, that you would like to stop betting money but didn't think you could?

In the past 12 months, have you ever hidden from your family or friends any betting slips, I.O.U.'s, lottery tickets, money that you've won, or other signs of gambling?

In the past 12 months, have you had money arguments with family or friends that centered on gambling?

In the past 12 months, have you borrowed money to bet and not paid it back?

In the past 12 months, have you ever skipped or been absent from school or work due to betting activities?

Have you ever borrowed or stolen money in order to bet or cover gambling debts in the past 12 months?

---

revised DSM-IV-MR-J was modeled very closely on the adult version DSM-IV criteria for pathological gambling), with several significant adaptations. One major difference pertains to where individuals acquire their money. For example, it refers to supporting their gambling from money allocated for "school lunch" and "bus transportation." With respect to committing crimes, it specifies theft from home, theft from outside the family, and shoplifting rather than the adult examples of forgery, fraud, and embezzlement. The DSM-IV-J comprised nine dimensions of pathological gambling: progression and preoccupation, tolerance, withdrawal and loss of control, escape, chasing, lies and deception, illegal acts, and family and academic disruptions. The revised scale, DSM-IV-MR-J, questions the appropriateness of using yes/no responses in non-clinical situations while retaining the original 9 dimensions (12 items). Rather than merely having a yes/no format, the revised version incorporates a qualitative range on several questions (e.g., never, once or twice, sometimes, often; or never, less than half the time, more than half the time, every time), with only the more frequent responses being scored as an endorsement. Identification of four out of nine dimensions is suggestive of probable pathological gambling. Internal consistency reliability was acceptable (Cronbach's alpha = .075), with one principal factor being found.

Massachusetts Adolescent Gambling Screen (MAGS)

The Massachusetts Adolescent Gambling Screen (MAGS) (Shaffer et al., 1994) assesses the prevalence of problem and pathological gambling amongst a general population of adolescents. It is described as a brief clinical screening instrument that yields indices of pathological and non-pathological gambling. Incorporated within the MAGS are the DSM-IV criteria for pathological gambling in a set of survey questions. The MAGS in conjunction with the DSM-IV criteria is a 26-item scale, including two subscales, designed to provide clinicians and researchers with a method of identifying individuals with gambling difficulties. The scale includes a DSM-IV subscale which yielded a Chronbach alpha of .87 while the MAGS subscale yielded an alpha of .83. Validity data and discriminant analyses were found to be effective predictors of pathological gambling. The scale assesses the biological, psychological, and social problems found amongst youth with excessive gambling problems. Once identified as a probable pathological gambler on the MAGS, Shaffer et al. suggest further diagnostic in-treatment clinical assessments to provide more detailed information about specific gambling behaviors.

Gamblers Anonymous Twenty Questions (GA-20)

A widely utilized screen for pathological gambling with adults, the Gamblers Anonymous Twenty Questions (GA-20) has also been used with adolescents and young adults. This instrument was based upon the difficulties experienced by Gamblers Anonymous members. It was designed to be a self-administered tool for problem gamblers to assess the severity of their gambling problems and to decide whether help would be required. The twenty items identify particular situations and behaviors that are typical of pathological gamblers. Questions address the financial correlates of continued gambling, the personal consequences of excessive gambling (e.g.,

Table 3. Diagnostic Statistical Manual-IV-MR-J

DSM-IV-MR-J items[1]

Think about gambling all the time

Spend more and more money on gambling

Become tense, restless, when trying to cut down

Gamble as a way of escaping from problems

Chase losses

Lie to family and friends about gambling behavior

Use other money (e.g. lunch money) for gambling

Taken money from family to gamble without telling them

Stolen money from outside family to gamble

Fallen out with family because of gambling behavior

Skip school more than 5 times to gamble in past year

Sought help for serious money worry caused by gambling

[1] Scoring of bolded responses on the DSM-IV-MR-J: Item 1—never/ once or twice/sometimes/often; Items 2 & 12—yes/no; Items 3 & 4—never/once or twice/sometimes/often; Item 5—never/less than half the time/more than half the time/every time; Items 6–11—never/once or twice/sometimes/often.

Table 4. Massachusetts Gambling Screen (MAGS)

Subscale Items[1]

Have you ever experienced social, psychological or financial pressure to start gambling or increase how much you gamble?

How much do you usually gamble compared with most other people?

Do you feel that the amount or frequency of your gambling is "normal"?

Do friends or relatives think of you as a "normal" gambler?

Do you ever feel pressure to gamble when you do not gamble?

Do you ever feel guilty about your gambling?

Does any member of your family ever worry or complain about your gambling?

Have you ever thought that you should reduce or stop gambling?

Are you always able to stop gambling when you want?

Has your gambling ever created problems between you and any member of your family or friends?

Have you ever gotten in trouble at work or school because of your gambling?

Have you ever neglected your obligations (e.g., family, work or school) for two or more days in a row because you were gambling?

Have you ever gone to anyone for help about your gambling?

Have you ever been arrested for gambling?

[1] All items require dichotomous answers (i.e., yes or no) except question two which has a 3 point response scale: less, about the same or more.

Table 5. Gamblers Anonymous Twenty Questions (GA-20)

GA-20 Items
Do you ever gamble longer than you planned?
After a win, do you have a strong urge to return and win more?
After losing do you feel you must return as soon as possible and win back your losses?
Do you ever feel remorse after gambling?
Do you often gamble until your last dollar is gone?
Do you have an urge to celebrate good fortune by a few hours of gambling?
Do you ever borrow to finance your gambling?
Do you ever gamble to escape worry or trouble?
Do arguments, disappointments, or frustrations create within you an urge to gamble?
Are you reluctant to use "gambling money" for normal expenditures?
Does gambling affect your reputation?
Do you lose time from school or work due to gambling?
Does gambling cause a decrease in your ambition (motivation) or efficiency?
Does gambling cause you to have difficulty sleeping?
Do you ever consider self-destruction as a result of your gambling?
Does gambling make your home life unhappy?
Do you ever commit or consider committing illegal acts to finance your gambling?
Does gambling make you careless about the welfare of your family?
Do you ever sell anything to finance gambling?
Do you ever gamble to get money with which to pay debts or to otherwise solve financial problems?

difficulty sleeping, remorse for excessive gambling, decreased ambition), and social correlates associated with excessive behavior (difficult home life, arguments associated with gambling). Individuals endorsing seven of the twenty items are considered to have a pathological gambling problem (Custer & Custer, 1978). While developed by compulsive gamblers, a number of items are significantly different from the DSM-IV diagnostic criteria.

Perspectives on the Prevalence Data

While the current screening instruments have been widely used, the discrepant variability of reported prevalence rates of youth problem gambling within the scientific literature is troubling (see Derevensky, Gupta & Winters, 2003 for a comprehensive discussion). The reported variability amongst studies of adolescents is in general considerably greater compared to the variability reported for adult prevalence rates of problem gambling (see the findings of the National Research Council, 1999). As well, questions regarding the comparability of findings using different instruments have been raised and the validity of reported prevalence rates has been seriously questioned (Ladouceur, 2001; Ladouceur et al., 2000), with Ladouceur and his colleagues suggesting that the reported rates of serious gambling problems among adolescents being over-estimated and inflated.

Derevensky et al. (2003) have argued that differences in prevalence rates are likely affected by a number of situational and measurement variables. Such variables might include sampling procedures (e.g., telephone surveys vs. school-based screens, community vs. convenience samples), use of different instruments and measures, varying cut-point scores associated with different instruments, the use of abridged and/or modified instruments, the inconsistency of availability and accessibility of gambling venues, gender distributions within each of the studies, the age of the population being assessed, cultural differences, as well as the distinct possibility that adolescent reports may be more variable than their adult counterparts (for a more thorough explanation see the reviews by Derevensky & Gupta, 2000a, 2000b; Stinchfield, 2002; Volberg, 2001; and Winters, 2001).

Compounding the issue of variability amongst adolescent studies is the wide variety of terms used to identify adolescents who have serious gambling and gambling-related problems (e.g., pathological gamblers, probable pathological gamblers, compulsive gamblers, problem gamblers, Level 3, disordered gamblers). This has prompted a number of researchers to call for standardization of nomenclature, terminology and definitions (Cunningham-Williams, 2000; Shaffer & Hall, 1996; Shaffer et al., 2004). Volberg (2001) has argued that while some standardization may be desirable, there is considerable value in our continued discussions and debate over the definition of problem and pathological gambling. Such discussions will ultimately help stimulate the development of new criteria and refinements of instruments. Volberg (2001) has also highlighted the need for research to examine the clustering of symptoms of problem and pathological gambling within particular timeframes. Still further, others have argued that pathological gamblers are not a homogenous group (see Nower & Blaszczynski, in this volume) which might necessitate the development of different criteria and/or assessment tools.

Estimation of Adolescence Prevalence Rates

The assumption that the prevalence rates of adolescent gambling problems are not accurate has serious social policy and public health policy implications. Those questioning the validity of the reported rates generally suggest that the current reported rates are over-estimated. As such, a brief examination of arguments made to support their contention is important. Derevensky et al. (2003) identified five arguments proposed for the inflated rate perspective: (a) given the reported prevalence rates of gambling problems among adolescents with gambling problems, more adolescents would present themselves for treatment, (b) youth misunderstand and fail to adequately comprehend many of the questions on problem gambling screens and have a preset bias toward false-positive responses, (c) the discrepancy between prevalence rates of pathological gambling for adults and youth makes little sense given that adults have in general more financial resources and greater availability and easier accessibility of high-stakes gambling, (d) there are common scoring errors in certain instruments, in particular the DSM-IV-J, which have resulted in over-estimates, and (e) current screening instruments for youth lack sufficient construct validity. A brief discussion of each of these arguments follows (see Derevensky et al., 2003 for a more comprehensive discussion).

I. The lack of adolescents seeking treatment is inconsistent with reported prevalence rates.

The assumption underlying this argument is that more adolescents should be presenting themselves for treatment given the high rates of pathological gambling. While it is accurate that few clinicians see adolescents for problem gambling (Gupta & Derevensky, 2000), Derevensky et al. (2003) suggested that the process by which any individual seeks professional help is a complex one, and is affected by a large number of individual and health service delivery factors. The following plausible reasons have been proposed to account for the failure of youth with serious gambling problems to seek treatment: (a) adolescents generally have a perceived sense of invulnerability and invincibility, (b) in the absence of significant financial difficulties adolescents either believe they do not have a problem or firmly believe that they have the ability to stop gambling whenever they want, (c) few readily available and easily accessible treatment centers for adolescent gambling problems exist, (d) adolescents, in general, have a distrust for treatment providers and are more likely to seek peer support or from others whom they believe are more trustworthy, (e) there is a general failure by clinicians/treatment providers to ask pertinent questions about gambling behaviors when youth are seen for other addictive or mental health problems), (f) some, or many, youth may experience natural recovery, (g) youth committing delinquent acts, especially those stealing from home, are often not brought through the court system as they are frequently bailed out of financial trouble by friends and family members, (h) the negative consequences associated with gambling problems may be attributed to other problems or normal adolescent risk-taking tendencies, (i) denial concerning having a gambling problem, and (j) adolescence is a developmental period marked by high-risk taking behaviors with few seeking professional help for a wide range of problems (Derevensky et al., 2003; Griffiths, 2001; Gupta & Derevensky, 2000; Hardoon, Derevensky & Gupta, 2000; Hardoon, Derevensky, & Gupta, 2002; Hodgins, Makarachuk, el-Guebaly & Peden, in press; Jessor, 1998; Stinchfield, 1999).

Derevensky et al. (2003) further contend that this should not be misinterpreted that adolescent problem gambling is unique as an under-referred behavioral problem. Adolescents, as a group, similarly don't readily seek treatment for other behavioral problems, including alcohol and drug abuse and dependence despite their appreciable rates (Johnston, O'Malley & Bachman, 2001; SAMSHA, 2001). While many of the barriers to seeking treatment are also relevant to adults, adolescents generally have fewer external influences and pressures such as a spouse or peer requiring or strongly encouraging them to seek treatment; accessibility and travel to treatment programs can be more difficult for a young person; and adolescents generally have less self-insight resulting from their egocentricity and developmental immaturity. As such, Derevensky et al. (2003) contend that youth problem gamblers may have to overcome more service delivery barriers compared to adult problem gamblers.

II. Youth misinterpret items on gambling screens and have a preset bias toward positive responses.

Ladouceur et al. (2000) have suggested that youth fail to understand the meaning of several questions on a number of adolescent gambling screens and as such over-estimate the prevalence rates of pathological gambling. These assertions emanate from a series of empirical studies. In one study, Ladouceur and his colleagues administered the SOGS-RA to children age 9–12 (grades 4, 5, & 6). They reported that on average 27% of the SOGS-RA items were misunderstood by the children and that after clarification fewer children (a 73% reduction) met criteria for problem/ pathological gambling. While there is a consensus and evidence that children as young as age 9 are gambling for money (Derevensky, Gupta, & Della-Cioppa, 1996; Wynne, Smith & Jacobs, 1996), Derevensky et al. (2003) argued that from a clinical perspective it is difficult to conceive of elementary school age children as having pathological gambling problems given that the severity of the negative behaviors associated with gambling problems are atypical at this developmental level. In a second study, using older high school age adolescents,

Ladouceur and his colleagues noted a significant decrease on total SOGS-RA scores between the first (M = 2.14; SD = 2.32) and second administration (M = 1.51; SD = 2.29) (after clarification of items on the SOGS-RA). A careful examination of these findings reveals that this decrease actually represents a decrease of less than one item (.63). While this *may* have decreased the overall scores by 29% (no data is presented by to support this claim) and possibly reaches statistical significance, this finding is not clinically significant given the small decrease overall. Of significant concern is that this study was likely done using a French translation of the SOGS-RA. A third study using the SOGS with adults also reported confusion over the meaning of several items. However, in two separate studies by Thompson, Walker, Milton and Djukic (2001), using adults in Australia, they failed to replicate and substantiate Ladouceur et al.'s findings. It may well be that vocabulary and cultural variability issues are not easily addressed. Replications of such findings are essential.

It is important to note that measurement errors may also be under-estimating prevalence rates given most adolescent school-based studies use a convenience sample of students, failing to account for school dropouts. The acquiescence bias that Ladouceur et al. (2000) cite as a primary reason respondents initially over-endorsed certain items is questionable. Derevensky et al. (2003) contend that there is no psychological *a priori* reason suggesting why respondents are inclined to bias responses in a positive direction when faced with an ambiguous item, although Ladouceur and his colleagues contend that when uncertain of the exact meaning of a question gamblers may be more motivated to exaggerate their gambling exploits. However, it is equally plausible that adolescent pathological gamblers under-report their gambling involvement given the evidence that gamblers in treatment frequently deny the extent of their gambling problems (Dickerson & Hinchey, 1988).

III. Since adult prevalence rates of pathological gambling are considerably lower, youth prevalence rates must be over-estimated.

The assumption underlying this argument is that typical youth behaviors include participating in multiple risk-taking behaviors and with maturity most ultimately mature out of their adolescent risky behaviors (see Jessor, 1998 for a comprehensive examination of adolescent risky behaviors). As such, youth pathological gambling may be only a transient state and adolescents with gambling problems would experience natural recovery as they mature into adulthood (Derevensky et al., 2003). This is an interesting argument, however, there is a paucity of prospective studies to assess the validity of this argument. While Winters, Stinchfield, Botzet and Anderson (2002) have published a prospective study, their sample of problem gamblers is too small to draw meaningful conclusions. Gupta and Derevensky (2000) have argued that this may also be the result of a cohort effect such that this is the first generation of youth that will spend their entire lives in an environment in which gambling is widely accepted, endorsed, promoted, and often owned at least partially by the government (e.g., government controlled lottery). Derevensky et al. (2003) suggest that this extensive exposure may result in less "maturing-out" as can be expected with other adolescent high-risk behaviors. Inevitably, only longitudinal research and prospective studies with adequate sample sizes will determine whether rates of problem gambling change over time (Volberg, 2001).

IV. There are common scoring errors made on certain instruments.

Such scoring errors have been reported by a number of researchers using the DSM-IV-J as there was some confusion as to whether or not the scoring criteria was originally 4 of the 12 items or 4 of the 9 domains. Fisher (personal communication) confirmed that her intention was that an adolescent was required to score 4/9 categories rather than 4/12 items on the DSM-IV-J in order to meet the criteria for probable pathological gambling. The establishment of 4/9 categories was recommended and developed to both parallel the DSM-IV criteria for pathological gambling and to distinguish between gambling-related delinquent behaviors and non-gambling-related delinquent antisocial behaviors. Derevensky et al. (2003) recalculated the prevalence rates of four data sets in which scoring on the DSM-IV-J were inaccurate, representing over 5,000 adolescents. These recalculations yielded no meaningful, appreciable or statistically significant differences in prevalence rates. Item analyses revealed that endorsed items focusing upon preoccupation, spending increasing amounts of money on gambling, becoming tense and/or restless when gambling, using gambling as a way of escaping problems, and chasing losses were the predominant responses of problem gamblers. The items that lead to more positive cases (probable pathological gamblers) are more behavioral indices and important indicators of problematic gambling related behaviors. Most of the probable pathological gamblers far exceeded the minimum criteria (four items) to be classified. Nevertheless, it is important for researchers to report the item endorsement rates independent of instrument used.

V. Our nomenclature is confusing and current instruments lack good reliability and construct validity.

The issue of nomenclature, reliability estimates and construct validity of youth problem gambling measures are both significant and important and should be carefully addressed in the development of new screening measures. While nomenclature issues are important and scientific standards are essential, the existing screening instruments represent our current state of knowledge and best estimates of adolescent pathological and problem gambling. Nevertheless, the reliability and validity evidence for the measures most often used by researchers in the field are consistent with acceptable psychometric standards, with one importune exception–the lack of adequate criterion validity (Derevensky et al., 2003). If the field had a *gold standard* criterion measure, then a criterion validity study would be warranted. However, in the absence of such a standard we must use a "best estimate" procedure. Within this procedure, diagnostic (or criterion) decisions are finalized on the basis of findings from either a well-established structured or semi-structured interview, or in the absence of such interviews, from a detailed clinical interview conducted by at least one diagnostic expert (Leckman, Scholomskas, Thompson, Belanger, & Weisman, 1982; Kosten & Rounsaville, 1992). Given that none of the youth problem gambling prevalence studies have used instruments that have achieved this standard of establishing criterion validity (Winters, 2001), and given the proclivity of screening tools to over-identify positive cases, the current body of prevalence data merits further investigation.

Are screening instruments comparable?

As previously discussed, different instruments examine somewhat different constructs and criterion. The National Research Council (1999), when examining the issue of adolescent prevalence rates interpreted comparability data with extreme caution. Derevensky and Gupta (2000a) sought to address this issue in a study using a school-based sample of 980 youth, age 16–20 (mean age = 18.5 years, s.d. = 1.69), in a direct comparison of three measures (DSM-IV-J, SOGS-RA and the GA-20 Questions). Derevensky and Gupta (2000a) reported a fairly high degree of agreement between, with a relatively small classification error. Using the recommended criteria, the DSM-IV-J identified 3.4%, the SOGS-RA identified 5.3%, and the GA-20 identified 6.0% of this age group of youth as probable pathological gamblers. Their data suggested much greater agreement amongst the instruments for identifying male problem gamblers. The inter-correlation matrix for the three instruments revealed correlation coefficients in the moderate range (.61—.68), with correlations being much higher for males (range between .75—.84) than females (range between .31—.50), an expected finding given the lower variability of severity of female gambling problems. Derevensky and Gupta reported a high concordance rate for the identification of problem gamblers amongst these instruments. Equally important was the relatively small false negative and false positive rates between instruments. Youth identified as probable pathological gamblers were found to have endorsed *all* items more frequently. While the MAGS was not included in their comparative study, results by Volberg (1998) examining adolescent prevalence rates of problem gambling in New York State found the MAGS to be a more conservative measure than the SOGS-RA and approximating what one would expect using the DSM-IV-J.

A closer examination of all the four most commonly used scales reveals considerable overlap. Yet, differences, which are fundamental to the perceived behavioral characteristics and negative outcomes associated with pathological gambling also exist. Shaffer et al. (2004) contend that most screening instruments use uni-dimensional scaling criteria (merely summing the total number of endorsed responses) to represent a multidimensional state, a totally inadequate procedure. They argue that the summing of endorsed items on screening instruments assumes that all dimensions exist on the same continuum and that each of these dimensions is equally predicative of gambling disorders. Our clinical and research experience would disagree with the supposition that all items are of equal weighting.

When examining item differences for adolescents reaching the criteria for pathological gambling, significant differences were found. For example, the two most endorsed questions on the DSM-IV-J among adolescent pathological gamblers refer to a preoccupation with gambling (constantly thinking about gambling) and lying about gambling activities (Derevensky & Gupta, 2000a). Only the DSM-IV-MR-J *directly* measures preoccupation and both the DSM-IV-MR-J and the SOGS-RA assess lying and deceptive behavior associated with gambling. All scales assess loss of control, illegal acts and/or borrowing money to gamble, familial problems resulting from excessive gambling, and occupational/school problems. While some scales are concerned with the level of financial loss, other scales do not view this as particularly important.

The development of items appears dependent upon one's perspective of the importance of specific negative behavioral consequences associated with excessive gambling. While the DSM-IV-MR-J, in contrast to the DSM-IV-J, now includes differential multiple response options on several questions (e.g., never, once or twice, sometimes, and often; or never, less than half the time, more than half the time, every time) with only certain responses being scored positively, only the MAGS has two questions with a similar multiple level response-format. On all scales, equal weighting is placed on all questions yet there is ample evidence that differential responses differentiate problem and pathological gamblers (see Derevensky & Gupta, 2000a). The most highly endorsed items on the DSM-IV-J by

Table 6. Comparison Between Instruments

Assessment Items	DSM-IV-J	SOGS-RA	MAGS	GA 20
Preoccupation	x			
Tolerance	x			
Withdrawal	x			
Escape	x			x
Chasing Losses	x	x		x
Lying/Secretiveness	x	x		
Loss of Control	x	x	x	x
Illegal Acts/Borrowing Money	x	x	x	x
Risked Significant Relationships	x		x	x
Bailout		x		x
Family Problems	x	x	x	x
Guilt /Remorse		x	x	
Occupational/School Problems	x	x	x	x
Pressure to Gamble			x	
Help-Seeking	x		x	
Frequency of Gambling Compared to Others			x	
Self-perception of Gambling			x	
Difficulty Sleeping				x
Celebratory Gambling				x
Reputation				x
Financial concerns				x
Concern and Criticism from Others		x	x	
Parents' Gambling		x		
Amount of Money Gambled		x		
Self-destructive Thoughts				x
Dissociative Reaction				x

pathological gamblers related to preoccupation (90.9%), chasing losses (84.8%), lying to family members and friends (69.7%), withdrawal (becoming tense and irritable when trying to reduce gambling) (60.6%), using other money (e.g., school lunch money) (60.6%), tolerance (wagering increasing amounts of money) (57.6%), escape (51.5%), skipping school (27.3%), stealing from family (24.2%), sought help for money issues (24.2%), risked job, education relationships (21.2%), and stolen money from outside the home (12.1%); all of which are related to their gambling behavior.

Our Current Conceptualization of Pathological Gambling

Pathological gambling is currently conceptualized as a preoccupation with gambling, a lack of adequate control over one's behavior, and an inability to stop playing in spite of one's desire to do so (American Psychiatric Association, 1994). It is accompanied by guilt associated with the gambling behavior, withdrawal symptoms are frequently present, and difficulties in social relations and occupational/educational difficulties often ensue. Rosenthal (1992) has suggested that pathological gambling is in fact a progressive disorder (not single trial learning) accompanied by continuous and/or periodic episodes of loss of control over gambling, preoccupation, irrational thinking, and a continuation of the behavior in spite of repeated losses and negative adverse consequences. These characteristics are generally represented in most adolescent screening instruments and are present in youth problem gamblers who seek treatment (see Gupta & Derevensky, in this volume).

There is concern that our current instruments are inadequate. Shaffer et al. (2004) have suggested three fundamental limitations associated with assessing severity of gambling problems: (a) the dimensions within each of the screens are arbitrary, (b) the utility of different self-report timeframes causes confusion (i.e., past six months, past year, lifetime), and (c) general problems associated with self-report measures. The lack of weighting of importance of items represents a serious shortcoming. As Nower and Blaszczynski (in this volume) and Gupta and Deverensky (in this volume) have argued, there may be multiple pathways for adolescent problems gamblers with different aetiologies and behavioral characteristics. By extension, this may necessitate alternative assessment strategies and treatments paradigms.

While self-report scales for adolescents generally incorporate a past year time framework, some have argued that this may be confusing (i.e., past 12 months vs. calendar year). Clearly, the scope and intent of the instrument needs to be addressed. Most adolescent instruments provide a snapshot in time. And, while it is readily agreed upon that individuals can move between pathological gambling and non pathological gambling states, one should not under-estimate the long-term negative impact resulting from excessive gambling, including delinquency, school dropout, academic failure, and disrupted peer and familial relations (see Gupta & Derevensky, 2000; Ladouceur & Mireault, 1988).

Any self-report measure is subject to the individual reporting accurate information. While there is evidence that individuals scoring within the pathological gambling range on screening instruments fail to view themselves as having a significant gambling problem (Hardoon, Derevensky

& Gupta, 2003), this problem is not unique to gambling screens but to many psychometric measures. Epidemiological studies of problem and pathological gamblers among both adults and adolescents have been plagued with serious methodological limitations and biases including problems specific to survey instruments, non-responses and refusal biases, the exclusion of institutionalized populations, exclusion of specific groups, and difficulties associated with telephone surveys (Lesieur, 1994).

Of critical importance in the measurement of adolescent pathological gambling are the constructs used to assess gambling problems and severity. Derevensky and Gupta (2002) recently suggested that that youth gambling problems may not be a unitary construct or trait but rather represent a constellation of disorders (Figure 1). This perceived constellation of constructs may also be a contributing factor as to why youth with gambling problems are not presenting for gambling-related treatment. Other disorders may be more evident and have become the focus of intervention and treatment. Nevertheless, the issue remains as to which construct represents the primary disorder.

Future Directions

Clearly, discrepancies in prevalence research results can stem from a multitude of parameters—theoretical, conceptual, methodological, environmental, structural, cultural, linguistic, and economic (Derevensky et al., 2003). There is no doubt that our current screening instruments need refinement and that psychometrically sound, comprehensive instruments need to be developed that better approach a gold standard for defining youth problem gambling. The field remains plagued by nomenclature issues and multiple terminologies used to identify adolescents who have serious gambling and gambling-related problems (e.g., pathological gamblers, probable pathological gamblers, compulsive gamblers, problem gamblers, subclinical, Level 3, disordered gamblers). However, there is a consensus amongst gambling researchers, clinicians, and educators that there is a need for continued awareness of this potential source of health risk among youth, and continued attention toward developing relevant and effective prevention and treatment programs. As well, additional research designed to identify the underlying risk and protective factors that can help prevent youth gambling and mental health problems is needed. In several recent papers we argued for a better understanding of youth gambling problems within the context of adolescent high-risk behaviors (e.g., Derevensky, Gupta, Dickson & Deguire, 2001; Dickson, Derevensky & Gupta, 2002; 2004). The development of new instruments needs to be sensitive to these factors.

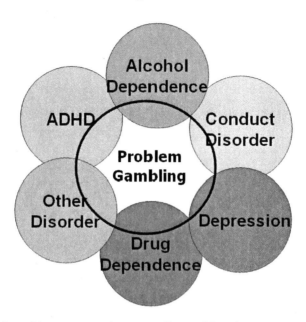

Figure 1. Youth gambling represented as a constellatoin of disorders.

While there is a clear danger in becoming an alarmist and over-exaggerating the prevalence rate of youth gambling problems, there is an equal danger in minimizing these problems. If gambling venues continue to increase, and the gambling activities become more interesting and entertaining for youth (e.g., the use of video-game technology on electronic gaming machines, and Internet gambling), and accessibility by underage youth remains widespread, there is little doubt that more youth will be engaging in these behaviors quite early. Given that a substantial amount of time is necessary between initial onset of gambling behavior and pathological gambling to occur (Australian Productivity Commission, 1999; Tavares, Zilberman, Beites & Gentil, 2001), it is conceivable that the issue of youth problem gambling may continue to present even more serious concerns over time.

Despite the fact that refinement of instrumentation and nomenclature issues still require resolving, the reported rates of problem gambling among youth are quite provocative and are cause for concern. There is ample evidence that gambling related problems amongst youth result in numerous psychological, social, economic, health and interpersonal difficulties that can be long lasting.

Researchers and clinicians need to establish whether to strive to develop an instrument either for the purpose of identification of prevalence rates of problematic gambling in a general population or whether it should also have clinical utility. While the two purposes may not be mutually exclusive there may be some fundamental differences. It is important to note that our current screening tools are designed to be simple, quick and efficient and are not expected to measure the subtleties and complexities associated with a multi-dimensional behavioral disorder. Effective screening measures, in some settings, should err on the side of caution by way of encouraging item endorsements minimizing the number of false-negatives (Anastasi, 1976).

The range of money spent gambling by youth varies considerably and should not be the overriding determinant of a gambling problem. Nevertheless, an analysis of the available data clearly points to the issues of preoccupation, chasing losses, lying to family members and peers, and the need to escalate wagers as symptomatic of a significant problem. The underlying reasons which prompt their gambling behavior (see Gupta & Derevensky 1998a, 1998b) and their treatment implications (see Gupta & Derevensky, 2000, in this issue) have only begun to be addressed.

There is little doubt that an effective screening tool designed to measure the prevalence of youth problem gambling and to help identify individuals at-risk for developing a problem must include behavioral items describing not only the frequency and severity of the problem but their natural psychological, sociological, and financial consequences. Such a measure must be age-appropriate and incorporate the contextual environment within which the identified population resides. Gambling researchers and treatment providers need to work together to help develop a psychometrically and clinically sound instrument for the identification of youth problem gambling. Shaffer et al. (2004) have suggested that the epidemiological study of gambling has reached a crossroads. While prevalence studies are numerous, incidence studies, which can provide valuable information concerning the nature and progression of gambling related problems, are extremely scarce and necessary. Ultimately, Shaffer and his colleagues contend that movement toward understanding the determinants of disordered gambling will result in the development of better psychometric tools. Until such time as new instruments are developed our current measures should suffice.

References

American Psychiatric Association (1980). *DSM-III: Diagnostic and statistical manual* (3rd Edition). Washington, DC: American Psychiatric Association. American Psychiatric Association (1987). *DSMIII-R: Diagnostic and statistical manual* (3rd Edition-Revised). Washington, DC: American Psychiatric Association.

American Psychiatric Association (1994). *DSM-IV: Diagnostic and statistical manual* (4th Edition). Washington, DC: American Psychiatric Association.

Anastasi, A. (1976). *Psychological testing* (4th edition). New York: MacMillan Publishing.

Australian Productivity Commission (1999). *Australia's gambling industries, Vol.1.* Commonwealth of Australia.

Cunningham-Williams, R. (2000, Dec.). *Assessments of pathological gambling: Apples and oranges?* Paper presented at the First Annual Research Synthesis Conference on Pathological Gambling, Las Vegas, NV.

Custer, R. L, & Custer, L. F. (1978, December). *Characteristics of the recovering compulsive gambler.* Paper presented at the Fourth Annual Conference on Problem Gambling, Reno, Nevada.

Derevensky, J., & Gupta, R. (2000a). Prevalence estimates of adolescent gambling: A comparison of the SOGS-RA, DSM-IV-J, and the G.A. 20 Questions. *Journal of Gambling Studies, 16,* 227–251.

Derevensky, J., & Gupta, R. (2000b). Youth gambling: A clinical and research perspective. *e-Gambling: The Electronic Journal of Gambling Issue, 2,* 1–10.

Derevensky, J., & Gupta, R. (2002, June). Youth gambling and problem gambling: Intrepreting the numbers. Paper presented at the annual meeting of the National Council on Problem Gambling, Dallas.

Derevensky, J., Gupta, R., & Della-Cioppa, G. (1996). A developmental perspective on gambling behavior in children and adolescents. *Journal of Gambling Studies, 12,* 49–66.

Derevensky, J., Gupta, R., Dickson, L., & Deguire, A-E. (2001). *Prevention efforts toward minimizing gambling problems.* Report prepared for the National Council on Problem Gambling and SAMHSA.

Derevensky, J., Gupta, R., & Winters, K. (2003). Prevalence rates of youth gambling problems: Are the current rates inflated? *Journal of Gambling Studies, 19,* 405–425.

Dickerson, M. G., & Hinchy, J. (1988). The prevalence of excessive and pathological gambling in Australia. *Journal of Gambling Behavior, 4,* 135–151.

Dickson, L., Derevensky, J., & Gupta, R. (2002). The prevention of gambling problems in youth: A new conceptual framework. *Journal of Gambling Studies, 18,* 97–160.

Dickson, L., Derevensky, J., & Gupta, R. (2004). Harm reduction for the prevention of youth gambling problems: Lessons learned from adolescent high-risk prevention programs. *Journal of Adolescent Research, 19,* 233–263.

Ferris, J., Wynne, H., & Single, E. (1999). *Measuring problem gambling in Canada: Final Report-Phase I.* The Inter-Provincial Task Force on Problem Gambling, CCSA, Ottawa.

Fisher, S. E. (1992). Measuring pathological gambling in children: The case of fruit machines in the U.K. *Journal of Gambling Studies, 8,* 263–285.

Fisher, S. E. (2000). Developing the DSM-IV-MR-J criteria to identify adolescent problem gambling in non clinical populations. *Journal of Gambling Studies, 16,* 253–273.

Griffiths, M. (2001). Why don't adolescent gamblers seek treatment? *e-Gambling: The Electronic Journal of Gambling Issues, 5.*

Gupta, R., & Derevensky, J. L. (1998a). Adolescent gambling behavior: A prevalence study and examination of the correlates associated with problem gambling. *Journal of Gambling Studies, 14,* 319–345.

Gupta, R., & Derevensky, J. L. (1998b). An empirical examination of Jacobs' General Theory of Addictions: Do adolescent gamblers fit the theory? *Journal of Gambling Studies, 14,* 17–49.

Gupta, R., & Derevensky, J. L. (2000). Adolescents with gambling problems: From research to treatment. *Journal of Gambling Studies, 16,* 315–342.

Hardoon, K., Derevensky, J., & Gupta, R. (2000, June). *Social influences operant in children's gambling behavior.* Poster presented at the annual meeting of the Canadian Psychological Association, Ottawa.

Hardoon, K., Derevensky, J., & Gupta, R. (2002). An examination of the influence of familial, emotional, conduct and cognitive problems, and hyperactivity upon youth risk-taking and adolescent gambling problems. Report prepared for the Ontario Problem Gambling Research Centre, Ontario.

Hardoon, K., Derevensky, J., & Gupta, R. (2003). Empirical vs. perceived measures of gambling severity: Why adolescents don't present themselves for treatment. *Addictive Behaviors, 28,* 933–946.

Hodgins, D., Makarchuk, K., el-Guebaly, N., & Peden, N. (in press). Why problem gamblers quit gambling: A comparison of methods and samples. *Addiction Theory and Research.*

Jessor, R. (1998). New perspectives on adolescent risk behavior. In R. Jessor (Ed.), *New perspectives on adolescent risk behavior.* Cambridge, UK: Cambridge University Press.

Johnston, L. D., O'Malley, P. M., & Bachman, J. G. (2001). *Monitoring the future: National results on adolescent drug use, overview of key findings, 2000.* Washington: National Institute on Drug Abuse.

Kosten, T.A., & Rounsaville, B.J. (1992). Sensitivity of psychiatric diagnosis based on the best estimate procedure. *American Journal of Psychiatry, 149,* 1225–1227.

Ladouceur, R. (2001, December). *Conceptual issues in screening and diagnostic instruments: Implications for treatment and prevention of gambling disorders.* Paper presented at the Toward Meaningful Diagnosis of Gambling Disorders: From Theory to Practice Conference, Las Vegas.

Ladouceur, R., Bouchard, C., Rhéaume, N., Jacques, C., Ferland, F., Leblond, J., et al. (2000). Is the SOGS an accurate measure of pathological gambling among children, adolescents and adults? *Journal of Gambling Studies, 16,* 1–21.

Ladouceur, R. & Mireault, C. (1988). Gambling behaviors amongst high school students in the Quebec area. *Journal of Gambling Studies, 4,* 3–12.

Leckman, J. F., Scholomskas, D., Thompson, W. D., Belanger, A., & Weisman, M. M. (1982). Best estimate of lifetime psychiatric diagnosis: A methodological study. *Archives of General Psychiatry, 39,* 879–883.

Lesieur, H. R. (1994). Epidemiological surveys of pathological gambling: Critique and suggestions for modification. *Journal of Gambling Studies, 10,* 385–398.

Lesieur, H. R., & Blume, S. B. (1987). The South Oaks Gambling Screen (SOGS): A new instrument for the identification of pathological gamblers. *American Journal of Psychiatry, 144,* 1184–1188.

Lesieur, H. R., & Klein, R. (1987). Pathological gambling among high school students. *Addictive Behaviors, 12,* 129–135.

National Research Council (1999). *Pathological gambling: A critical review.* Washington, DC: National Academy Press. Rosenthal, R. J. (1992). Pathological gambling. *Psychiatric Annals, 22,* 72–78.

SAMHSA (2001). *Uniform facility data set (UFDS): 1999. Data on substance abuse treatment facilities.* Washington, DC: Department of Health and Human Services, Substance Abuse and Mental Health Services Administration.

Shaffer, H. J., & Hall, M. N. (1996). Estimating prevalence of adolescent gambling disorders. A quantitative synthesis and guide toward standard gambling nomenclature. *Journal of Gambling Studies, 12,* 193–214.

Shaffer, H. J., Hall, M. N., & Vander Bilt, J. (1997). *Estimating the prevalence of disordered gambling behavior in the United States and Canada: A meta-analysis.* Boston: Harvard Medical School.

Shaffer, H. J., LaBrie, R., LaPlante, D., Nelson, S., & Stanton, M. (2004). The road less travelled: Moving from distribution to determinants in the study of gambling epidemiology. *Canadian Journal of Psychiatry, 49,* 159–171.

Shaffer, H. J., LaBrie, R., Scanlan, K. & Cummings, T. (1994). Pathological gambling among adolescents: Massachusetts Gambling Screen. *Journal of Gambling Studies, 10,* 339–362.

Steinberg, M. A. (1997). *Connecticut High School Problem Gambling Surveys 1989 & 1996.* Guilford, Conn.: Connecticut Council on Problem Gambling.

Stinchfield, R. (1999). *Relevance of resilience to adolescent gambling: Implications for intervention.* Proceedings of the International Think Tank on Youth and Gambling, Winnipeg, Manitoba.

Stinchfield, R. (2002). Youth gambling: How big a problem? *Psychiatry Annals, 32,* 197–202.

Tavares, H., Zilberman, M., Beites, F., & Gentil, V. (2001). Gender differences in gambling progression. *Journal of Gambling Studies, 17,* 151–160.

Thompson, A., Walker, M., Milton, S. & Djukic, E. (2001). *Explaining the high false positive rates of the South Oaks Gambling Screen.* Unpublished manuscript.

Volberg, R. (1994). The prevalence and demographics of pathological gamblers: Implications for public health. *American Journal of Public Health, 84,* 237–241.

Volberg, R. (1998). *Gambling and problem gambling among adolescents in New York.* Report to the New York Council on Problem Gambling. Albany, NY.

Volberg, R. A. (2001). *Measures to track gambling rates, behaviors and related factors.* Report prepared for the National Council on Problem Gambling and SAMSHA, Washington DC.

Volberg, R., & Steadman, H. J. (1992). Accurately depicting pathological gamblers: Policy and treatment implications. *Journal of Gambling Studies, 8,* 402–412.

Westphal, J. R., Rush, J. A., & Stevens, L. (1997). *Statewide baseline survey for pathological gambling and substance abuse among Louisiana adolescents.* Baton Rouge: Louisiana department of Health and Hospitals, Office of Alcohol and Drug Abuse.

Winters, K.C. (2001, December). *Screening, assessment and diagnosis of gambling disorders: Are adolescents different?* Paper presented at the Toward Meaningful Diagnosis of Gambling Disorders: From Theory to Practice Conference, Las Vegas.

Winters, K. C., Stinchfield, R. D., Botzet, A., & Anderson, N. (2002). A prospective study of youth gambling behaviors. *Psychology of Addictive Behaviors, 16,* 3–9.

Winters, K.C., Stinchfield, R.D., & Fulkerson, J. (1993). Toward the development of an adolescent gambling problem severity scale. *Journal of Gambling Studies, 9,* 371–386.

Wynne, H. J., Smith, G, J., & Jacobs, D. F. (1996). Adolescent gambling and problem gambling in Alberta. Prepared for the Alberta Alcohol and Drug Abuse Commission. Edmonton, AB: Wynne Resources Ltd.

Chapter **8**

A Dynamic Process Perspective on Gambling Problems

Carlo C. DiClemente, Ph.D., Janine Delahanty, M.A. and Debra Schlundt, B.S.

Many perspectives have been used to understand how people become addicted and how they change (Glantz & Pickens, 1992; Orford, 1985; Rotgers, Keller & Morgenstern, 1996). A review of these explanatory models reveals that becoming addicted usually involves multiple determinants representing very different domains of human functioning. Some influences come from inside the individual and include biological and psychological vulnerabilities. Others are related to societal influences. The search for a single explanatory construct at a single point in the life of an individual that would explain how that individual becomes addicted appears futile. Similarly, once a person has developed an addiction, it is difficult to pinpoint a single factor explaining how cessation or recovery occurs.

Numerous studies have sought to identify the characteristics and risk factors of individuals that make them vulnerable to pathological gambling. Some have identified parental gambling (Govoni, Rupich & Frisch, 1996); others have identified behavior similar to Attention Deficit Disorder (ADD) (Lopez Viets, 1998). There is some evidence pointing to the involvement of impulsivity (Vitaro, Ferland, Jacques & Ladouceur, 1998) or video arcade games (Fisher & Griffiths, 1995; Gupta & Derevensky, 1996). Others have found a connection between gambling and substance abuse (Cunningham-Williams, Cottler, Compton & Spitznagel, 1998; Feigelman, Wallisch &

Lesieur, 1998; Gupta & Deverensky, 2000; Lesieur & Blume, 1991; McCormick, 1994; Winters & Anderson, 2000) and psychiatric comorbidity (Crockford & el-Guebaly, 1998). In one review Spunt, Dupont, Lesieur, Liberty and Hunt (1998) highlight sex differences in gambling initiation indicating that males are encouraged by the thrill of winning while females are more likely to seek escape from personal problems (see the reviews by Deverensky & Gupta, 2004; Dickson, Derevensky, & Gupta, 2004; and Stinchfield, this volume for an examination of risk factors associated with youth gambling problems). These data create a complex, complicated collage of factors contributing to the initiation of gambling problems that involve biological, psychological, and sociological determinants. There is substantive evidence to support the involvement of each of these areas of influence on gambling problems. Blum, Cull, Braverman and Comings (1996) have found evidence for the influence of genetics and neurotransmitters. Moore and Ohtsuka (1997) found that *Theory of Reasoned Action* variables and some personality characteristics accounted for some of the variance in gambling behavior. Reinforcement schedules, access and availability have also been shown to influence gambling behavior (Emerson & Laundergan, 1996; Gupta & Derevensky, 1996; Shaffer, 1996). Gambling behavior is multi-determined in origin in a manner that is similar to other addictive behaviors (DiClemente, 2003; Glantz & Pickens, 1992).

It can be helpful to draw on knowledge regarding the initiation of abuse and dependence on alcohol, illegal drugs, and nicotine when seeking to understand the causes of problem and pathological gambling (DiClemente, 1999; DiClemente, Story, & Murray, 2000; Glantz & Pickens, 1992). As one reviews the research and theoretical perspectives proposed to understand gambling and other addictive behaviors (e.g., Huba & Bentler, 1982; Jessor & Jessor, 1977; Moore & Ohtsuka, 1997; Tarter & Mezzich, 1992; Vitaro, Ferland, Jacques & Ladouceur, 1998), it becomes clear that no one developmental model or singular historical path can explain acquisition of and recovery from addictions (Chassin, Presson, Sherman & Edwards, 1991; Jessor, Van Den Bos, Vanderryn, Costa, & Turbin, 1995; Schulenberg, Maggs, Steinman, & Zucker, 2001). To explain any addictive behavior as having a single causative or curative factor is naive. Gambling and other addictive behaviors begin and develop within the context of familial, societal, cultural, genetic, and biochemical influences, and personal circumstances. Individual and societal factors can help us understand initiation. However, in order to accurately portray the initiation and cessation processes these factors must be viewed within the context of the individual and group-level variability of those who move through experimentation and social engagement to more problematic and pathological forms of gambling behavior and then from pathological gambling to remediation or recovery.

The Transtheoretical Model (TTM) of Intentional Behavior change has been used to provide a conceptual framework that integrates divergent perspectives by focusing on how rather than why individuals change behavior. It is the personal pathway and not simply the type of person or environment that appears to be the best way to integrate and understand the multiple influences involved in the acquisition and cessation of addictions. The TTM model identifies key dimensions involved in this process (DiClemente, 2003; DiClemente & Prochaska, 1998; Prochaska & DiClemente, 1984). Beginning and stopping an addictive behavior involves unique decisional considerations. Individuals' choices influence and are influenced by both character and social forces. For each individual, acquiring or leaving an addiction, there is an interaction between risk and protective factors and personal decision-making that helps determine the outcome. Transitions into and out of addictions do not occur without the active participation of the individual. The TTM views addiction through the perspective of a process of change and the personal journey through this intentional change process influenced at various points by the host of risk and protective factors.

This chapter offers a view of the process of initiation and cessation of gambling problems using the basic elements of the Transtheoretical Model of Intentional Behavior Change. The acquisition and cessation of addictive behaviors will be best understood as movement through a series of stages of change. Conflicting information about the determinants of initiation may be the result of a simplistic dichotomous (on/off) view of pathological gambling. This stage model provides a multi-step perspective for examining how environmental influences, thoughts, and expectancies interact with experimentation, which, in turn, leads to increased involvement from occasional recreational gambling to planned regular patterns of engagement that can become problematic and eventually result in maintained addiction (DiClemente, 2003). However, at the outset, it is important to note that experimentation does not always lead to or promote pathological gambling involvement. In fact, many individuals who engage in gambling behaviors do so more or less regularly without significant problems, with adherence to present limits and acceptable financial losses (e.g., gambling losses that occur are within tolerable limits). The vast majority of youth who engage in gambling do so without becoming pathological gamblers or experience significant problems.

Research into recovery from gambling problems, although in its infancy, also suggests that many individuals recover from gambling problems and that natural recovery may be the rule rather than the exception (Slutske, Jackson & Sher, 2003). However, the notion of natural recovery has not been explored with adolescent problem gamblers. Although prevalence of problem gambling during the past-year and lifetime were rather stable across time in Slutske et al.'s study, problem gambling seems to be episodic with individuals moving into and out of problem gambling over time. Nevertheless, there is ample support that treatment can be helpful. In a recent review of controlled studies, cognitive-behavioral treatment interventions received empirical support (Toneatto & Ladouceur, 2003). Although there are some differences that are intriguing, the process of recovery from gambling problems appears similar to other types of addictions. Similarities and differences make gambling a very interesting addictive behavior to examine in light of this dynamic process perspective (DiClemente, Story & Murray, 2000) (for a similar and more extensive discussion of adolescent initiation of gambling see DiClemente, Story, & Murray, 2000).

Transtheoretical Model of Intentional Behavior Change

The Transtheoretical Model is an integrative perspective that has attempted to characterize both the process of initiation of addictive behaviors and that of recovery (modification or cessation) from these behaviors (DiClemente, 2003; DiClemente, 1994; Prochaska, DiClemente & Norcross, 1992). Paths leading into addictive behaviors as well as those stopping their behaviors are best understood within a complex change process. This process of change provides an informative, overview that can help make sense of initiation and cessation of gambling as well as other addictive behaviors across variations in individual and group level characteristics (DiClemente, 2003).

The four dimensions identified in the Transtheoretical Model represent distinct aspects of the process of intentional behavior change. Patterns of behavior are not usually created, modified, or stopped in a single moment in time. There are steps or segments to the process labeled *Stages of Change*. These stages depict the motivational and dynamic fluctuations of the process of change over time. Each stage represents specific tasks that must be accomplished and goals that need to be achieved if the individual is to move forward from one stage to the next (DiClemente, 2003). Individuals move from the *Precontemplation* stage (not considering initiating or absence of a desire to change a behavior), where the task is arousing some interest or concern that would support consideration of change to *Contemplation* (seriously considering it) where a risk-reward analysis leads to a decision to change. From there, individuals move on to *Preparation* (preparing to change) where commitment and planning are critical tasks, to *Action* (performing the actual behavior) with the goal of establishing a new pattern of behavior. Finally, individuals will seek to move to *Maintenance* (sustaining the behavior change over time) where the task is to integrate the new behavior into the individual's lifestyle. The second dimension, *Processes of Change,* represents the engine (activities and experiences) that helps individuals move through the various stages. There are identifiable sets of cognitive/experiential and behavioral processes gleaned from various theories of therapy that act as the engine for movement through the specific stages (Prochaska & DiClemente, 1982). A holistic perspective is needed in order to understand fully the process of human intentional behavior change. The third dimension, *Context of Change,* represents areas of functioning where issues, problems, resources or liabilities can facilitate or hinder successful change of a given pattern of behavior. The five areas of functioning identified in the TTM are current life situation, beliefs and attitudes, interpersonal relationships, family/social systems and enduring personal characteristics (DiClemente, 2003; DiClemente & Prochaska, 1998; Prochaska & DiClemente, 1984). Issues and problems in any one of these areas of functioning can act as facilitating or restraining factors that may moderate or mediate movement through the stages of change for any given behavior.

The final dimension is perceived to be *Markers of Change.* Two related constructs have been examined consistently in research using the Transtheoretical Model: *Decisional Balance* and *Self-Efficacy.* Decisional balance identifies the relationship between the positive and negative motives for change (Janis & Mann, 1977) and has emerged as an important marker of movement through the early stages of change (Prochaska et al., 1994; Velicer, DiClemente, Prochaska & Brandenberg, 1985). On the other hand, Self-Efficacy, Bandura's concept describing an individual's confidence to perform a specific behavior, emerged as an important predictor of action and long-term success (Bandura, 1977, 1997; DiClemente, Carbonari, Montgomery & Hughes, 1994; DiClemente, Fairhurst & Piotrowski, 1995; DiClemente, Prochaska & Gibertini, 1985; Velicer, DiClemente, Rossi & Prochaska, 1990). These four dimensions form the basic constructs of the model that are used to understand the process of change, interacting in a predictable manner and representing constructs that are empirically verifiable.

This overview of the process of intentional behavior change has been used to characterize the initiation of behaviors that protect and promote health behaviors (e.g., exercise, mammography, etc.), as well as those that create health-related problems (e.g., smoking, illegal drugs, etc.). This same change perspective has been used to characterize modification and cessation of problem behaviors (e.g., alcohol abuse and dependence, obesity, anxiety, etc.) (DiClemente, 1999; DiClemente & Prochaska, 1998). Clearly, there are specific differences and unique considerations for each of the behaviors studied as well as differences between initiation and cessation that must be considered. However, there does appear to be an underlying process of change that is similar for both initiation and cessation that applies across behaviors (DiClemente, 2003; DiClemente & Prochaska, 1998; Prochaska et al., 1994). Informed appreciation of the similarity in the process can enrich our theory and enhance our prevention and intervention efforts (Werch & DiClemente, 1994).

The Process of Initiation of Gambling

Even those individuals who become pathological gamblers began initially as pre-contemplators at some point in time. Precontemplators are not considering change of a current behavior pattern or adoption of a new one. The individual in precontemplation does not perceive the need to move toward gambling. This new behavior is either viewed as irrelevant, unwanted, not needed, or unacceptable. These individuals may have moved into contemplation and considered engaging in the behavior before returning to precontemplation or may simply be in precontemplation by virtue of lack of interest or opportunity. Whatever the reason, individuals in precontemplation are not considering the specific changes that would move them from the current pattern of behavior to one that includes gambling (Werch & DiClemente, 1994). Surveys of youth indicate that the majority of youth move out of this precontemplation stage for the first time in early adolescence (some by age 10) with over 60% reporting gambling by high school (Arcuri, Lester & Smith, 1985; Gaboury & Ladouceur, 1993; Gupta & Derevensky, 1997). Most pathological gamblers, in particular, began gambling early in life (Gupta & Derevensky, 1998a; National Research Council, 1999; Shaffer & Hall, 1996; Winters, Stinchfield & Fulkerson, 1993). One early study found that 37% of pathological gamblers began gambling by ten years of age, 47% between 11 and 18, and only 14% initiated gambling after the age of 18 (Dell, Ruzicka & Palasi, 1981).

Although many pathological gamblers report starting young, the converse is also true as many recreational gamblers also started gambling at a young age but fail to become pathological gamblers. Many youth move out of precontemplation but never move along the path that leads to becoming pathological gamblers. Understanding how and why certain individuals follow the paths through the process of change to different outcomes is the goal of the Transtheoretical Model.

Contemplation is the stage wherein attitudes and expectancies are developed as the individual considers the pros and cons of gambling. Consideration of change allows for an exploration of the positive and negative aspects of the current status quo and of the positive and negative expectations associated with the potential new behavior pattern. Although human behavior does not always appear rational or logical, individuals require a rationale to leave the status quo and begin a new behavior. While information and modeling offer important data for decision-making, experimentation is the way an individual gathers first-hand information about the pros and cons of engaging in a new behavior. Therefore, in the contemplation stage individuals who will move forward in the initiation process begin to develop at least some positive attitudes toward gambling and engage in initial experimentation with gambling.

Being prepared to engage in regular gambling activities requires some plan of premeditated action and the dedication to follow through with that plan. To make any change, the individual needs to focus attention and energy on breaking or leaving an old pattern of behavior and creating a new one. Planning involves organizing the environment and developing strategies that enable the individual to make the changes in the current behavior pattern that would be needed to create a new pattern of behavior. These tasks of reorganizing the environment and of implementing effective change strategies require energy. One of the most frequent reasons given by individuals for not changing is the lack the time, resources and energy required. Finding the time and energy is really a matter of commitment. Once an individual has had a gambling experience and likes it, the decisional balance becomes tipped toward engaging in the behavior again. This may occur as a result of winning or losing (Gupta & Derevensky, 1996). The individual subsequently begins to find ways to gain greater access to gambling activities. Although gambling often appears to be an activity that is spontaneous, impulsive, and not planned, many elements that are required for engaging in gambling behavior require forethought (access, financial resources, opportunity). Individuals in the preparation stage are prepared to engage and are open to opportunities to participate in this potentially high-risk behavior. This planning and commitment moves individuals from contemplation to preparation and ultimately to action.

The actual implementation of one's plan represents the *Action* stage of change. Modification or elimination of an old pattern of behavior and beginning to engage in the new behavior comprises the action step. In general, it may take weeks rather than days to establish a new pattern of behavior, and months rather than weeks to make it habitual. Three to six months is usually the suggested duration for the *Action* stage for behaviors that have a high frequency of occurrence, such as smoking which is practiced on a daily basis (DiClemente & Prochaska, 1998). This period may be longer for behaviors like gambling or cocaine use that often occur in a less than daily pattern, or shorter if the reinforcers are particularly potent for an individual. Once the new behavior pattern is solidly established, the task becomes sustaining or continuing the behavior, which occurs during the Maintenance stage. Two paths constitute action toward the maintenance stage. The first path involves actively engaging in gambling and establish a pattern of gambling behavior that is non-problematic and under self-regulation. For these individuals gambling is a leisure past-time and form of entertainment engaged in with limit-setting and without loss of control, although engaged in repeatedly (e.g. small betting on lottery scratch cards). The second path would comprise more problematic gambling. Here, individuals experience negative consequences and gambling-related problems, ignore them, and have impaired self-regulation.

Maintaining a new behavior pattern requires that the behavior becomes integrated into the lifestyle of the individual (which is the primary goal of the Maintenance stage of change). During the maintenance stage the new behavior pattern becomes engraved and requires little thought and effort to sustain it. The changed behavior pattern becomes the normative behavior pattern that is a familiar and integral part of the individual's behavioral repertoire. For the self-regulated gambler, the pattern is one of occasional or regular participation in lottery, card playing, sports betting, video-lottery playing or casino visits remains enjoyable, exciting and a form of relaxation. For the problematic gambler, the pattern becomes one of regular excessive engagement in gambling behaviors with significant negative consequences that accumulate over time. The well maintained patterns of both the self-regulated gambler and of the problematic gambler become a part of the individual's life and both patterns become highly resistant to change.

The maintenance stage for initiation of gambling has all the characteristics referred to as defining symptoms in the diagnostic categorization of compulsive gambling—recurrent engagement despite problems, failure to stop, preoccupation, and disruption in other areas of life (American Psychological Association, 1994). Lack of financial resources can make smaller losses problematic and can encourage illegal activities to obtain money for gambling. In many cases, engagement in gambling is already an illegal activity for some, depending on age and existing laws. Responsible, self-regulated gambling may be more difficult to achieve for regular adolescent gamblers. Thus, the path through action more easily moves into a problem and/or pathology track. Longitudinal studies of adolescents are needed to understand how adolescents move through this process of initiation of pathological gambling, to identify the critical markers of the transitions from one stage to another, and to delineate the loss of self-regulation.

This sequence of stages, as proposed in the model, identifies the critical experiences or tasks that accompany movement from one thinking or behavior pattern to another. According to the model, movement from an absence of gambling behavior at one extreme to regular problematic gambling at the other would follow a path of change characterized by this sequence of stages. This assumption is based on initiation patterns of other addictive and health-related behaviors (DiClemente & Prochaska, 1998; Prochaska et al., 1994; Werch & DiClemente, 1994). However, strictly linear movement through these stages in a short period of time appears to be the exception and not the norm (Carbonari, DiClemente, & Sewell, 1999). Individuals can stay in a single stage, like contemplation, for a long period of time. At times they move backward as well as forward through early stages (precontemplation, contemplation, and preparation), while being influenced by peers, their environment, and opportunity. Finally, many move into action, begin to experience negative consequences that shift the decisional balance against regular gambling, and then they return to an earlier stage in the process of change. Movement through the stages of change is typically more cyclical and circuitous than the linear description of movement presented above. However, some individuals may move more quickly through the stages than others. Some adolescent pathological gamblers appear to move through these stages rather quickly, aided by biological factors, social setting, parental example, and other risk factors (Cunningham-Williams et al.,1998; Feigelman et al., 1998; Gupta & Derevensky, 1997; 1998a; Winters, Bengston, Dorr & Stinchfield, 1998)

The Problem Gambler and the Change Process

As individuals reach the maintenance stage of problematic, pathological gambling, their behavior becomes highly resistant to change. The well-maintained addictive behavior is integrated into the lifestyle of the individual and has become a significant source of reinforcement for that individual. The individual is no longer characterized as gambling but has become a gambler. Some basic patterns of life get organized around gambling, as gambling becomes a core or central activity for that individual. Compulsive gamblers can also be characterized as precontemplators for changing their gambling behavior. The same behavior change process characterized by the five stages of change (precontemplation, contemplation, preparation, action and maintenance) can be used to understand how problematic and compulsive gamblers move away from problem gambling into successful modification or cessation of their gambling behaviors.

There is a similar set of stages of change for cessation of problematic or pathological gambling once it has become established as a recurrent and habitual pattern of behavior. Precontemplators for stopping or modifying gambling behaviors must develop a decisional balance that favors the change (Contemplation), create and nurture the commitment and action plan (Preparation), successfully implement this action plan (Action), and finally maintain the behavioral change over a significant period of time (Maintenance). Many who make an attempt at stopping will relapse and return to problematic gambling before they are able to successfully change (Echeburua, Fernandez-Montalvo, & Baez, 2000; Marlatt & Gordon, 1985). Movement through these stages of change often presents more of a cyclical and spiral pattern than a linear one (DiClemente & Prochaska, 1998; Prochaska et al., 1992). Problematic and pathological gamblers would conceivably move through the same stages of precontemplation, contemplation, preparation, action and maintenance in the recovery process as they did for the initiation of gambling behavior. Again, as in the case with initiation, cyclical movement through the stages is more normative than strictly linear movement.

As has been described elsewhere (DiClemente & Prochaska, 1998), individuals attempting to modify a problem behavior move from not considering change (Precontemplation) to seriously considering change (Contemplation) and then committing to a plan (Preparation) before they take Action and are able to sustain the change over time (Maintenance). Once an adolescent has become a compulsive gambler, the challenge shifts from preventing initiation to promoting cessation or, at minimum, significant modification of the gambling behavior. The compulsive gambler must become convinced that the negative consequences associated with the gambling behavior outweigh the positive ones, make a firm decision to stop, develop a viable plan, take effective action, and sustain that action over time. It is these tasks that are delineated in the various stages of change that become the focus of any intervention. Which task becomes the primary focus depends on where the compulsive gambler is in the cycle of the stages of recovery.

Often compulsive gambling in adolescents is associated with other emotional and behavioral problems (Cunningham-Williams et al., 1998; Feigelman et al., 1998; Winters et al., 1998; Yoeman & Griffiths, 1996). Drinking and drug use, illegal activities, and family problems promote problematic engagement in and complicate recovery from gambling. The complexity of multiple problems creates additional challenges for treatment both of adolescents and adults. There are, however, two important considerations that need to be addressed. The first is that readiness and the process of change for each of the associated problems can be viewed through the same perspective of the stages of change. Unwillingness to change drinking behavior, for example, may realistically limit the amount of sustained change of gambling behavior that can be accomplished. Moving individuals through the process of change for two behaviors simultaneously is a daunting challenge but can be accomplished. The second consideration is that working to resolve problems in other areas of life functioning may necessitate establishing priorities and can have a positive impact upon movement through the stages for modifying the compulsive gambling. For a 40 year-old gambler who began gambling as an adolescent, the span of time separating early motivations from current considerations may lessen the importance of etiology. However, for the adolescent compulsive gambler, the short time span between initiation and current behavior preserves the importance of associated problems that also played a role in initiation. Without losing sight of the central focus on compulsive gambling, interventions could be targeted first at associated problems (academic, interpersonal, familial, or psychological) and then at the gambling behavior, should research indicate this approach seems to work best (see Gupta & Derevensky, in this volume). This approach is more likely to be successful with gambling problems than with substance use behaviors. Interestingly, although there are very few controlled trials of treatment efficacy, the components that have proven helpful in treatment of problem gambling address thinking patterns, problem solving skills, social skills, and preventing relapse (Sylvain, Ladouceur, & Boisvert, 1997). Treatment approaches that are gaining support are typically multi-modal and cognitive-behavioral (Gupta & Derevensky, in this volume; Lopez Viets & Miller, 1997; Nower & Blaszczynski, in this volume).

One of the most important discoveries about the process of change is that the stages of change interact with the processes of change in a predictable manner (DiClemente & Prochaska, 1998; Perz, DiClemente, & Carbonari, 1996; Prochaska, Velicer, DiClemente, Guadagnoli & Rossi, 1991). In the earlier stages the cognitive and experiential processes of change are more salient, while in the later stages the behavioral processes of change are more relevant. Treatment should not be uniform throughout the change process or consist of simply doing more of the same at latter stages but rather should consist of doing the right thing at the right time in the process of change (Perz et al., 1996; Velasquez, Maurer, Crouch & DiClemente, 2001). In practice this goal has led clinicians and researchers to develop techniques that are more motivational in nature and concentrate on decision making for individuals in the early stages of change (Miller & Rollnick, 1991; Miller, Zweben, DiClemente, & Rychtarik, 1992). Behavioral strategies, like counterconditioning, stimulus control, reinforcement management and self-liberation, are most important during the later stages from preparation to action and maintenance (DiClemente & Prochaska, 1998). Sequencing and shifting intervention strategies to meet the needs of the client moving through the stages of change, either linearly or cyclically, lie at the core of the Transtheoretical Model of intentional behavior change (DiClemente, 2003; DiClemente & Prochaska, 1998).

Tailoring Prevention Interventions to the Stages of Initiation

If initiation of problematic gambling involves a process of change that occurs over time and requires a sequence of different tasks that are reflected in the stages of change, then prevention efforts of necessity must be flexible and targeted. All individuals are not equally and simultaneously vulnerable to engaging in gambling behavior. An individual's behavior depends on where he or she is in the process of initiation, along with the influence of past experiences, expectations, and social context. The same individual may react differently to the identical situation depending on where in the process of change this experience occurs. Different strategies would be required in schools or communities where most individuals are in precontemplation for initiation versus those where many people have moved forward into preparation and action stages of initiation (i.e., those seeking treatment). Prevention specialists can tailor programs to specifically target individuals and groups. In order to do this they should first track the process of change that constitutes the initiation of self-regulated or pathological gambling among the target population. Interventions can then be tailored to address the stages of initiation for those receiving the prevention program initiatives.

The initial challenge for prevention is to assess and identify the distribution of the population across the stages of initiation. This requires a stage-based epidemiology rather than a simple count of the number of individuals who have ever engaged in gambling behavior or have done so in the past month. The initial step is to identify how many in the population are in action or maintenance mode, either for self-regulated or for problematic gambling. For those not in action or maintenance, some assessment of attitudes and intentions related to gambling can be used to classify them into the precontemplation, contemplation, and preparation stages of change. Thus, estimates can be generated for the entire population that categorize individuals into one of these stages of change. In one community there might be a distribution of 2% in maintenance and another 3% in action for pathological gambling with 30% in action or maintenance for self-regulated gambling and the rest distributed throughout the earlier stages of precontemplation (25%), contemplation (20%) and preparation (20%) for initiation. Another group of adolescents could present a very different picture with a distribution of 10% in action or maintenance for pathological gambling and 50% in action or maintenance for self-regulated gambling with only 10% in precontemplation, 10% in contemplation and 20% in preparation for initiation. These two groups would be considered very different, requiring different types of prevention. Not only would they have different amounts of gambling, these two different communities would exhibit different norms and social influences regarding gambling by virtue of the distribution across the stages. Consequently, different types of prevention and treatment efforts should be presented. In the first case, efforts could be focused on keeping individuals from moving into action. In the case of the second group, increases in treatment options and aggressive responsible gambling campaigns may well be the intervention of choice (DiClemente, 1999; Werch & DiClemente, 1994).

Both at the level of the individual and of the community, it makes a difference where individuals lie in the process of gambling initiation. The more individuals there are in earlier stages, the more primary prevention efforts are needed. Once individuals become engaged in gambling behavior and move into the later stages of initiation, secondary prevention, harm reduction, and early treatment programs are warranted. When the focus of the intervention is on those in the action stage, and the goal is to promote responsible and controlled use; prevention addresses an at-risk population and tries to facilitate the transition to maintained, self-regulated use. Individuals already well into the action stage of change should be considered already in difficulty and require programs to prevent movement to a continued addiction. However, once individuals have reached the Maintenance stage of addiction, programmatic shifts using the stages of recovery are needed. There is no "one size fits all" prevention strategy that could be effective with every individual or with every community across the spectrum of the stages of initiation. Some individuals and communities have greater access to gambling and more risk and less protective factors, all of which would promote movement through these stages. Prevention programs should be multidimensional and sustained over time.

Tailoring Treatments and Interventions to the Stages of Change

As is true with the stages of initiation, assisting individuals in moving away from pathological gambling requires some knowledge of their current stage and how to engage the appropriate strategies that can move them toward successfully maintaining change. Convincing youth that their gambling behavior is problematic and requires modification is the first step to moving from precontemplation. Motivational interventions that avoid argumentation and concentrate on the individual's decisional considerations would be useful for engaging the person in the process of change. Coping skill assessment and development are critical during the preparation stage to ensure that they have all the psychological equipment to carry through on the action plan. Behavioral strategies that include viable substitutes, stimulus control of the environment to avoid cues and people associated with gambling, and developing contingencies that support change are needed in the action and maintenance stages. Skills related to money management and anxiety management could complement the action strategies. Relapse prevention strategies would be most relevant for the person who had achieved some measure of success. Treatment programs are needed that can track the process of change for problem and pathological gamblers and assist them to make their way through the steps needed to achieve recovery. Recent research supports the need for multi-component, skills-based treatment programs (Gupta & Derevensky, 1998a, 1998b, in this volume; Ladouceur, Boisvert & Dumont, 1994; Lopez Viets & Miller, 1997; McCormick, 1994; Sylvain et al., 1997). Incorporating a process of change perspective in the application of these programs represents a next logical step in creating treatments for gamblers.

Initial investigations into the treatment for pathological gambling appear to parallel treatment research in other areas of addictive behaviors and make an argument for understanding the process of change model. Toneatto and Ladouceur (2003) conducted a review of eleven empirically based studies on the treatment of compulsive gambling. The studies examined treatments from several different perspectives, including behavioral, cognitive, pharmacological, and self-help. Multi-component, multidimensional treatments appeared more effective overall. Although they found little discussion about the process of change model, they did present studies that demonstrated an effect for brief, self-help interventions that were motivational in nature and seemed to work best for individuals with less severe gambling problems (Hodgins, Currie, & el-Guebaly, 2001). As is often the case, even individuals assessed in the wait list control group showed some improvement. Over 80% of the sample demonstrated reduced gambling behavior during the one-year period after treatment. It is not clear how much of this may be simply a reflection of the natural fluctuations in gambling behavior over time or the process of natural recovery. Another small study has begun to examine the processes of change in recovery from gambling addiction. Hodgins (2001) incorporated a modified version of the Processes of Change Questionnaire (Prochaska, Velicer, DiClemente & Fava, 1988) to measure the 10 processes that have been reliably found in studies of recovery with other addicted populations. Gamblers who did not receive treatment were found to less likely experience cognitive experiential processes of change including consciousness-raising, self-reevaluation, helping relationship, environmental reevaluation and dramatic relief compared to their treatment-seeking counterparts. Similarly non-treatment seeking gamblers appeared to engage in less stimulus control activity and experience less social liberation. Treatments seem to be related to process of change activity although the results of this study must be interpreted cautiously as it was a retrospective report from a small number of individuals. Nevertheless, these studies suggest a need to better understand the process of recovery and how self-help, treatment, and the processes of change interact.

Recommendations Based on a Process Analysis

Although prevention and treatment of gambling behavior represent a rather new field of research and clinical practice, there is a substantial body of research and practice with other addictive and health compromising behaviors. While there are discussions about whether to classify gambling as an impulsive, compulsive, or addictive behavior, there is no question that there are similarities in etiology as well as in emotional and behavioral aspects of gambling with other addictive behaviors including substance abuse and dependence (DiClemente 2003; Glantz & Pickens, 1992). Examining parallels and prior research can be instructive and offer both promising directions and paths to avoid. Initiation of gambling is most similar to initiation of alcohol consumption. There could be important advantages to examining the similarities and differences among multiple addictive behaviors when seeking answers to prevention of and intervention with gambling behavior.

Prevention of gambling problems should focus on achievable goals. Prevalence data suggests that it may be impossible to prevent exposure and experimentation for the majority of adolescents. Currently, there are too many activities, venues, and opportunities to gamble. However, we can influence the expectancies about the odds and the rewards of gambling as well as teaching self-control. More realistic expectancies can help adolescents in their decision considerations and lead to attempts to moderate and self-regulate their gambling behavior. In addition, individuals most vulnerable to move into the Action stage for compulsive gambling can be identified. These vulnerable individuals can be targeted with interventions to reduce risk and increase protective factors. For the group of adolescents who are already reaching sustained problematic gambling, treatment strategies must be initiated.

A similar array of treatment approaches has been proposed for treatment of gambling behavior as has been used for other addictive behaviors (Lopez Viets, 1998). However, readiness to change has often proved to be a better predictor of outcome than type of treatment program (Project MATCH, 1997; 1998). A treatment program that utilizes established change strategies and is applied skillfully with sensitivity to motivational considerations can produce significant change despite differences in treatment philosophy (Project MATCH, 1997). Research on interventions for gambling should focus on the process of change rather than replicate the competitive, treatment comparison studies that have been done with other addictive behaviors. An array of treatments should be provided to those who have already become problem or pathological gamblers recognizing the important role of motivation, decision-making, skills development, action and maintenance.

There are significant implications for policy makers and politicians that flow from this analysis. Increasing opportunity to gamble brings with it the obligation to understand the development of problematic gambling so that legislation and social policies can be developed to lessen the probability of young adolescents gaining access to gaming venues and to promote responsible gambling.

Extreme gambling is a risky behavior for society as well as for the individual. Serious economic, personal, familial, and social consequences are an integral part of widespread gambling. However, gambling problems and their negative consequences may not be immediate or uniform between individuals. Problematic, compulsive gambling involves a process of initiation and modification that needs to be explicated and better understood. Armed with a better this understanding of the process for initiation of and recovery from compulsive gambling, prevention and treatment professionals will be empowered to create more effective interventions.

References

American Psychiatric Association (1994). *Diagnostic and Statistical Manual of Mental Disorders* (4th ed.). Washington, DC: American Psychiatric Association.

Arcuri, A. F., Lester, D., & Smith, F. O. (1985). Shaping adolescent gambling behavior. *Adolescence, 20,* 935–938.

Bandura, A. (1977). The anatomy of stages of change. [Editorial] *American Journal of Health Promotion, 12,* 8–10.

Bandura, A. (1997). *Self-Efficacy: The Exercise of Control.* New York: W.H. Freeman & Company.

Blum, K., Cull, J. G., Braverman, E. R., & Comings, D. E. (1996). Reward deficiency syndrome: Addictive, impulsive and compulsive disorders including alcoholism, attention-deficit disorder, drug abuse and food bingeing may have a common genetic basis. *American Scientist, 84,* 132–145.

Carbonari, J. P., DiClemente, C.C. & Sewell, K. B. (1999). Stage transitions and the transtheoretical "stages of change" model of smoking cessation. *Swiss Journal of Psychology, 58,* 134–144.

Chassin, L., Presson, C.C., Sherman, S.J. & Edwards, D.A. (1991). Four pathways to young-adult smoking status: Adolescent social-psychological antecedents in a midwestern community sample. *Health Psychology, 10,* 409–418.

Crockford, D.N. & el-Guebaly, N. (1998). Psychiatric comorbidity in pathological gambling: A critical review. *Canadian Journal of Psychiatry, 43,* 43–50.

Cunningham-Williams, R. M., Cottler, L. B., Compton, W. M., & Spitznagel, E. L. (1998). Taking chances: Problem gamblers and mental health disorders—Results from the St. Louis Epidemiological Catchment Area (ECA) Study. *American Journal of Public Health, 88,* 1093–1096.

Derevensky, J., & Gupta, R. (2004). Adolescents with gambling problems: A review of our current knowledge. *e-Gambling: The Electronic Journal of Gambling Issues, 10,* 119–140.

Dell, L. J., Ruzicka, M. F., & Palasi, A. T., (1981). Personality and other factors associated with the gambling addiction. *The International Journal of the Addictions, 16,* 149–156.

Dickson, L., Derevensky, J., & Gupta, R. (2004). Harm reduction for the prevention of youth gambling problems: Lessons learned from adolescent high-risk prevention programs. *Journal of Adolescent Research, 19,* 233–263.

DiClemente, C. C. (1994). If behaviors change, can personality be far behind. In T. Heatherton & J. Weinberger (Eds.), *Can personality change* (pp. 175-198). Washington, DC: American Psychological Association.

DiClemente, C. C. (1999). Prevention and harm reduction for chemical dependency: A process perspective. *Clinical Psychology Review, 19,* 473–486.

DiClemente , C. C. (2003). *Addiction and change: How addictions develop and addicted people recover.* New York: Guilford Press.

DiClemente, C.C., Carbonari, J.P., Montgomery, R., & Hughes, S. (1994). The Alcohol Abstinence Self-Efficacy Scale. *Journal of Studies on Alcohol, 55,* 141–148.

DiClemente, C. C., Fairhurst, S. K., & Piotrowski, N. A. (1995). The role of self-efficacy in the addictive behaviors. In J. Maddux (Ed.), *Self-efficacy, adaptation and adjustment: Theory, research and application.* New York: Plenum Press.

DiClemente, C. C. & Prochaska, J. O. (1998). Toward a comprehensive, transtheoretical model of change: Stages of change and addictive behaviors. In W. R. Miller & N. Heather (Eds.), *Treating Addictive Behaviors* (2nd Ed., pp. 3–24). New York: Plenum.

DiClemente, C. C., Prochaska, J. O., & Gibertini, M. (1985). Self-efficacy and the stages of self-change smoking. *Cognitive Therapy and Research, 9,* 181–200.

DiClemente, C.D., Story, M., Murray, K. (2000). On a roll: The process of initiation and cessation of problem gambling among adolescents. *Journal of Gambling Studies, 16,* 289–313.

Echeburua, E., Fernandez-Montalvo, J. & Baez, C (2000). Relapse prevention in the treatment of slot-machine pathological gambling : Long-term outcome. *Behavior Therapy, 3,* 351–364.

Emerson, M. O., & Laundergan, J. C. (1996). Gambling and problem gambling among adult Minnesotans: Changes 1990 to 1994. *Journal of Gambling Studies, 12,* 291–304.

Feigelman, W., Wallisch, L. S., & Lesieur, H. R. (1998). Problem gamblers, substance users, and dual-problem individuals: An epidemiological study. *American Journal of Public Health, 88,* 467–470.

Fisher, S., &. Griffiths. M. (1995). Current trends in slot machine gambling: Research and policy issues. *Journal of Gambling Studies, 11,* 239–247.

Gaboury, A., & Ladouceur, R. (1993). Evaluation of a prevention program for pathological gambling among adolescents. *The Journal of Primary Prevention, 14,* 21–28.

Glantz, K., & Pickens, R. (1992). *Vulnerability to drug abuse.* Washington, DC: American Psychological Association.

Govoni, R., Rupcich, N., & Frisch, G. R. (1996). Gambling behavior of adolescent gamblers. *Journal of Gambling Studies, 12,* 305–317.

Gupta, R., & Derevensky, J. L. (1996). The relationship between gambling and video-game playing behavior in children and adolescents. *Journal of Gambling Studies, 12,* 375–394.

Gupta, R., & Derevensky, J. (1997). Familial and social influences on juvenile gambling behavior. *Journal of Gambling Studies, 13,* 179–192.

Gupta R., & Derevensky, J. (1998a). Adolescent gambling behavior: A prevalence study and examination of the correlates associated with excessive gambling. *Journal of Gambling Studies, 14,* 319–345.

Gupta, R., & Derevensky, J. (1998b). An empirical examination of Jacobs' general theory of addictions: Do adolescent gamblers fit the theory? *Journal of Gambling Studies, 14,* 17–49.

Gupta, R., & Derevensky, J. (2000). Adolescents with gambling problems: From research to treatment. *Journal of Gambling Studies, 16*, 315–342.

Hodgins, D. C. (2001). Processes of changing gambling behavior. *Addictive Behaviors, 26*, 121–128.

Hodgins, D. C., Currie, S. R., & el-Guebaly, N. (2001). Motivational enhancement and self-help treatments for problem gambling. *Journal of Consulting and Clinical Psychology, 69*, 50–57.

Huba, G. & Bentler, P. (1982). A developmental theory of drug use: derivation and assessment of a causal modeling approach. In P. Baltes & O. Brim (Eds.) *Life-span development and behavior* (Vol. 4, pp. 147–203). San Diego, CA: Academic Press.

Janis, I.L., & Mann, L. (1977). *Decision making*. New York: Free Press.

Jessor, R. & Jessor, S. (1977). *Problem behavior and psychosocial development: A longitudinal study of youth*. San Diego, CA: Academic Press.

Jessor, R., Van Den Bos, J., Vanderryn, J., Costa, F.M., & Turbin, M. S. (1995). Protective factors in adolescent problem behavior: Moderator effects and developmental change. *Developmental Psychology, 31*, 923–933.

Ladouceur, R, Boisvert J.-M., & Dumont J. (1994). Cognitive-behavioral treatment for adolescent pathological gamblers. *Behavior Modification, 18*, 230–242.

Lesieur, H. R., & Blume, S. B. (1991). Evaluation of patients treated for pathological gambling in a combined alcohol, substance abuse, and pathological gambling treatment unit using the Addiction Severity Index. *British Journal of Addiction, 86*, 1017–1028.

Lopez Viets, V. C. (1998). Treating pathological gambling. In W. R. Miller & N. Heather (Eds.), *Treating Addictive Behaviors* (2nd ed., pp. 259–270). New York: Plenum Press.

Lopez Viets, V. C., & Miller, W. R. (1997). Treatment approaches for pathological gamblers. *Clinical Psychology Review, 17*, 689–702.

Marlatt A., & Gordon, J. (1985). *Relapse Prevention*. New York: Guilford.

McCormick, R. A. (1994). The importance of coping skill enhancement in the treatment of the pathological gambler. *Journal of Gambling Studies, 10*, 77–86.

Miller, W. R., & Rollnick, S. (1991). *Motivational interviewing: Preparing people to change addictive behavior*. New York: Guilford Press.

Miller, W., Zweben, A., DiClemente, C. C., & Rychtarik, R. G. (1992). Motivational enhancement therapy manual: A clinical research guide for therapists treating individuals with alcohol abuse and dependence. *National Institute on Alcohol Abuse and Alcoholism Project MATCH Monograph Series, 2* (Department of Health and Human Services Publication No. (ADM) 92–1894. Bethesda, MD: National Institute on Alcohol Abuse and Alcoholism.

Moore, S. M., & Ohtsuka, K. (1997). Gambling activities of young Australians: Developing a model of behaviour. *Journal of Gambling Studies, 13*, 207–236.

National Research Council (1999). *Pathological gambling: A critical review*. Washington, DC: National Academy Press.

Orford, J. (1985). *Excessive appetites: A psychological view of addictions*. New York: John Wiley & Sons.

Perz, C. A., DiClemente, C. C., & Carbonari, J. P. (1996). Doing the right thing at the right time? Interaction of stages and processes of change in successful smoking cessation. *Health Psychology, 15*, 462–468.

Prochaska, J. O., & DiClemente, C. C. (1982). Transtheoretical therapy: Toward a more integrative model of change. *Psychotherapy: Theory, research and practice, 19*(3), 276–288.

Prochaska, J. O., & DiClemente, C. C. (1984). *The Transtheoretical approach: Crossing the traditional boundaries of therapy*. Malabar, FL: Krieger.

Prochaska, J. O., DiClemente, C. C., & Norcross, J. C. (1992). In search of how people change: Applications to addictive behaviors. *American Psychologist, 47*, 1102-1114.

Prochaska, J. O., Velicer, W. F., DiClemente, C. C., Guadagnoli, E., & Rossi, J.S. (1991). Patterns of change: Dynamic typology applied to smoking cessation. *Multivariate Behavioral Research, 26,* 83-107.

Prochaska, J. O., Velicer, W. F., DiClemente, C. C. & Fava, J. (1988). Measuring processes of change: Applications to the cessation of smoking. *Journal of Consulting and Clinical Psychology, 56,* 520-528.

Prochaska, J. O., Velicer, W. F., Rossi, J. S., Goldstein, M. G., Marcus, B. H., Rakowski, W., et al. (1994). Stages of change and decisional balance for 12 problem behaviors. *Health Psychology, 13,* 39-46.

Project MATCH Research Group. (1997). Matching alcoholism treatments to client heterogeneity: Project MATCH post-treatment drinking outcomes. *Journal of Studies on Alcohol, 58,* 7-29.

Project MATCH Research Group. (1998). Matching alcoholism treatments to client heterogeneity: Project MATCH three year drinking outcomes. *Alcoholism Clinical and Experimental Research, 22,* 1300-1311.

Rotgers, F., Keller, D.S. & Morgenstern, J. (1996). *Treating substance abuse: Theory and technique.* New York: Guilford Press.

Schulenberg, J., Maggs, J.L., Steinman, K.J., and Zucker, R.A. (2001). Development matters: Taking the long view on substance abuse etiology and intervention during adolescence. In P. M. Monti, S.M. Colby and T.A. O'Leary (Eds.), *Adolescents, alcohol and substance abuse.* (pp. 19-57). New York: Guilford Press.

Shaffer, H. J. (1996). Understanding the means and objects of addiction: Technology, the internet, and gambling. *Journal of Gambling Studies, 12,* 461-469.

Shaffer, H. J., & Hall, M. N. (1996). Estimating the prevalence of adolescent gambling disorders: A quantitative synthesis and guide toward standard gambling nomenclature. *Journal of Gambling Studies, 12,* 193-214.

Slutske, W.S., Jackson, K.M., & Sher, K. J. (2003). The natural history of problem gambling from age 18 to 29. *Journal of Abnormal Psychology, 112,* 263-274.

Spunt, B., Dupont, I., Lesieur, H., Liberty, H. J., & Hunt, D. (1998). Pathological gambling and substance misuse: A review of the literature. *Substance Use and Misuse, 33,* 2535-2560.

Sylvain, C., Ladouceur, R., &. Boisvert, J.-M. (1997). Cognitive and behavioral treatment of pathological gambling: A controlled study. *Journal of Consulting and Clinical Psychology, 65,* 727-732.

Tartar, R.E. & Mezzich, A.C. (1992). Ontogeny of substance abuse: Perspectives and Findings. In M. Glantz & R. Pickens. (Eds.), *Vulnerability to drug abuse* (pp. 149-178). Washington DC: American Psychological Association.

Toneatto, T. & Ladouceur, R. (2003). Treatment of pathological gambling: A critical review of the literature. *Psychology of Addictive Behaviors, 17,* 284-292.

Velasquez, M.M., Maurer, G.G., Crouch, C. & DiClemente, C.C. (2001). *Group treatment for substance abuse: A stages of change therapy manual.* New York: Guilford Press.

Velicer, W.F., DiClemente, C.C., Prochaska, J.O. & Brandenburg, N. (1985). A decisional balance measure for assessing and predicting smoking status. *Journal of Personality and Social Psychology, 48,* 1279-1289.

Velicer, W.F., DiClemente, C.C., Rossi, J. & Prochaska, J.O. (1990). Relapse situations and self-efficacy: an integrative model. *Addictive Behaviors, 15,* 271-283.

Vitaro, F., Ferland, F., Jacques, C., & Ladouceur, R. (1998). Gambling, substance use, and impulsivity during adolescence. *Psychology of Addictive Behaviors, 12,* 185-194.

Werch, C. E., & DiClemente, C. C. (1994). A multi-component stage model for matching drug prevention strategies and messages to youth stage of use. *Health Education Research: Theory & Practice, 9,* 37-46.

Winters, K. C., & Anderson, N., (2000). Gambling involvement and drug use among adolescents. *Journal of Gambling Studies, 16,* 175–198.

Winters, K. C., Bengston P., Dorr D., & Stinchfield, R. (1998). Prevalence and risk factors of problem gambling among college students. *Psychology of Addictive Behaviors, 12,* 127–135.

Winters, K. C., Stinchfield, R. D. & Fulkerson, J. (1993). Patterns and characteristics of adolescent gambling. *Journal of Gambling Studies, 9,* 371–386.

Yoeman, T. & Griffiths, M. (1996) Adolescent machine gambling and crime. *Journal of Adolescence, 19,* 183–188.

Chapter 9

A Treatment Approach for Adolescents with Gambling Problems

Rina Gupta, Ph.D. and Jeffrey L. Derevensky, Ph.D.

As indicated in previous chapters, it is not uncommon for an adolescent to be participating in one form of gambling or another, be it the lottery, card playing for money, sports wagering, or gambling on electronic gambling devices. The results of the National Research Council's (NRC) (1999) review of empirical studies suggest that 85% of adolescents (the median of all studies) report having gambled during their lifetime, with 73% of adolescents (median value) reporting gambling in the past year. This raises serious mental health and public policy concerns (Derevensky, Gupta, Messerlian & Gillespie, in this volume; NRC, 1999).

Meta-analyses (Shaffer & Hall, 1996) and a review of more recent studies (see Jacobs, in this volume) confirm that between 4–8% of youth are experiencing very serious gambling-related problems, with another 10–15% at-risk for the development of a gambling dependency. More recent debates have raised the question as to the accuracy of prevalence rates of problem gambling amongst youth. Some have recently argued that our current instruments and screens are not accurately assessing pathological gambling amongst adolescents but are over-estimating the prevalence rates (i.e, Ladouceur et al., 2000; Jacques & Ladouceur, 2003). Yet, in a comprehensive discussion of the arguments, Derevensky, Gupta and Winters (2003) and Derevensky and Gupta (in this volume) suggest that many of the assertions raised have little merit. Nevertheless, while this debate plays itself out in the research community and the search for the *gold standard* instrument continues, it remains clear that a small but identifiable number of youth actually develop serious gambling-related problems. While the need for treatment of youth who gamble problematically is evident, little progress has been made in understanding the treatment needs of this population, a conclusion also reached by the NRC (1999) review. Treatment studies reported in the literature have generally been case studies with small sample sizes (Knapp & Lech, 1987; Murray, 1993; Wildman, 1997) and have been criticized for not being subjected to rigorous scientific standards (Blaszczynski & Silove, 1995; Nathan, 2001; National Gambling Impact Study Commission, 1999; NRC, 1999).

A critical review of treatment issues pertaining to pathological gambling highlights the stringent and rigorous criteria that treatment outcome studies must meet in order to be considered an *Empirically Validated Treatment* (EVT) approach (Toneatto & Ladouceur, 2003) or falling within the parameters of *Best Practices*. Both models base their criteria upon recommendations put forward by the American Psychological Association (Kazdin, 2001), SAMSHA and CSAT. Along with replicability of findings, randomization of patients to an experimental group, the inclusion of a matched control group, and the use of sufficiently large enough samples are viewed as the minimum requirements necessary to validate effective treatment paradigms. Unfortunately, the treatment of adolescent pathological gamblers has not yet evolved to the point that treatment evaluation studies have met the criteria for EVT or Best Practices.

There are several reasons to explain why more stringent criteria, scientifically validated methodological procedures, and experimental analyses concerning the efficacy of treatment programs for youth have not been implemented. Primarily, these reasons include the fact that there exist very few treatment programs prepared to include young gamblers amongst their clientele and few underage problem gamblers actually present themselves for treatment in centers with trained personnel. This small number of young people seeking treatment in any given centre results in the difficulty of obtaining matched control groups. Matched controls are even more difficult to obtain when considering that young gamblers often present with a significant number and variety of secondary psychological disorders. Another obstacle to treatment program evaluation is that treatment approaches may vary within a center and may be dependent upon the gamblers specific profile, developmental level, or therapist's training orientation. Given the lack of empirically based treatment in the field of pathological gambling, this therapy issue is relatively new compared to existing treatment models for youth with other addictions and mental health disorders. There nevertheless remains a growing interest in identifying effective treatment strategies to help minimize youth gambling problems.

Existing Treatment Approaches

Treatment paradigms used for adults have in general been based upon a number of theoretical approaches. These paradigms fundamentally include one or more of the following orientations: psychoanalytic or psychodynamic (Bergler, 1957; Miller, 1986; Rosenthal, 1987; Rugle & Rosenthal, 1994), behavioral (Blaszczynski & McConaghy, 1993; Walker, 1993), cognitive and cognitive-behavioral (Bujold, Ladouceur, Sylvain, & Boisvert, 1994; Ladouceur & Walker, 1998; Toneatto & Sobell, 1990; Walker, 1993), pharmacological (Grant, Chambers & Potenza, in this volume; Grant, Kim & Potenza, 2003; Haller & Hinterhuber, 1994; Hollander, Frenkel, DeCaria, Trungold, & Stein, 1992; Hollander & Wong, 1995), physiological (Blaszczynski, McConaghy, & Winters, 1986; Carlton & Goldstein, 1987), biological/genetic (Comings, 1998; DeCaria, Hollander & Wong, 1997; Hollander et al., 1992; Saiz, 1992), addiction-based models (Lesieur & Blume, 1991; McCormick & Taber, 1988), or self-help (Brown, 1986, 1987; Lesieur, 1990) (For a more comprehensive overview of these models the reader is referred to the reviews by Griffiths, 1995; Lesieur, 1998; NRC, 1999; Rugle, Derevensky, Gupta, Winters & Stinchfield, 2001).

The resulting treatment paradigms have in general incorporated a rather restrictive and narrow focus depending upon one's theoretical orientation of treatment (see Blaszczynski & Silove, 1995 for their analyses of the limitations of each approach). The application of theory and research findings to clinical practice has been similarly limited. Ladouceur and his colleagues have long argued for a cognitive-behavioral approach to treating both adults and youth with gambling problems (Bujold et al., 1994; Ladouceur, Boisvert & Dumont, 1994; Ladouceur, Sylvain, Letarte, Giroux & Jacques, 1998; Ladouceur & Walker, 1996, 1998). The central assumption underlying the cognitive-behavioral approach is that pathological gamblers will continue to gamble in spite of repeated losses given they maintain an unrealistic belief that losses can be recovered. As such, this perspective assumes that a number of erroneous beliefs (including a lack of understanding of independence of events, perceived level of skill in successfully predicting the outcome of chance events, and illusions of control) result in their persistent gambling behavior (Ladouceur & Walker, 1998).

In one of the few empirically-based treatment studies with adolescents, Ladouceur et al. (1994), using four adolescent male pathological gamblers, implemented a cognitive-behavioral therapy program. Within their treatment program five components were included: information about gambling, cognitive interventions, problem-solving training, relapse prevention, and social skills training. Cognitive therapy was provided individually for approximately 3 months (mean of 17 sessions). Ladouceur and his colleagues reported clinically significant gains resulting from treatment, with 3 of the 4 adolescents remaining abstinent three and six months after treatment. They further concluded that the treatment duration necessary for adolescents with severe gambling problems was relatively short compared to that required for adults, and that cognitive therapy represents a promising new avenue for treatment for adolescent pathological gamblers. This therapeutic approach is predicated upon the belief that adolescents (a) persist in their gambling behavior in spite of repeated losses primarily as a result of their erroneous beliefs and perceptions, and (b) that winning money is central to their continued efforts. However, their limited sample (four adolescents) while somewhat informative, is not sufficiently representative to depict a complete picture.

Research with adolescents suggests that the clinical portrait of adolescent problematic gamblers is much more complex than merely that of erroneous beliefs and the desire to acquire money. Our earlier research demonstrates strong empirical support for Jacobs' *General Theory of Addictions* for adolescent problem gamblers (Gupta & Derevensky, 1998a). Adolescent problem and pathological gamblers were found to have exhibited abnormal physiological resting states (resulting in a tendency toward risk-taking), greater emotional distress in general (i.e., depression and anxiety), reported significantly higher levels of dissociation when gambling, and had higher rates of comorbidity with other addictive behaviors. More recently, a series of studies have uncovered that adolescent problem and pathological gamblers differ on their ability to successfully cope with daily events, adversity and situational problems (Gupta & Derevensky, 2001; Gupta, Derevensky & Marget, in press; Hardoon, Gupta & Derevensky, in press). The empirical knowledge of the correlates and risk-factors associated with adolescent problem gambling has been described in more detail elsewhere (Derevensky & Gupta, 2004; Griffiths & Wood, 2000; Hardoon & Derevensky, 2002; Stinchfield, in this volume). Furthermore, contrary to common beliefs and the tenets of the cognitive-behavioral approach, our research and clinical work suggests money is not the predominant reason why adolescents with gambling problems engage in these behaviors (see Gupta & Derevensky, 1998b). Rather, it appears that money is often perceived as a means to enable these youth to continue gambling.

Blaszczynski and Silove (1995) further suggest that there is ample empirical support that gambling involves a complex and dynamic interaction between ecological, psychophysiological, developmental, cognitive and behavioral components. Given this complexity, each of these components needs to be adequately incorporated into a successful treatment paradigm (to achieve abstinence and minimize relapse). While Blaszczynski and Silove addressed their concerns with respect to adult problem gamblers, a similar multidimensional approach appears to be necessary to successfully address the multitude of problems facing adolescent problem gamblers.

This chapter serves to add to the growing body of literature focused upon youth gambling problems. In particular, we seek to provide an example of our treatment approach which is conceptually linked to, based upon, and derived from existing empirical research. Nonetheless, it is important to note that we have not empirically tested our approach to the standards set forth by SAMSHA or APA due to the lack of a sufficiently large control group. It is our contention that placing youth requesting treatment on a waiting list for an extended period of time is problematic due to the high level of distress evidenced by these youth, the belief that if they remain in a control group their problems will escalate, and the concern that they will no longer seek treatment after waiting in a control group. As such, to date, we have elected to provide immediate treatment to all youth requesting services.

Finding a Treatment Population

Adolescents with gambling problems in general tend not to present themselves for treatment. There are likely many reasons that they fail to seek treatment including (a) fear of being identified, (b) the belief that they can control their behavior, (c) adolescent self-perceptions of invincibility and invulnerability, (d) the negative perceptions associated with therapy by adolescents, (e) guilt associated with their gambling problems, (f) a lack of recognition and acceptance that they have a gambling problem despite scoring high on gambling severity screens, and (g) their inherent belief in natural recovery and self-control (for a more detailed explanation see Derevensky, Gupta & Winters, 2003; Derevensky & Gupta, 2004).

Referrals from parents, friends, teachers, the court system, and the local *Help/Referral Line* are the primary sources through which we acquire our treatment population. As part of an effective outreach program, posters and brochures are distributed to schools, media exposure and media campaigns are frequent, and workshops are provided for school psychologists, guidance counselors, social workers, teachers, and directly to children and adolescents. As a result of this outreach program, we receive a number of calls from adolescents directly requesting treatment. Interestingly, our Internet site has generated several inquiries for on-line help and assistance.

Research and our clinical experience suggests that adolescent problem gamblers develop a social network consisting of other peers with gambling problems (Wynne, Smith & Jacobs, 1996). This results in clients recommending their friends for treatment. Once an adolescent accepts and realizes that he/she has a serious gambling problem, they become astutely aware of gambling problems amongst their friends. Eventually, some successfully convince their peers to seek help as well.

Since adolescents with gambling problems have little access to discretionary funds and many initially seek treatment without parental knowledge, treatment is provided without cost. While this is not practical for treatment providers in independent practice, State or Provincial funding (or support by insurance providers when available) appears to be fundamental when treating these adolescents.

The location of the treatment facility plays an important role in successfully working with youth. Concerns about being seen entering an addiction center, mental health facility or hospital may discourage some youth from seeking treatment. Accessibility by public transportation is essential since most young clients do not own cars or have money for taxi fare. Although our clinic is adjacent to a University counseling centre, it operates as a self-contained facility exclusively for work with youth experiencing gambling problems.

The McGill Treatment Paradigm

This treatment approach has been refined through our continued work over a seven-year period with over 50 young problem gamblers, ranging in age from 14–21. While not a sufficiently large number of clients upon which to draw firm conclusions, it nevertheless has provided us with sufficient diversity of experience to appreciate the broad applicability of our approach considering the variability of the age range of clients and the concomitant co-occurring problems often accompanying their gambling problems. Based upon empirical findings and our clinical observations with these individuals, their reported success in remaining abstinent, and their improvement in their overall psychological well-being, the approach adopted in our clinic is generally successful in assisting youth to resume a healthy lifestyle.

The criterion by which to evaluate success differs from one treatment facility and approach to the next. In a recent review of treatment literature, Toneatto and Ladouceur (2003) suggest that several different outcome measures have traditionally been used when assessing treatment effectiveness; these being personal ratings of urges, reduction of gambling involvement, and gambling cessation. Our treatment philosophy is predicated upon the assumption that sustained abstinence is necessary for these youth to recover from their gambling problem and that their general overall psychological well-being and mental health must be improved (this also includes improvement in their coping skills and adaptive behaviors). During the past seven years, we have observed a large percentage of youth in treatment who initially had as their primary goal controlled gambling. Our clinical work suggests that while controlled gambling (ability to respect self-imposed limits) can be an interim goal, abstinence is eventually necessary. Attempts are made to closely monitor these youth for at least one-year post treatment, however it becomes difficult to maintain contact with many of these youth after this point in time. Several youth call periodically beyond the one-year follow-up period to report their progress, but we remain acutely aware that youth who may have relapsed may be unwilling to contact the treatment centre unless they are prepared to re-enter treatment. There is also some recent evidence with adults that pathological gamblers who have successfully completed treatment and who have relapsed often fail to return to the same treatment centre for assistance but are more likely to seek treatment elsewhere (Chevalier, Geoffrion, Audet, Papineau & Kimpton, 2003).

For the most part, our treatment philosophy is predicated upon the work of Jacobs' *General Theory of Addictions* and the work of Blaszczynski and his colleagues' *Pathways Model* (see Nower & Blaszczynski, in this volume, for a comprehensive discussion of the model and an adaptation of the *Pathways Model* for youth problem gambling). This model presupposes that there are three different subtypes of pathological gamblers—each subtype having a different etiology and different accompanying pathologies. It is further assumed that these different subtype pathological gamblers would by necessity require different types of intervention (with different emphases) and that the duration for treatment will likely differ. While there is some overlap between the two models, with both describing the etiology, trajectory and psychology of the addicted gambler, Jacobs' model primarily describes the *Pathway 3* gambler articulated by Nower and Blaszczynski. The commonalities lie in the belief that these youth have a combination of emotional and/or psychological distress coupled with a physiological predisposition toward impulsively seeking excitement. This subset of problem gamblers represents our most typical young clients who seek therapy: those tending to gamble impulsively primarily for purposes of escape and as a way of coping with their stress, depression, and/or daily problems. Longitudinal data recently published following young boys aged 11 to 16 suggests that early indicators of gambling problems include indices of anxiety and impulsivity (Vitaro, Wanner, Ladouceur, Brendgen & Tremblay, 2004). Recent research has also replicated earlier findings that adolescent problem gamblers are more likely to be exposed to peer and parent gambling, are more susceptible to peer pressure, are more likely to exhibit conduct problems and antisocial behaviors, engage in substance use, and have suicide ideation and indicate more suicide attempts (Langhinrichsen-Rohling, Rhode, Seeley, & Rohling, 2004). Such a constellation of correlates and risk-factors are sure to result in different profiles of young problem gamblers.

A General Profile of Youth Seeking Treatment

It has been suggested that those individuals who present themselves for treatment are distinct, representing a minority of young pathological gamblers. It is important to note that while our clients voluntarily come for treatment a number may be less than motivated to participate at first. A considerable number attend because of parental pressure, mandatory referrals from the judicial system, or are strongly encouraged by significant others (i.e., boyfriends, girlfriends) and comply for fear of losing relationships.

The youth that do present for treatment tend to share a similar constellation of behaviors. Other than the psychological variables of depression, anxiety, impulsivity and poor coping abilities previously mentioned, it is not uncommon to see youth who have a history of academic difficulties (usually due to a learning disability and further compounded by their gambling preoccupation and gambling behavior), stressed interpersonal relationships with family members and old friends, involvement with unhealthy peer groups, and are engaging in delinquent criminal behaviors to support their gambling (e.g., shoplifting, cheque forgery, credit card scams). Despite these commonalities, individual differences exist resulting in three distinct profiles.

The following represents a brief synopsis profile of the three predominant types of young gamblers we have treated in our practice, with those fitting in Nower and Blaszczynski's Pathway 3 being most representative of the majority of youth with whom we have worked.

Pathway 1: Behaviorally-Conditioned Problem Gamblers

Joe, a 17-year-old male, is primarily a blackjack casino player (in spite of legal prohibitions). On one of his early visits to the casino, Joe reportedly won over $200 leading him to believe that gambling could provide a good and easy source of revenue. Personal accounts suggest he played, on average, between $300–$500 per week before seeking treatment. Joe also revealed that he had lost up to $2,000 on several visits to the local casino. He attends a post secondary business school, but was failing due to his problem gambling and preoccupation with gambling debts. He presents with occasional drug use and antisocial behaviors related to his gambling behaviors.

Motivation for gambling. Joe reports that gambling is very rewarding as it makes him feel exceptionally good. He revealed that gambling is highly exciting and he perceives it to be the ultimate challenge to outsmart the casino, recoup his losses, and to win large amounts of money.

Financial resources. Joe works part-time in father's company while attending school. He takes money from the company coffers, steals money from family members, and has even stolen and cashed alimony checks sent to his mother to enable him to gamble. He reportedly has borrowed money from friends and while he does his best to repay them he remains in constant debt.

Therapeutic objectives. Joe entered treatment reporting that he could stop gambling by himself but likes the support and supervision therapy provides. He acknowledged his need for an outlet to deal with the frustration and agitation resulting from his gambling withdrawal. The primary therapeutic objectives were to gradually help him reduce his gambling participation by setting frequency, time, and money limits on his activities while simultaneously addressing his erroneous beliefs about wagering and winning. Restructuring his time was essential to ensure he had minimal free time to think about gambling. This included helping him prioritize school work, seeking and developing healthy peer relationships, and minimizing his use of drugs.

Pathway 2: Emotionally Vulnerable Problem Gamblers

Candice, a 17-year-old female, primarily wagers on sports and casino playing (blackjack was her preferred game of choice). She reported wagering on average between $500–$1,500 per week. She generally plays until all her funds are depleted. She readily understood that the gambling cycle involves wins and losses, with the casino holding the edge over the player. Upon entry into treatment she was enrolled in the first year of CEGEP (Junior College), but was rarely attending as she spent much of her time at the casino. She also held a part-time job that she approached in a responsible manner.

Motivation for gambling. Candice reports gambling primarily to make herself feel special, impress friends, become closer to her father (also a pathological gambler), and as a way of dealing with depression, low self-esteem, agitation, and anxiety. She indicates that she had always experienced academic difficulties and preferred to spend time at the casino versus attending class and completing assignments.

Financial resources. Since all of her expenses were paid by her family (pocket money, car expenses, clothing, cell phone), the money Candice earned from her job was used almost exclusively for gambling. In addition, she would regularly take cash advances on her credit card (approximately $300 per week), which was readily paid by her father.

Therapeutic objectives: The primary goals established for Candice focused upon the identification of her underlying stressors and unresolved issues, addressing the underlying depression and anxiety, and improving her coping skills and adaptive behavior. There was also a need to directly address her gambling behavior and determine her willingness to abstain from gambling. This was accomplished through the gradual introduction of limit setting (money spent, time and frequency spent at the casino).

Pathway 3: Antisocial Impulsivist Problem Gamblers

Sonny, an 18-year-old male, is primarily a casino card player. He reports playing on average between $300–$600 per week depending on his success at the casino. He acknowledges being a thrill-seeker and was diagnosed with Attention Deficit Hyperactivity Disorder (ADHD) at the age of 12. He frequently engages in drug use, primarily cannabis to "take off the edge." Sonny has a family history of depression, meets the criteria for a mild chronic depression (dysthymia), and reports having repeated suicidal ideations.

Motivation for gambling. Sonny reports that while he is unhappy about his inability to control his gambling it provides him with such a thrill and escape that he can't stop. He has also calculated that the casino "owes" him $7000, and that it would be easier to stop once he wins back that money (a frequent form of logic seen with our clients). When explained that he would be unlikely to recoup the money lost, he acknowledged that most people lose money over time when gambling but that he is the exception to the rule. His erroneous belief system about his ability to control the outcomes of random events was pervasive. Sonny gambled primarily for escape, excitement, and to recoup lost money.

Financial resources. Sonny has little access to gambling funds as he was attending school and only holds a small part-time job. His parents are divorced and he works in his father's company on the weekend. His psychological profile indicates antisocial tendencies, often stealing money from his father's company. He also reports repeatedly lying to and manipulating his mother and friends to obtain money to gamble.

Therapeutic objectives. Sonny's impulsivity was underlying his inability to control his gambling. Thus, controlling impulsive tendencies (ADHD) and finding more appropriate ways to channel them were primary objectives. Sonny also met the criteria for a mild depression that required treatment and monitoring. His lying, stealing and manipulation of his family and friends were without remorse, representing an important treatment goal. Sonny's peers were perceived to be a negative influence and as such fostering a healthier choice of peers was important. The treatment plan also included a gradual reduction of his gambling participation and modifying erroneous cognitions.

The Treatment Procedure

Intake Assessment

The intake procedure includes a semi-structured interview using the DSM-IV criteria for pathological gambling as well as other pertinent gambling behaviors (e.g., preferred activities, frequency, wagering patterns, accumulated losses, etc.). Current familial situation and relationships, academic and/or work status, and social functioning are ascertained. Information concerning alcohol or drug use, the presence of other risk-taking behaviors, self-concept, coping skills, and selected personality traits are ascertained through a variety of instruments and clinical interviews. An evaluation for clinical depression as well as a history of suicide ideation and attempts is included.

An explanation of our procedures, requirements and goals are provided to each client in order to avoid any misconceptions. Client expectations and personal goals are also ascertained. Many youth report that they desperately want their unbearable situation to improve. However, approximately 60% of clients are initially ambivalent about abstinence.

Tenets of Therapy

A staff psychologist provides all therapy individually. Initially, therapy is provided weekly, however if the therapist deems more frequent sessions are required, appropriate accommodations are made. All clients are provided with a pager or cell phone number for emergency contacts. The number of sessions varies significantly with the motivation and degree of gambling severity of the client and the concomitant disorders. The number of therapy sessions generally range between 20—50 sessions.

The basic therapeutic process includes the following components:

Establishing mutual trust and respect. Mutual trust and respect are fundamental to the therapeutic relationship. Total honesty is emphasized and a non-judgmental therapeutic relationship is provided. This results in the adolescent not fearing reactions of disappointment if weekly personal goals are not achieved. However, since treatment is provided without cost, clients are required to respect the therapist's time. This involves calling ahead to cancel and reschedule appointments, punctual attendance at sessions, and a commitment to complete 'homework' assignments.

Assessment and setting of goals. Since the emphasis of different therapeutic objectives is tailored to the individual, a more detailed profile of the client is required. This is accomplished through comprehensive clinical interviews (beyond intake assessment), usually taking place over the first three sessions. The initial interview consists of the completion of several instruments primarily designed to screen for gambling severity, impulsivity, conduct problems, depression, antisocial behaviors, and suicide ideation and attempts. Their responses to these measures are followed up through more in-depth diagnostic interviews over the next few sessions and more details about the consequences associated with their gambling (i.e., academic and/or occupational status, peer and familial relationships, romantic and inter-personal relationships, legal problems, etc.) are obtained.

This comprehensive evaluation allows for the therapeutic goals to be established. For example, an adolescent who presents with serious depression will not be approached in the same manner as one who does not evidence depressive symptomatology. If a client presents with a severe depression, this becomes the initial therapeutic objective while the gambling problem becomes a secondary objective. Interestingly, for many youth, once gambling has stopped depressive symptomatology actually increases as youth report that their primary source of pleasure, excitement and enjoyment has been eliminated. It is therefore important to periodically screen for depressive symptomatology throughout the therapeutic process.

Assessment of readiness to change. An important factor influencing the therapeutic approach relates to the client's current willingness to make significant changes in their life. Our experience suggests that most adolescents experiencing serious gambling related problems are reluctant and are not convinced that they really want to stop gambling completely. Rather, most state that they believe in *controlled gambling* and hold onto this belief for some time in spite of our reluctance. Some individuals seek basic information but remain open to the idea of making more permanent changes. Others have decided that they really must stop gambling but are unable to do so without therapeutic assistance and support. Finally, some adolescents have made the decision to stop gambling and do so prior to their first session but require support in maintaining abstinence. These three examples depict adolescents in different stages of the process of change (see chapter by DiClemente, Delahanty & Schlundt, in this volume, for a comprehensive discussion of the Stages of Change Model).

While there are a multiplicity of approaches taken depending upon one's severity of gambling problems, underlying psychological disorders or problems, age, and risk factors, the overall therapeutic philosophy remains similar, with different weightings of therapeutic goals placed where most needed.

Goals of Therapy

DiClemente, Story and Murray (2000) initially proposed a *Transtheoretical Model of Intentional Behavior Change* for adolescent gambling problems whereby they contend that paths leading from addiction to recovery involve interactions between biological, psychological, sociological and behavioral elements in a person's life (see also the chapter by DiClemente, Delahanty & Schlundt, in this volume). As such, a multimodal, multi-goaled therapeutic approach is necessary. Within our treatment philosophy, the overall framework is to address multiple therapeutic goals simultaneously over time, tailoring the time allocated to each goal to the client. Some will require more emphasis on psychological issues, others on their physiological impulses, others on environmental /social factors while others will require examining their motivations to change. Nevertheless, each client receives individualized therapeutic attention in all areas to ensure they are achieving a balanced lifestyle.

The goals of therapy can be conceptualized as follows:

1) Understanding the motivations for gambling

Adolescents experiencing serious gambling problems continue gambling in the face of repeated losses and serious negative consequences as result of their need to dissociate and escape from daily stressors. Without exception, youth with gambling problems report that when gambling they enter a "different world," a world without problems and stresses. They report that while gambling, they feel invigorated and alive, they are admired and respected, that time passes quickly, and all their problems are forgotten, be they psychological, financial, social, familial, academic, work-related, or legal. As such, gambling becomes the ultimate escape.

Adolescents are required to write a short essay on why it is they feel they gamble, entitled, "What gambling does for me." We contend that the youth must be benefiting in some way from their gambling experiences, albeit temporarily, to continue playing despite serious negative consequences. This exercise is important for two reasons. First, it enables us, in a general way, to understand the individual's perceptions of the reasons underlying why they are gambling excessively. Second, and more importantly, it enables them to articulate and understand the underlying reasons why they gamble. The following are excerpts from their writings; the first one highlighting difficulties with interpersonal relationships and poor coping/adaptive skills, while the second example illustrates an individual's gambling to alleviate a depressed state and as a form of psychological escape:

> I always had trouble making friends, and never had a girlfriend. Gambling has now become my best friend and my one true love. I can turn to her in good times and bad and she'll always be there for me. (Male, age 18)

> Gambling, well, it's strange to talk about the positive side because of how upside down it has turned my life, but I guess the pull of it is how it makes me feel so alive, so happy, and so much like I belong, but only when I am gambling. The low I feel after I realize what I did, and how much I have lost, is worse than anything I can explain. I guess I just need to feel good from time to time, it lets me escape the black hole that is my life. (Male, age 17)

2) *Analysis of gambling episodes*

Self-awareness is essential to the process of change. If individuals understand the underlying motivations prompting certain behaviors they begin to feel empowered to gain control and make change. Every person who repeatedly engages in a self-injurious pattern of excessive behavior can be guided through an analysis of their behavioral patterns. An awareness of their gambling triggers, their psychological and behavioral reactions to those triggers, as well as the consequences which ensue from this chain reaction is important to achieve. This type of analysis empowers the individual to make long-term successful changes to their behaviors. The following model provides an overview of the framework:

Triggers➤Emotional Reactions and Rationalizations➤Behavior➤Consequences

Triggers. These can consist of places, people, times of day, activities, particular situations, and/or emotions. While initially many individuals are unaware of their specific triggers, they can be identified through discussions of prior experiences, as well as by examining written journals (i.e., a component within the therapeutic process). Once identified, avoiding or effectively dealing with the triggers becomes possible. For example, one of the most common triggers for gamblers is the handling of large sums of money. We therefore help them adopt strategies to minimize the exposure to this trigger, such as arranging for payment of something to be made by a third party, or to have the money replaced by a cheque, and limiting access to cash withdrawals from bank machines. In one case, a parent who was financially supporting his son made daily deposits into his account rather than weekly deposits. Other examples of triggers include gambling advertisements or landmarks, personal anxiety or depressed feelings, interpersonal difficulties, enticement of peers, stressful situations (i.e., exams), the need to make money quickly, or quite simply daydreaming of engaging in gambling. Sometimes, just having the awareness of one's triggers provides a person with a better ability to deal with gambling urges. Additional research is needed to better understand the relationship between triggers and mechanisms of self-control.

Gambling-free times. It is also important to properly understand the times in a person's day when they do not seem to have the urge to gamble. Identifying the circumstances, time of day, who they are with, their emotional state, activity levels, physical location, etc. is essential. By understanding the circumstances in which the urge to gamble is less or absent, it provides a set of guidelines by which the therapist can help recreate similar situations at other times in the day. For example, we have noted that many of the young gamblers undergoing treatment often report that when actively engaged in playing sports with friends, bicycling, physical activity in gym, or rollerblading they felt better and had their minds clear of their gambling desires both during and after the activity. As a result, for these youth, when helping them to structure and organize their week, we attempt to include similar types of activities on a daily basis.

3) Establishing a baseline of gambling behavior and encouraging a decrease in gambling

Once the motivations for gambling are understood and an analysis of gambling patterns has been made, efforts are focused on making changes to the adolescent's gambling behavior. In order to set goals and measure improvements, it is useful and important to initially establish a baseline of gambling behavior. Adolescents are required to record their gambling behaviors in terms of frequency, duration, time of day, type of gambling activity, amount of money spent, losses and wins. When establishing goals for a decrease in gambling participation, individuals are guided to establish *reasonable* goals for themselves. Some elect to target multiple factors such as frequency and duration and amount spent simultaneously, while others may focus on one form of behavior (e.g., frequency or duration). For these individuals we encourage a decrease in frequency or duration of each gambling episode versus initially focusing on amount wagered. Some meet their goals immediately at which point we generally support decisions to maintain this decrease for several weeks while setting new goals immediately. Others struggle to meet their goals at which point goals are generally modified.

4) Addressing cognitive distortions

It has been well established that individuals with gambling problems experience multiple cognitive distortions (Ladouceur & Walker, 1998; Langer, 1975). They are prone to have an illusion of control and perceive that they can control the outcome of gambling events, they underestimate the amount of money lost and over-estimate the amount won, they fail to utilize their understanding of the laws of independence of events, and they believe that if they persist at gambling they will likely win back all money lost (chasing behavior). Addressing these cognitive distortions remains an important treatment goal. Furthermore, the analysis of their gambling behavior usually reveals the rationalizations they make to justify their gambling behavior, and these rationalizations need to be addressed, as they too represent distortions of reality. An example of a rationalization for gambling is, "If I gamble now, I will be in a good mood and I will be more able to have fun at my friend's party tonight," or "By gambling now, the urge will be out of my system and I'll be more able to focus on studying for my exam." The overarching goal would be to ensure the individual comprehends that the gambling episode will likely result in a bad mood if they were to lose money, thus a negative mood at their party; or an inability to focus on studying for their exam. Ultimately, the goal of addressing many of the cognitive distortions is to highlight how their thinking is self-deceptive, to provide pertinent information about randomness, to encourage a realization that they are incapable of controlling outcomes of random events and games, payout rates, etc.

5) Establishing the underlying causes of stress and anxiety

In light of empirical research (Gupta & Derevensky, 1998a; Jacobs, 1998; Jacobs, Marsten & Singer, 1985) and clinical findings, a primary treatment goal is to identify and treat any underlying problem that results in increased stress and/or anxiety. These in general include one or more of the following problems: personal (e.g., low self-esteem, depression, ADHD, oppositional defiant disorders), familial, peer, academic, vocational, and legal. Through traditional therapeutic techniques these problems are addressed and alternative approaches to problem solving are supported while sublimation, projection, repression and escape are discouraged. For example, Candice was initially struggling with chronic depression, a learning disability, and poor coping skills. The combination of these factors resulted in significant anxiety when faced with school assignments and exams; all of which resulted in a poor self-esteem affecting her ability to establish and maintain healthy peer relationships. As a result of a clinical evaluation, Candice's depression and learning problems were addressed. Candice gained insight as to the reasons she needed to escape through her excessive gambling. Ultimately, she was relieved to have her primary problems addressed, her self-esteem gradually improved, and she was encouraged to develop a healthier lifestyle and more effective coping skills. In time, Candice found developed a very good friendship with someone in whom she could confide about her struggles with gambling. This friend assisted her in overcoming her gambling urges, kept her occupied with healthy activities, and became a good study partner. This friendship also helped Candice develop a stronger sense of self-worth and she came to better understand her value and potential.

6) Evaluating and improving coping abilities

The need to escape one's problems usually occurs more frequently among individuals who have poor coping and adaptive skills. Using gambling, or other addictive activities to deal with daily stressors, anxiety or depression represents a form of maladaptive coping. Recent research efforts have confirmed these clinical observations, where adolescents who meet the criteria for pathological gambling demonstrated poor coping skills as compared to same age peers without a gambling problem (Gupta, Derevensky & Marget, in press; Marget, Gupta & Derevensky, 1999; Nower, Gupta & Derevensky, 2000). A primary therapeutic goal involves building and expanding the individual's repertoire of coping abilities. This happens best by using examples of situations in the individual' life that were dealt with inappropriately and suggesting more appropriate ways of handling them. As adolescents begin to comprehend the benefits of effective coping abilities and their repertoire of coping responses expands, they are more apt to apply these skills to their daily lives. Examples of healthy coping skills include honest communication with others, seeking social support, and learning to weigh the benefits or costs associated with potential behaviors. Also included in the discussions and role playing exercises are ways to improve social skills (e.g., learning to communicate with peers, developing healthy friendships, being considerate of others, and developing trust).

7) Rebuilding healthy interpersonal relationships

Common consequences of a serious gambling problem involve impaired and severed relationships with friends and family members. Helping the adolescent rebuild these crucial relationships constitutes an important therapeutic goal. Often through lies and manipulative behaviors resulting from their gambling problem, friends and family members become alienated, leaving unresolved negative feelings. Once a youth has been identified as being a liar or a thief, it becomes difficult to earn back the trust of others and to resume healthy relationships. One needs to explain to family members and friends that these deceptive actions are part of the constellation of problematic behaviors exhibited by individuals who cannot control their gambling. Consequently, once the gambling is under control, family member and friends can anticipate being treated with more respect. Family members, peers, and significant others become important support personnel to help ensure abstinence and can take an active role in relapse prevention. We contend that youth with gambling problems will be happier and are more likely to abstain from gambling if they feel they belong to a peer group and are supported by family and friends. As a result, the occasional inclusion of family members and friends in therapy sessions can prove to be very beneficial.

As an example, Sonny, having stolen from his father's company, and having manipulated his mother with lies in order to obtain funds for gambling faced a difficult challenge in regaining the trust of his parents. Both parents perceived him as being ruthless and were convinced that his anti-social criminal behaviors would not stop. Once he regained control of his gambling and was abstinent for several months, he came to understand how his behaviors were hurtful. As a result, he experienced significant remorse. Through inclusion of his parents in the therapeutic process, concomitant with improved communication skills and his willingness to accept responsibility for the emotional distress he caused his parents, he slowly regained the support and trust of his family members and peers. This process remains ongoing and often takes considerably longer than the client wants.

8) Restructuring free time

Adolescents struggling to overcome a gambling problem experience more positive outcomes when not faced with large amounts of unstructured time. Some adolescents in treatment are still in school and/or have a job, and as such their free time consists mainly of evenings and weekends. Others have dropped out of school and may have a part-time job while others are not working. For these youth, structuring their time becomes paramount as they initially find it exceedingly difficult to resist urges to gamble when they are bored. We frequently ask adolescents to carry an agenda with them where we have helped articulate ways of spending time with friends, family, school or work related activities. Other activities can involve participating in organized sports activities, engaging in a hobby, and performing volunteer work. The *success* of their week is evaluated on how they achieve their weekly goals as agreed upon, with their gambling-related goals (reduction or abstinence) being one part of the program. Thus, if an individual fails to meet their goals surrounding their gambling behavior, they still may achieve success in other areas. This approach tends to keep the young gamblers from being discouraged and motivates them to keep trying to attain a balanced lifestyle.

9) Fostering effective money management skills

These skills are typically lacking in adolescents who have a gambling problem. Therapeutic goals involve educating them as to the value of money (as they tend to lose perspective after gambling large sums), building money management skills, and helping them develop effective and reasonable debt repayment plans.

10) Relapse prevention

Despite a lack of strong empirical evidence, our clinical work suggests that abstinence from gambling is necessary in order to prevent a relapse of pathological gambling behaviors. It should be noted that small, occasional relapses throughout the treatment process are to be expected. However, once gambling has ceased for an extended period of time (i.e., 4–6 months), an effective relapse prevention program should help these individuals remain free of gambling. Relapse prevention includes continued access to their primary therapist, the existence of a good social support network, engagement in either school or work, the practice of a healthy lifestyle, and avoidance of powerful triggers. Youth are contacted periodically via telephone for one year post treatment to ensure they are maintaining their abstinence and doing well in general. Support is offered if required. Gamblers representative of Pathways 2 and 3 are more apt to need additional support after the termination of therapy.

Concluding Remarks

The authors acknowledge that the treatment program's efficacy has not been empirically validated using the standards necessary for a rigorous, scientifically controlled study (i.e., no random assignments to a control group matching for severity of gambling problems and other mental health disorders, controlling for age, SES, frequency and type of gambling activity preferred, etc.). As such, more clinical research is necessary before definitive conclusions can be drawn. Nevertheless, based upon clinical criteria established for success (i.e., abstinence for six months post treatment, return to school or work, not meeting the DSM criteria for pathological gambling, improved peer and family relationships, improved coping skills, and no marked signs of depressive symptomatology, delinquent behavior or excessive use of alcohol or drugs), the McGill University treatment program appears to have reached its objectives in successfully working with youth with serious gambling problems.

The description of our treatment philosophy and approach were elaborated upon to provide clinicians and treatment providers with a better understanding of the different components necessary when working with young problem gamblers. Treating youth with severe gambling problems requires clinical skills, a knowledge of adolescent development, an understanding of the risk factors associated with problem gambling, and a thorough grounding in the empirical work concerning the correlates associated with gambling problems. By no means should this chapter substitute for proper training.

While we did not elaborate upon how to treat youth with multiple addictions in this chapter, it is clear that gamblers with concomitant substance abuse problems pose a greater challenge for treatment (Ladd & Petry,

2003). Youth with clinical levels of depression, high levels of impulsivity, and anxiety disorders are often referred to psychiatry to simultaneously undergo pharmacological treatment while undergoing our therapy. The use of serotonin re-uptake inhibitors tend to be effective in helping these youth manage their depression and anxiety, and preliminary research suggests that they may be useful in lowering levels of impulsivity which often underlie pathological gambling behavior (Grant, Chambers & Potenza, in this volume; Grant, Kim & Potenza, 2003).

The finding that several youth enter treatment immediately after stopping their gambling on their own, requesting assistance in maintaining abstinence and in dealing with the concomitant gambling-related problems and underlying issues, raises an interesting research and clinical question. Would these youth have maintained abstinence without intervention?

While the incidence of severe gambling problems amongst youth remains relatively small, the devastating short-term and long-term consequences to the individual, their families, and friends are significant. One adolescent, when discussing the severity of his gambling problem responded, "It's an all-encompassing problem that invades every facet of my life. I wouldn't wish this problem on my worst enemy, for it's way too harsh a punishment."

The vast majority of the youth seen in our clinic have a wide array of problems. Merely treating the gambling problem without examining the individual's overall mental health functioning will likely have limited results. The following is a text written by a young pathological gambler we treated, one year post-treatment:

> Gambling is an extremely addictive activity which can get unbelievably out of control. It can lead to a very horrible reality, one in which just getting out of bed can seem unthinkable. Unfortunately, I have lived this reality. I was eighteen when I began to fight for my life back. My future did not look very good. I was severely depressed, anxious and overweight, I wanted to disappear. Thankfully, with the support of an amazing team I have managed to overcome my addiction, lose thirty pounds and continue my schooling. I feel like I am relearning how to live. This continues to be a very long and emotionally painful process, however it does get easier with time. My memories of the gambling, the lies and unhappiness are slowly fading away . . . becoming part of the past. However I will never forget my struggle or how easy it was to lose control. In my gambling years I have seen and experienced first hand an incredible amount of heartache. I hope to never witness such avoidable pain again. Now at twenty years old, I am beginning a journey which holds an endless amount of opportunity. My dream to be a health-care professional seems closer than ever. Please let my story be a source of hope for anyone in a similar situation. I understand how bad life can seem, I've been there, believe me. You are not alone. Get the help you need, be true to yourself and start your own journey.

While it appears as though large numbers of adolescents who gamble problematically appear to resolve their gambling problems without therapeutic intervention (natural recovery), providing support for those in need remains essential. Our governments, private corporations, and charitable organizations, recipients of the revenues generated from gambling, need to help address this issue by providing funding for the establishment of treatment centers and training of professionals. Problem gambling, even for adolescents, can have devastating short-term and long-term consequences.

The youth briefly described, Joe, Candice, and Sonny, are all doing relatively well and are living happy productive lives. Joe has channeled his energies into starting his own business, always taking significant but well reasoned risks. Candice has successfully returned to her studies, and although she was unable to enter into the health science university program (she always envisioned herself as attending medical school) as a result of academic failures during her excessive gambling days, she nevertheless is happily enrolled in an alternative, related program. She remains highly motivated and committed toward building her career. Sonny has learned to manage his ADHD and his depression and has integrated full-time into the workforce. He has built a solid peer network of social support for himself and is working on repairing broken relationships with friends and family members.

In spite of gains in knowledge concerning the correlates and risk factors associated with severe gambling problems amongst youth during the past ten years a general lack of public and parental awareness exists. The fact that the prevalence rates for youth with severe gambling problems remain higher than that of adults is of significant concern. Whether maturation will result in individuals stopping their excessive gambling behavior by the time they become adults with additional responsibilities still remains an unanswered question (the issue of natural recovery remains a highly important issue in need of considerable research). As we have argued elsewhere, independent of whether or not individuals with severe gambling during adolescence become more responsible 'social gamblers' as adults, the personal costs and consequences incurred along the way often remain with them.

Gambling problems among youth will raise important public health and social policy issues in the 21st century. Greater emphasis on outreach and prevention programs is absolutely essential. Our governments must help fund more basic and applied research and be responsible for supporting and developing effective and scientifically validated prevention and treatment programs. The treatment of young problem gamblers is a complex, multi-modal process. While such an approach can take months or longer, the benefits to the individual and society outweigh the costs of funding such programs.

References

Bergler, E. (1957). *The psychology of gambling.* London: International Universities Press.

Blaszczynski, A. P., McConaghy, N., & Winters, S. W. (1986). Plasma endorphin levels in pathological gambling. *Journal of Gambling Studies, 2,* 3–14.

Blaszczynski, A. P., & McConaghy, N. (1993). A two to nine year treatment follow-up study of pathological gambling. In W. Eadington & J. A. Cornelius (Eds.), *Gambling behavior and problem gambling.* Reno, NV: Institute for the Study of Gambling and Commercial Gambling.

Blaszczynski, A. P., & Silove, D. (1995). Cognitive and behavioral therapies for pathological gambling. *Journal of Gambling Studies, 11,* 195–220.

Brown, R. I. (1986). Dropouts and continuers in gamblers anonymous: Life context and other factors. *Journal of Gambling Behavior, 2,* 130–140.

Brown, R. I. (1987). Dropouts and continuers in gamblers anonymous: IV. Evaluation and summary. *Journal of Gambling Behavior, 3,* 202–210.

Bujold, A., Ladouceur, R., Sylvain, C., & Boisvert, J. M. (1994). Treatment of pathological gamblers: An experimental study. *Journal of Behavioral Therapy and Experimental Psychiatry, 25,* 275–282.

Carlton, P. L., & Goldstein, L. (1987). Physiological determinants of pathological gambling. In T. Galski (Ed.), *Handbook on pathological gambling.* Springfield, IL: Charles C. Thomas.

Chevalier, S., Geoffrion, C., Audet, C., Papineau, É., & Kimpton, M-A. (2003). *Évaluation du programme experimental sur le jeu pathologique. Rapport 8-Le point de vue des usagers.* Montréal, Institut nationale de sante publique du Québec.

Comings, D. (1998, June). The genetics of pathological gambling: The addictive effect of multiple genes. Paper presented at the National Conference on Problem Gambling, Las Vegas.

DeCaria, C., Hollander, E. & Wong, C. (1997, August). Neuropsychiatric functioning in pathological gamblers. Paper presented at the National Conference on Problem Gambling, New Orleans.

Derevensky, J., & Gupta, R. (2004). Adolescents with gambling problems: A review of our current knowledge. *e-Gambling: The Electronic Journal of Gambling Issues, 10,* 119–140.

Derevensky, J., Gupta, R., & Winters, K. (2003). Prevalence rates of youth gambling problems: Are the current rates inflated? *Journal of Gambling Studies, 19,* 405–425.

DiClemente C. C., Story, M., & Murray, K. (2000). On a roll: The process of initiation and cessation of problem gambling among adolescents. *Journal of Gambling Studies, 16,* 289–314.

Grant, J.E., Kim, S.W., & Potenza, M.N. (2003). Advances in the pharmacological treatment of pathological gambling. *Journal of Gambling Studies, 19,* 85–109.

Griffiths, M. D. (1995). *Adolescent gambling.* London: Routledge.

Griffiths, M. D., & Wood R. T. (2000). Risk factors in adolescence: The case of gambling, video-game playing, and the internet. *Journal of Gambling Studies, 16,* 199–226.

Gupta, R., & Derevensky, J. (1998a). Adolescent gambling behavior: A prevalence study and examination of the correlates associated with excessive gambling. *Journal of Gambling Studies, 14,* 319–345.

Gupta, R., & Derevensky, J. (1998b). An empirical examination of Jacob's General Theory of Addictions: Do adolescent gamblers fit the theory? *Journal of Gambling Studies, 14,* 17–49.

Gupta, R., & Derevensky, J. (2001). *An examination of the differential coping styles of adolescents with gambling problems.* Report prepared for the Ontario Ministry of Health and Long-Term Care, Toronto.

Gupta, R., Derevensky, J., & Marget, N. (in press). Coping strategies employed by adolescents with gambling problems. *Child and Adolescent Mental Health.*

Haller, R., & Hinterhuber, H. (1994). Treatment of pathological gambling with carbamazepine. *Pharmacopsychiatry, 27,* 129.

Hardoon, K., & Derevensky, J. (2002). Child and adolescent gambling behavior: Our current knowledge. *Clinical Child Psychology and Psychiatry, 7,* 263–281.

Hardoon, K., Gupta, R., & Derevensky, J. (in press). Psychosocial variables associated with adolescent gambling: A model for problem gambling. *Psychology of Addictive Behaviors.*

Hollander, E., Frenkel, M., DeCaria, C., Trungold, S., & Stein, D. (1992). Treatment of pathological gambling with chlomipramine. *American Journal of Psychiatry, 149,* 710–711.

Hollander, E., & Wong, C. M. (1995). Body dismorphic disorder, pathological gambling, and sexual compulsions. *Journal of Clinical Psychiatry, 56,* 7–12.

Jacobs, D. F. (1998). *An overarching theory of addictions: A new paradigm for understanding and treating addictive behaviors.* Paper presented at the National Academy of Sciences Meeting, Washington, D.C.

Jacobs, D. F., Marsten, A. R., & Singer, R. D. (1985). Testing a general Theory of Addictions: Similarities and differences between alcoholics, pathological gamblers and compulsive overeaters. In J. J. Sanchez-Soza (Ed.), *Health and clinical psychology.* Amsterdam, Holland: Elcevier Publishers.

Jacques, C., & Ladouceur, R. (2003). DSM-IV-J Criteria: A scoring error that may be modifying the estimates of pathological gambling amongst youth. *Journal of Gambling Studies, 19,* 427–432.

Kazdin, A. (2001). Progress of therapy research and clinical application of treatment requires better understanding of the process. *Clinical Psychology: Science and Practice, 8,* 143–151.

Knapp, T. J., & Lech, B, C, (1987). Pathological gambling: A review with recommendations. *Advances in Behavior Research and Therapy, 9,* 21–449.

Ladd, G.T., & Petry, N.M. (2003). A comparison of pathological gamblers with and without substance abuse treatment histories. *Experimental & Clinical Psychopharmacology, 11,* 202–209.

Ladouceur, R., Boisvert, J. M., & Dumont, J. (1994). Cognitive-behavioral treatment for adolescent pathological gamblers. *Behavioral Modification, 18,* 230–242.

Ladouceur, R., Bouchard, C., Rhéaume, N., Jacques, C., Ferland, F., Leblond, J., et al. (2000). Is the SOGS an accurate measure of pathological gambling among children, adolescents and adults? *Journal of Gambling Studies, 16,* 1–24.

Ladouceur, R., Sylvain, C., Letarte, H., Giroux, I., & Jacques, C. (1998). Cognitive treatment of pathological gamblers. *Behaviour Research and Therapy, 36,* 1111–1120.

Ladouceur, R., & Walker, M. (1996). Cognitive perspectives on gambling. In P. M. Salkoviskis (Ed.), *Trends in cognitive therapy.* Chichester, UK: Wiley.

Ladouceur, R., & Walker, M. (1998). Cognitive approach to understanding and treating pathological gambling. In A.S. Bellack & M. Hersen (Eds.), *Comprehensive clinical psychology,* New York: Pergamon.

Langer, E. J. (1975). The illusion of control. *Journal of Personality and Social Psychology, 32,* 311–321.

Langhinrichsen-Rohling, J., Rhode, P., Seeley, J.R., & Rohling, M.L. (2004). Individual, family, and peer correlates of adolescent gambling. *Journal of Gambling Studies, 20,* 23–46.

Lesieur, H. R. (1990). Working with and understanding Gamblers Anonymous. *Working with self help.* Homewood, IL: Dorsey.

Lesieur, H. (1998). Costs and treatment of pathological gambling. *The Annals of the American Academy of Social Science, 556,* 153–171.

Lesieur, H. R., & Blume, S. B. (1991). Evaluation of patients treated for pathological gambling in a combined alcohol, substance abuse, and pathological gambling treatment unit using the Addiction Severity Index. *British Journal of Addictions, 86,* 1017–1028.

Marget, N., Gupta, R., & Derevensky, J. (1999, August). *The psychosocial factors underlying adolescent problem gambling.* Poster presented at the annual meeting of the American Psychological Association, Boston.

McCormick, R. A., & Taber, J. I. (1988). Attributional style in pathological gamblers in treatment. *Journal of Abnormal Psychology, 97,* 368–370.

Miller, W. (1986). Individual outpatient treatment of pathological gambling. *Journal of Gambling Behavior, 2,* 95–107.

Murray, J. B. (1993). Review of research on pathological gambling. *Psychological Reports, 72,* 791–810.

Nathan, P. (2001, Dec.). *Best practices for the treatment of gambling disorders: Too soon?* Paper presented at the annual Harvard–National Center for Responsible Gaming Conference, Las Vegas.

National Gambling Impact Study Commission (1999). National Gambling Impact Study Commission: Final Report.

National Research Council. (1999). *Pathological gambling: A critical review.* Washington, D.C.: National Academy Press.

Nower, L., Gupta, R., & Derevensky, J. (2000, June). *Youth gamblers and substance abusers: A comparison of stress-coping styles and risk-taking behavior of two addicted adolescent populations.* Paper presented at the 11th International Conference on Gambling and Risk-Taking, Las Vegas.

Rosenthal, R. J. (1987). The psychodynamics of pathological gambling: A review of the literature. In T. Galski (Ed.), *The handbook of pathological gambling.* Springfield, IL: Charles C. Thomas.

Rugle, L., Derevensky, J., Gupta, R., Winters, K., & Stinchfield, R. (2001). *The treatment of problem and pathological gamblers.* Report prepared for the National Council for Problem Gambling, Center for Mental Health Services (CMHS) and the Substance Abuse and Mental Health Services Administration (SAMHSA), Washington, D.C.

Rugle, L. J., & Rosenthal, R. J. (1994). Transference and countertransference in the psychotherapy of pathological gamblers. *Journal of Gambling Studies, 10,* 43–65.

Saiz, J. (1992). No hagen juego, senores (Don't begin the game). *Interviu, 829,* 24–28.

Shaffer, H. J., & Hall, M. N. (1996). Estimating prevalence of adolescent gambling disorders: A quantitative synthesis and guide toward standard gambling nomenclature. *Journal of Gambling Studies, 12,* 193–214.

Toneatto, T., & Ladouceur, R. (2003). Treatment of pathological gambling: A critical review of the literature. *Psychology of Addictive Behaviors, 17,* 284–292.

Toneatto, T., & Sobell, L. C. (1990). Pathological gambling treated with cognitive behavior therapy: A case report. *Addictive Behaviors, 15,* 497–501.

Vitaro, F., Wanner, B., Ladouceur, R., Brendgen, M., & Trembay, R.E. (2004). Trajectories of gambling during adolescence. *Journal of Gambling Studies, 20,* 47–69.

Walker, M. B. (1992). *The psychology of gambling.* New York: Pergamon.

Walker, M. B. (1993). Treatment strategies for problem gambling: A review of effectiveness. In W. Eadington & J. Cornelius (Eds.), *Gambling behavior and problem gambling,* Reno, NV: Institute for the Study of Gambling and Commercial Gaming.

Wildman, R. W. (1997). *Gambling: An attempt at an integration.* Edmonton, Alberta: Wynne Resources.

Chapter 10

A Pathways Approach to Treating Youth Gamblers

Lia Nower, J.D., Ph.D. and Alex Blaszczynski, Ph.D.

Pathological gambling among youth is a growing social concern. Studies suggest that 24–40% of adolescents gamble weekly, 10–14% are at risk for gambling problems, and 2–9% meet diagnostic criteria for pathological gambling (for extensive reviews of youth gambling see Griffiths, 1995; Jacobs, 2000, in this volume; National Research Council, 1999; Shaffer & Hall, 1996). The mean prevalence rate for adolescent pathological gambling has been reported to be 5%–three times the 1.5% average for adults (National Research Council, 1999).

Empirical findings suggest that gambling often begins at home, with youth modeling the betting behavior of their parents (Gambino, Fitzgerald, Shaffer, Renner & Courtage, 1993; Jacobs, 2000; Ladouceur & Mireault, 1988; Wood & Griffiths, 1998). In addition, early involvement in gambling has been shown to be highly predictive of gambling problems during adulthood (Griffiths, 1995; Jacobs, 2000). Both youth and adult problem and pathological gamblers typically experience significant adverse personal, familial, financial, professional, and legal consequences (National Research Council, 1999).

The psychological literature is replete with studies exploring risk factors that seem to predispose youth to gambling problems. Those factors include earlier age of onset, male gender, parental gambling, predisposition toward intensity seeking and impulsivity, depression and/or anxiety, comorbid substance abuse, antisocial behavior, low self-esteem, and

189

lack of social support (Gupta & Derevensky, 1998a; Stinchfield, in this volume; Vitaro, Arseneault & Tremblay, 1997; Vitaro, Ladouceur & Bujold, 1996; Wynne, Smith, & Jacobs, 1996). However, to date, no empirically validated theoretical model of pathological gambling has effectively incorporated the complex array of biological, psychological, and ecological factors into an etiological framework for youth gamblers (Blaszczynski, 1999; Brown, 1988; Ferris, Wynne, & Single, 1998; Shaffer & Gambino, 1989).

The Pathways Model (Blaszczynski, 1998; Blaszczynski & Nower, 2002) provides such a framework, suggesting that a multifaceted constellation of risk and protective factors differentially influences youth who may otherwise display similar phenomenological features to follow different and distinct pathways toward a gambling disorder. Within this chapter, we propose that the Pathways Model, originally applied to adult gamblers, can serve as an effective template for the development of early intervention, prevention, and targeted clinical management strategies for adolescent and young adult gamblers.

Theoretical Framework of the Pathways Model

Historically, there has been little consensus regarding classification of problem and pathological gamblers. In the youth gambling literature, classification schemes have included symptom count alone (Gupta & Derevensky, 1998b), frequency of gambling plus symptom count (Vitaro et al., 1997), self-report of gambling-related problems (Stinchfield, Cassuto, Winters, & Latimer, 1997), frequency of gambling plus money wagered (Vitaro et al., 1996) and multifactorial assessments (Govoni, Rupcich, & Frisch, 1996). Some researchers have suggested that the presence of harm rather than symptom count should define the gambling problem (Ferris et al., 1998; Victorian Casino and Gaming Authority, 1997).

In many cases, classification systems result from subjective value judgments, increasing Type I error (i.e., false positives), and expanding the pool of problem gamblers by misclassifying those for whom gambling is ego-syntonic with those for whom gambling is ego-dystonic (Blaszczynski & Nower, 2002; Walker, 1998). In the former group, gamblers report no impaired control though they experience negative interpersonal consequences for choosing to gamble rather than attending to family, monetary, employment, and other obligations. The latter group experiences negative consequences as well as a subjective sense of impaired control, defined by repeated unsuccessful attempts to control the gambling urge despite a reported genuine desire to cease gambling. Merging these two distinct types of gamblers into a single, heterogeneous group fosters confusion and contradiction in the research and clinical treatment literature (Blaszczynski & Nower, 2002). In fact, there is little agreement on typologies beyond the idea that there are at least two subgroups of gamblers; those chronically under stimulated, and the other, overstimulated (Jacobs, 1986; Blaszczynski, Winter, & McConaghy, 1986).

While accepted theories of pathological gambling postulate different explanations for impaired control, they each maintain that one model and set of theoretically-driven treatment applies to all pathological gamblers (Blaszczynski & Nower, 2002). However, no theory has successfully accounted for all permutations of problem gambling behavior. For example, learning theories, based on behavioral schedules of reinforcement, fail to account for the majority of gamblers who continue to exhibit control while cognitive theories fail to establish that distorted and irrational cognition are causal factors rather than secondary effects of cognitive dissonance (Blaszczynski & Nower, 2002).

Conceptually, pathological gambling is perceived either as an endpoint along a continuum of gambling involvement or as a categorical disorder. The dimensional view holds that pathological gamblers are qualitatively similar to social gamblers except for the amount of time and money spent gambling, identified by a variable cut-point (Walker, 1992). In contrast, a categorical perspective maintains that pathological gamblers are decidedly distinct from their non-impaired counterparts (Bergler, 1958; Rosenthal, 1992).

Increasingly, converging lines of research have begun identifying affective (Beaudoin & Cox, 1999; Blaszczynski, 1988; Getty, Watson, & Frisch, 2000), biochemical (Carrasco, Saiz-Ruiz, Hollander, Cesar, & Lopez-Ibor, 1994; Moreno, Saiz-Ruiz, & Lopez-Ibor, 1991) and genetic (Blum et al., 2000; Comings, Rosenthal, Lesieur, & Rugle, 1996) subtypes of gamblers, supporting a categorical approach to classification and tentatively linking receptor genes and neurotransmitter dysregulation to reward deficiency, arousal, impulsivity, and pathological gambling. Preliminary evidence supports the hypothesis that serotonin (mood regulation), norepinephrine (mediating arousal) and dopamine (reward regulation) may all play a role in impulsivity, mood disorders, and impaired control (Bergh, Eklund, Sodersten, & Nordin, 1997; De Caria et al., 1996; Lopez-Ibor, 1988; Moreno, et al., 1991; Roy, de Jong & Linnoila, 1989). In addition, genetic research suggests that possession of the dopamine D2A1 allele receptor gene results in deficits in the dopamine reward pathway, leading affected individuals to engage in pleasure-generating activities, thereby placing them at high risk for multiple addictive, impulsive, and compulsive behaviors including substance abuse, binge eating, sex addiction, and pathological gambling (Blum et al., 2000; Comings et al., 1996). Thus, in some sub-groups of problem and pathological gamblers, detrimental pleasure-seeking may be biologically prescribed, though the choice of behavior differs by individual (see Blaszczynski & Nower, 2002 for a discussion of biological correlates).

The Pathways Model (Blaszczynski, 1998; Blaszczynski & Nower, 2002) proposes that there are at least three subgroups of problem and pathological gamblers with distinct clinical features and etiological processes. *Behaviorally-conditioned* problem gamblers, Pathway 1, lack psychiatric pathology but fall prey to a highly addictive schedule of behavioral reinforcement. *Emotionally vulnerable* problem gamblers, Pathway 2, manifest both a biological and psychological vulnerability to pathology, characterized by high levels of depression and/or anxiety and a history of poor social support, low self-esteem, and emotional neglect by caregivers. Pathway 3, *antisocial impulsivist* problem gamblers, possess vulnerabilities similar to those in Pathway 2 but they are decidedly impulsive, antisocial, and often dually addicted.

Common Processes: Access, Availability, Acceptability, Conditioning & Cognitions

The Pathways Model asserts that each of the three major pathways leading to pathological gambling share certain common processes and symptomatic features. However, each pathway is distinguished by empirically testable differences in vulnerability factors, demographic features, and etiological processes. It is suggested that the biological, psychosocial, and environmental factors described in the literature can be incorporated effectively into a theoretical framework to help explain youth gambling behavior.

All three pathways share common ecological factors, including ease of access and social acceptability of gambling. Epidemiological surveys indicate that access to gambling facilities is associated with a higher incidence of pathological gambling (Abbott & Volberg, 1996; Grun & McKeigue, 2000; Volberg, 1996). Retrospective studies with both adults and youth have consistently reported that problem gamblers characteristically begin gambling before the age of 10 (Dell, Ruzicka, & Palisi, 1981; Griffiths, 1990; Gupta & Derevensky, 1997, 1998a). According to Jacobs (2000), the earliest gambling experiences among children occur in situations where there are opportunities to wager even small amounts of money, and the home environment facilitates and supports gambling. In a survey of children age 9–14, Gupta and Derevensky (1997) found that 81% of children reported gambling with family members, including parents (40%), siblings (53%), and other relatives (46%). Similarly, in examining a sample of 1,320 children between the ages of 8 to 13, Ladouceur, Dubé, and Bujold (1994), reported that 40% of the children gambled once a week or more, and that a majority of those gambled with parents on lotteries (59%), cards (53%) and sports (48%). In addition, Wood and Griffiths (1998) reported that parents of youth age 11—15 received lottery tickets (71%) and scratchcards (51%) purchased for them by their parents. Children of problem gamblers have also been found to be at increased risk of developing a gambling problem themselves (Jacobs et al., 1989).

Exposure to gambling at an early age is facilitated by the lack of responsible public policies and legislation that promotes and encourages gambling as a socially acceptable activity. In general, adults indicate that youth gambling, particularly the purchase of lottery tickets, is a harmless and condoned activity (Gupta & Derevensky, 1997; Winters, Stinchfield, & Kim, 1995). In most venues, public policy and regulatory legislation create and foster an environment in which gambling is socially accepted, encouraged, and actively promoted. Derevensky, Gupta, and Della Cioppa (1996) found that less than 1/3 of children aged 9—14 reported they were fearful of being caught gambling, and the incidence tended to decline with age. Similarly, Gupta and Derevensky (1997) reported that 44% of fourth graders (age 10–11) feared being caught gambling, but that by grade eight (age 13–14), that percentage had declined to only 10%. Wynne et al. (1996) cited four factors that may account for an inordinately high prevalence rate of problem youth gambling: (a) multiplicity of diverse gambling venues, (b) vendors who fail to require proof of age and enforce existing statutes, (c) advertising that tends to encourage gambling and minimize potential harmful effects, and (d) adult attitudes that minimize the dangers of youth gambling. Thus, access, availability, and acceptability function to foster youth gambling efforts.

After initial gambling, adolescents become influenced by the highly addictive schedules of behavioral reinforcement provided by gambling through classical and operant conditioning and thereby initiated into an increasingly frequent and habitual pattern of gambling (see Blaszczynski & Nower, 2002, for a discussion of the role of conditioning). A neo-Pavlovian perspective suggests that gambling causes repeated cortical excitation, creating a "neuronal model" of the habitual behavior, which is subsequently stimulated by gambling-related cues. In response to those cues, youth experience a seemingly uncontrollable drive to engage in the habitual behavior, and attempts at control are met with aversive states of arousal or compulsion. Similarly, intermittent wins delivered on a variable ratio reinforcement schedule produce states of arousal, which are classically conditioned to stimuli associated with the gambling environment. The excitement of gambling may also produce negative reinforcement by reducing prior-existing aversive anxiety states and depression. Such reinforcement fosters a habitual pattern of continued gambling.

Frequent gambling also produces biased and illogical cognitive schemas, suggesting that personal control or skill, superstitious beliefs, or erroneous evaluations about probabilities and odds will influence the gambling outcome (see Griffiths, 1995; Ladouceur & Walker, 1996 for a comprehensive review of these processes). These distorted cognitive belief structures increase in potency and pervasiveness with concomitant increasing levels of gambling involvement (Griffiths, 1990, 1995). Ultimately, gamblers feel pressured to chase losses in the face of mounting debts (Lesieur, 1984). At this point, individuals typically manifest clear diagnostic indicators of gambling pathology, which is commonly misconstrued to imply that all pathological gamblers belong to a homogenous group. The Pathways Model refutes this assumption by suggesting that gamblers follow three clinically distinct routes to developing pathology.

Pathway 1: Behaviorally-Conditioned Youth Problem Gamblers

Gamblers following Pathway 1 develop gambling problems as a result of conditioning rather than impaired control (Blaszczynski, 1998; Blaszczynski & Nower, 2002). They fluctuate between regular/heavy and excessive gambling resulting from habituation, distorted perceptions about winning, and/or a series of bad judgements or decisions. Despite intermittently meeting formal criteria for pathological gambling, they are characterized by an absence of premorbid psychopathology. As depicted in Figure 1, members of this subgroup may exhibit preoccupation with gambling and chase gambling losses. In addition, they may abuse alcohol and report high levels of depression and anxiety but only in response to the financial burden imposed by their behaviour. These symptoms are the consequence not the cause of their gambling excesses.

Pathway 2: Emotionally-Vulnerable Youth Problem Gamblers

Unlike Pathway 1 gamblers, these youth present with premorbid depression and/or anxiety, low self-esteem, poor coping and problem solving skills, a history of familial neglect or abuse, they lack social support, and exhibit other adverse developmental behaviors. The cumulative effect of these factors produces an "emotionally vulnerable gambler" who gambles as a way to decrease aversive affective states or meet specific psychological needs (Blaszczynski & Nower, 2002).

Support for the Pathway 2 gambler comes from a variety of sources. Several studies have implicated a family history of pathological gambling as a significant risk factor for youth (Jacobs, 1988; Gambino et al., 1993; Griffiths, 1995; Lesieur & Rothschild, 1989; Volberg, 1993; Wood & Griffiths, 1998). Children of problem gamblers report pervasive feelings of loss, existential feelings of emotional abandonment, and physical deprivation and

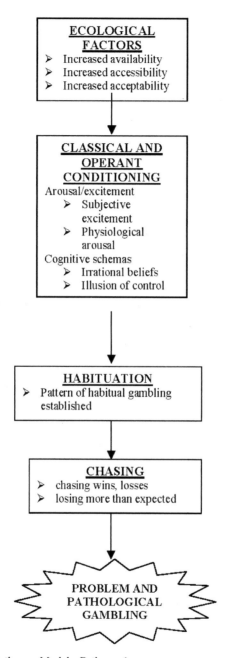

Figure 1. Integrated Pathways Model—Pathway 1

All figures adapted from Blaszczynski & Nower (2002) and reprinted by permission.

neglect due in part to the loss of the gambling parent (Darbyshire, Oster, & Carrig, 2001). In addition, studies have found that children of problem gamblers are significantly more likely to develop gambling problems themselves (Gupta & Derevensky, 1998b). In one study, youth with parents identified as problem gamblers were three times more likely to be problem gamblers; the risk increased 12-fold when both parents and grandparents were problem gamblers (Gambino et al., 1993).

According to Jacobs (1986), losses sustained as a result of a gambling parent and other adverse significant life events interact with personality variables and innately abnormal physiological states of arousal to lead to problem gambling. In his *General Theory of Addictions,* Jacobs (1986) proposes that pathological gamblers possess two interrelated sets of predisposing factors: an abnormal physiological resting states of hyper (anxiety) or hypo-arousal (depression), and a history of negative childhood experiences that result in feelings of inadequacy, low self-esteem, and low self-efficacy. These factors foster a need for wish-fulfillment and escape that lead the youth to seek chance encounters with substances or behaviors that promote dissociation and a feeling of being "alive" or "normal." Gambling maintains this fantasy, transforming anxiety into excitement and depression into relaxation and a sense of overall well-being.

Gupta and Derevensky (1998a) empirically tested Jacobs' theory with 817 high school students. Their study employed multivariate statistics and structural equation modeling to explore each model construct; depression and arousal (physiological resting state), self-worth, apprehension and childhood happiness (psychological distress), dissociation (need to escape), and frequency and severity of drug, alcohol and cigarette use as well as gambling (comorbid addictive behaviors). As predicted, adolescent problem and pathological gamblers exhibited higher levels of anxiety and depression, escape through dissociation, and cigarette, drug, and alcohol use than their peers. Dissociation proved a powerful predictor for both males and females, however, male problem gamblers were further distinguished by excitability (overactivity), and females, by depressed mood and use of stimulants.

The youth gambling literature offers much support for this sub-group of gamblers, which occupies an intermediary position in severity among the pathways. Several studies have noted that youth who gamble problematically report lower self-esteem (Gupta & Derevensky, 1998a; Peacock, Day, & Peacock, 1999), increased sexual activity (Stinchfield, 2000), higher rates of depression and anxiety (Gupta & Derevensky, 1998a; Stinchfield & Winters, 1998), a greater need to escape through dissociation (Jacobs, 1993; Kuley & Jacobs, 1988), poor coping skills (Nower, Gupta, & Derevensky, 2000), a lack of social support (Wynne et al., 1996), heightened risk of suicidal ideation and/or attempts (Gupta & Derevensky, 1998b; Stinchfield & Winters, 1998), and increased tobacco, drug and alcohol use (Volberg, 1993; Wynne et al., 1996). Because of their negative developmental history and poor coping skills, Pathway 2 gamblers are often too fragile to maintain sufficient control over their behavior to engage in controlled gambling.

Figure 2 illustrates the essential differences between the first two pathways. Pathway 1 gamblers initially gamble for entertainment or socialization, facilitated by access and availability. In contrast, Pathway 2 gamblers are more emotionally vulnerable as a result of psychosocial and biological factors, and gambling serves as a method of escape from aversive affective states. Once initiated, a habitual pattern of gambling fosters behavioral conditioning and dependence in both pathways. However, Pathway 2 gamblers are more resistant to change as a result of premorbid psychological dysfunction.

Pathway 3: Antisocial Impulsivist Youth Problem Gamblers

Youth in Pathway 3 are replete with psychopathology that is often evident from childhood and suggestive of neurological or neurochemical dysfunction. Similar to Pathway 2 gamblers, this subgroup possesses both psychosocial and biologically-based vulnerabilities. However, this group is distinguished by features of impulsivity, antisocial personality disorder, and attention deficit, which results in multiple maladaptive behaviors that impair overall psychosocial functioning (Blaszczynksi & Nower, 2002).

Clinically, impulsive youth engage in wide array of behavioral risk-taking and other misadventures wholly independent of their gambling. These youth often report a history of conduct disorder, sensation seeking, substance abuse, aggression, hyperactivity, and non-gambling related criminal behaviors. Impulsivity and disregard for consequences increases during times of stress and emotional upheaval. Pathway 3 gamblers exhibit difficulty maintaining healthy relationships; report emotional, physical or sexual abuse, or neglect by caregivers; and often endorse a family history of antisocial and alcohol problems. Gambling commences at an early age, rapidly escalates in intensity and severity, may occur in binge episodes, and is associated with early entry into gambling-related criminal behaviors. Dubbed the "anti-social impulsivist" subtype, these gamblers are typically non-motivated and non-compliant with treatment interventions (Blaszczynski, Steel, & McConaghy, 1997).

A number of studies have reported that problem youth gamblers demonstrate elevated levels of impulsivity (Vitaro, Arseneault, & Tremblay, 1997; 1999), sensation seeking (Gupta & Derevensky, 1998a; Powell, Hardoon, Derevensky, & Gupta, 1999), substance use (Ladouceur, Boudreault, Jacques, & Vitaro, 1999; Stinchfield et al., 1997) and antisocial behaviors (Vitaro

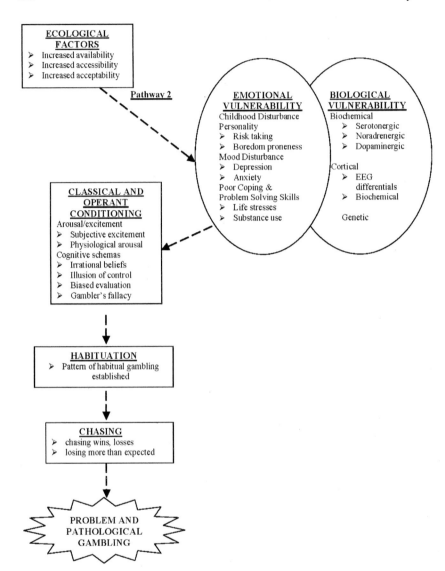

Figure 2. Integrated Pathways Model—Pathway 2

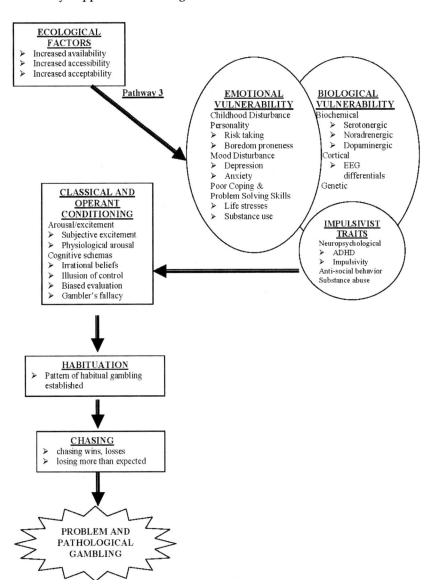

Figure 3. Integrated Pathways Model—Pathway 3

et al., 1996; Winters, Stinchfield, & Fulkerson, 1993). In a five-year longitudinal study of 154 boys, Vitaro and colleagues (1999) found that early impulsivity with a disregard for negative consequences was a significant predictor of problem gambling in late adolescence when controlling other personality
factors such as aggressivity and anxiety. Similarly, other studies have noted
that youth with serious gambling problems score high on the thrill and/or
adventure seeking, intensity-seeking, and disinhibition scales of sensation
seeking measures (Gupta & Derevensky, 1998a; Powell et al., 1999). This tendency toward risk taking would account for the finding that youth who
often play video games, which provide a high degree of neurological stimulation, are more likely than low-frequency players to be problem gamblers
(Gupta & Derevensky, 1996). These findings parallel similar results in the
adult gambling literature, which has found consistent correlations between
impulsivity, antisocial behaviors, sensation seeking, boredom proneness,
substance abuse and gambling problems (Gonzalez-Ibanez, Jimenez, &
Aymami,1999; McCormick, 1994; Steel & Blaszczynski,1996).

It is likely that many youth in this pathway exhibit features of the
hyperactive sub-type of attention deficit hyperactivity disorder (ADHD),
which is characterized by impulsivity beginning in childhood that is often
found to be associated with antisocial personality behaviors. Youth gambling research has yet to systematically evaluate the relationship between
ADHD and problem gambling. However, in a sample of adult pathological gamblers, Goldstein and his colleagues (Carlton et al., 1987; Goldstein, Manowitz, Nora, Swartzburg, & Carlton, 1985) found differential patterns of EEG activity and self-reported symptoms of childhood attention
deficit disorder. Rugle and Melamed (1993) administered several neuropsychological measures of attention deficits to 33 male pathological gamblers and a similar number of normal controls. The authors concluded that
gamblers differ from controls in exhibiting overactivity, destructibility, and
difficulty inhibiting conflicting behaviors. In addition, attention deficit-
related symptoms, reflecting impulsivity, are present in childhood and precede the onset of pathological gambling behavior. This biological vulnerability weakens behavioral control not only in the domain of gambling but
also in other areas of life. This gives rise to the hypothesis that impulsivity
is independent of gambling and functions as a good predictive factor for
severity of involvement in at least a subgroup of gamblers (Blaszczynski &
Nower, 2002).

In summary, Figure 4 illustrates the integrated pathways model. Gambling is initiated as a result of easy access and availability, proceeds through
one of three distinct pathways, and ultimately converges at the level of classical and operant conditioning that fosters habitual gambling, chasing, and
problem and pathological gambling behavior.

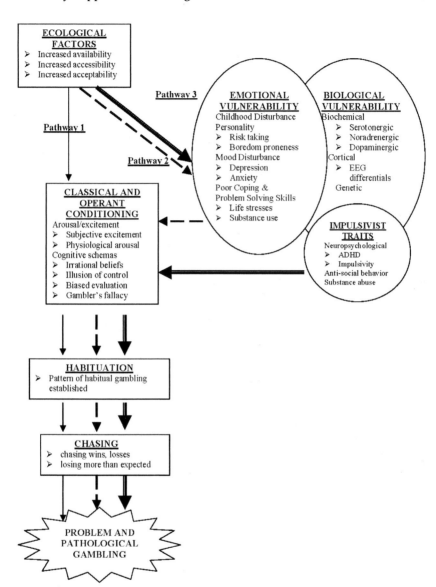

Figure 4. Integrated Pathways Model

Identification and Treatment Implications

Clinicians would be well advised to employ a comprehensive assessment battery to identify and assign youth to one of the three pathways, and rate them on each continuum. Typically, the assessment should include a general gambling questionnaire, exploring demographic variables, familial gambling behavior, age of onset, frequency and types of gambling, gambling locations, gambling peers, wagers, and cognitive perceptions about gambling (e.g., the Gambling Questionnaire by Gupta and Derevensky, 1996). All evaluations should screen for suicidality and homicidality to ensure identification of youth in need of immediate psychiatric intervention. In addition, assessments should be tailored to individual client needs, including assessment of some or all of the following:

- Youth gambling problem severity [e.g., DSM-IV-MR (Fisher, 2000) or the SOGS-RA (Winters et al., 1993) in the absence of a gold standard instrument]
- Personality and self-perception [e.g., High School Personality Questionnaire (Cattell, Cattell, & Johns, 1984) and Self-Perception Profile for Children (Harter, 1985)]
- Depression [e.g., Reynolds Adolescent Depression Scale (Reynolds, 1987)]
- Impulsivity [e.g., the narrow impulsiveness subscale of the Eysenck Impulsivity Scale (Eysenck & Eysenck, 1977)]
- Sensation seeking [e.g., Sensation Seeking Scale (Zuckerman, 1994) or the Arnett Inventory of Sensation Seeking (Arnett, 1994)]
- Stress-coping [e.g., COPE (Carver, Scheier, & Weintraub, 1989) or Coping Inventory of Stressful Situations (CISS) (Endler & Parker, 1990)]
- Substance use and abuse [e.g., Personal Experience Screening Questionnaire (Winters, 1992)]

Pathway 1 Youth Gamblers

Entry into this pathway may occur at any age, possibly due to family or peer involvement in gambling activities and socialization that encourages magical thinking regarding luck, chance, and superstition. This subgroup of youth report the least severe gambling and gambling-related problems of any of the three pathways, and manifest no significant symptoms of premorbid psychopathology, substance abuse, impulsivity, or disorganized behavior.

Identifying youth in Pathway 1 may be difficult, as they may constitute a rather small group of problem gamblers. In studies of youth gamblers to date, much attention has been directed at identifying common risk factors including factors such as impulsivity and risk-taking. However, there have been no systematic investigations of youth who manifest no such pathology yet who meet diagnostic criteria, reporting preoccupation, chasing, and frequent gambling of large amounts of money with significant negative consequences. In the adult population, Pathway 1 gamblers are often seniors or "empty nesters" that enjoy relatively healthy lifestyles until life span milestones such as retirement or death/abandonment by a spouse left them lonely and in search of the fellowship and excitement satisfied by gambling. In youth, Pathway 1 gamblers are conspicuous by their absence of premorbid signs or symptoms. They may have intact, supportive families, get good grades, and excel in sports. However, peer or family influences introduce the Pathway 1 youth to the exciting and seemingly harmless form of entertainment, which initially provides an opportunity for excitement, skill-testing, peer bonding, and satisfaction for competitive drives. It is likely that these youth are identified only when the conditioning effects have become so resistant to extinction that they begin borrowing, stealing, skipping school, failing classes, and manifesting other such symptoms characteristic of pathological gamblers.

These youth may fluctuate between heavy and problem gambling and are motivated to enter treatment and comply with instructions. It is proposed that counselling and minimal intervention programs benefit this subgroup. Successful treatments often employ cognitive-behavioral therapy and education to challenge distorted cognitions. When possible, supportive family members and peer supports should be invited to participate in the treatment plan (see Gupta & Derevensky, 2000, in this volume, for specific treatment interventions and techniques for youth gamblers).

Pathway 2 Youth Gamblers

Youth in this pathway are more easily identifiable and likely constitute the largest group of pathological youth gamblers. However, premorbid psychopathology makes this group more resistant to change and necessitates treatment that addresses the underlying vulnerabilities as well as specific gambling behaviors. Often depressed or anxious, youth in Pathway 2 may experience academic difficulties and have little social support at home. Unless affectively withdrawn, they are typically eager to pursue peer relationships and engage in risk taking behaviors. This tendency may sometimes result in difficulties with the law or school administrators, but their behaviors are the result of a desire for socialization rather than an innate impulsiveness or disregard for the rights of others. On standardized measures, they report elevated levels of depression and anxiety, low self-esteem and self-efficacy, and familial patterns of neglect, abuse or abandonment. However, these youth are unlikely to exhibit serious pathology. They may use or abuse substances. However, a thorough interview will reveal that such use is designed to escape unpleasant realities at home, counter feelings of anxiety or depression, combat issues of grief and loss, or ensure peer approval.

Treatment for Pathway 2 youth gamblers should be multi-modal, consisting of cognitive restructuring for disordered gambling-related cognitions and supportive therapy to heal grief and loss issues. The prudent clinician will devote significant effort to rapport and trust-building to ensure compliance and continued attendance. It is also necessary with this group to obtain a detailed familial history, identifying developmental deficits that may have manifested in behavioral pathology. If levels of depression and/or anxiety are elevated, the youth may require referral for a psychiatric evaluation to determine the appropriateness of medication management. Likewise, substance abuse issues should be addressed with specialized treatment or attendance at a 12-step group when necessary. It is likely that Pathway 2 gamblers will display a lifelong inability to cope with stress in active ways. Instead, they will avoid stressors by mentally disengaging (gambling, watching television, playing video games) or physically disengaging (shopping, sleeping, partying) from the stressor. For that reason, treatment should include assessment of stress-coping and problem-solving styles and instruction in the use of active, problem-focused strategies.

Pathway 3 Youth Gamblers

These gamblers are the most difficult to treat. Compliance is typically poor and relapse rates are very high. Like Pathway 2 gamblers, their assessments will reveal a host of emotional vulnerabilities–depression, anxiety, self-injurious behavior, low-self esteem, and an extensive history of physical and emotional losses. Unlike Pathway 2 gamblers, this subgroup does not merely seek emotional solace from gambling but also craves high levels of arousal and intense stimulation, likely precipitated by a combination of biochemical or genetic deficits, personality pathology, and poor stress-coping and problem-solving skills. Gambling onset will be early, and these youth often present with a long history of antisocial and impulsive behavior and comorbid addiction, particularly substance abuse. Initial motivation for treatment is low, therefore, clinicians should focus initially on establishing a therapeutic alliance that offers some narcissistic reward for compliance (e.g., "get my parents off my back").

Treatment strategies should be similar to those for Pathway 2. However, if it appears that biological correlates have contributed to the etiology of the disorder. Clinicians should attend to problems related to attention and organizational deficits, emotional lability, stress intolerance, and poor problem solving and coping skills. It is also important to highlight issues of compliance and attrition from treatment since Pathway 3 gamblers are typically inconsistent, unreliable, and intolerant of boredom. These gamblers may require intensive, long-term cognitive behavioral treatment targeting impulse control, and they may benefit from group therapy which fosters peer support for recovery. Like Pathway 2 gamblers, these youth may require medication to balance their neurochemical imbalances and treatment for comorbid addictions.

Conclusion

The Pathways Model identifies clinically distinct subgroups of gamblers who exhibit common, overt cardinal symptoms, but who, at the same time, differ significantly with respect to premorbid psychopathology, childhood history, and neurobiological functioning. The model proposes a conceptual framework that integrates research data and clinical observation to provide a structure to assist clinicians in identifying and separating distinct subgroups of gamblers that require different management strategies. While all youth gamblers are subject to ecological variables, operant and classical conditioning and cognitive processes, differences between subgroups have significant implications for diagnosis and treatment. *Pathway 1* youth gamblers are essentially normal in character but simply lose control over gambling in response to effects surrounding the probability of a win. In contrast, *Pathway 2* gamblers are characterized by disturbed family and personal histories, affective instability, and poor coping and problem-solving skills. They gamble as a means of emotional escape and mood regulation. Finally, *Pathway 3* gamblers exhibit biological vulnerability toward impulsivity and arousal-seeking, early onset of gambling, attentional deficits, antisocial traits, and poor response to treatment. Empirical research is needed to determine the relative proportion of youth in each pathway. However, identifying the appropriate pathway for youth gamblers by the characteristics presented should provide a practical and useful clinical guide that will ultimately improve the effectiveness of treatment interventions by refining diagnostic processes.

References

Abbott, M. W., & Volberg, R. (1996). The New Zealand national survey of problem and pathological gambling. *Journal of Gambling Studies, 12,* 43–160.

Arnett, J. (1994). Sensation seeking: A new conceptualization and a new scale. *Personality and Individual Differences, 16,* 289–296.

Beaudoin, C. M., & Cox, B. J. (1999). Characteristics of problem gambling in a Canadian context: A preliminary study using a DSM-IV-based questionnaire. *Canadian Journal of Psychiatry, 44,* 483–487.

Bergh, C., Eklund, T., Sodersten, P., & Nordin, C. (1997). Altered dopamine function in pathological gambling. *Psychological Medicine, 27,* 473–475.

Bergler, E. (1958) *The psychology of gambling.* New York: Hill and Wang.

Blaszczynski, A. (1998). *Overcoming compulsive gambling.* London: Robinson Publishing.

Blaszczynski, A. (1999). Pathological gambling: An impulse control, addictive or obsessive-compulsive disorder? *Anuario de Psicologia, 30,* 93–109.

Blaszczynski, A., & Nower, L. (2002). A pathways model of pathological gambling. *Addiction, 97,* 487–500.

Blaszczynski, A., Steel, Z., & McConaghy, N. (1997). Impulsivity in pathological gambling: The antisocial impulsivist. *Addiction, 92,* 75–87.

Blaszczynski, A., Winter, S. W., & McConaghy, N. (1986). Plasma endorphin levels in pathological gamblers. *Journal of Gambling Behavior, 2,* 3–14.

Blum, K., Braverman, E. R., Holder, J. M., Lubar, J. F., Monastra, V. J., Miller, D., et al. (2000). Reward deficiency syndrome: A biogenetic model for the diagnosis and treatment of impulsive, addictive, and compulsive behaviours. *Journal of Psychoactive Drugs, 32,* 1–112.

Brown, R. I. (1988). Models of gambling and gambling addictions as perceptual filters. *Journal of Gambling Behavior, 4,* 224–236.

Carlton, P. L., Manowitz, P., McBridge, H., Nora, R., Swartzburg, M., & Goldstein, L. (1987). Attention deficit disorder and pathological gambling. *Journal of Clinical Psychiatry, 48,* 487–488.

Carrasco, J. L., Saiz-Ruiz, J. Hollander, E., Cesar, J., & Lopez-Ibor, J. J. (1994). Low platelet monoamine oxidase activity in pathological gambling. *Acta Psychiatrica Scand, 90,* 427–431.

Carver, C. S., Scheier, M. F., & Weintraub, J. K. (1989). Assessing coping strategies: A theoretically based approach. *Journal of Personality and Social Psychology, 56,* 267–283.

Cattell, R. B., Cattell, E. S., & Johns, E. (1984). *Manual and norms for the High School Personality Questionnaire.* Champlain: IL: Institute for Personality and Ability Testing.

Comings, D. E., Rosenthal, R. J., Lesieur, H. R., & Rugle, L. (1996). A study of the dopamine D2 receptor gene in pathological gambling. *Pharmacogenetics, 6,* 223–234.

Darbyshire, P., Oster, C., & Carrig, H. (2001). The experience of pervasive loss: Children and young people living in a family where parental gambling is a problem. *Journal of Gambling Studies, 17,* 23–45.

De Caria, C., Hollander, E., Grossman, R., Wong, C., Mosovich, S., & Cherkasky, S. (1996). Diagnosis, neurobiology and treatment of pathological gambling. *Journal of Clinical Psychiatry, 57,* 80–84.

Dell, L. J., Ruzicka, M. E., & Palisi, A. T. (1981). Personality and other factors associated with gambling addiction. *International Journal of Addiction, 16,* 149–156.

Derevensky, J. L., Gupta, R., & Della Cioppa, G. (1996). A developmental perspective of gambling behaviors in children and adolescents. *Journal of Gambling Studies, 12,* 49–66.

Endler, N. S., & Parker, J. D. A. (1990). *Coping inventory for stressful situations (CISS): Manual.* Toronto, Canada: Multi Health Systems.

Eysenck, S. B. G., & Eysenck, H. J. (1977). The place of impulsiveness in a dimensional system of personality description. *British Journal of Social and Clinical Psychology, 16,* 57–68.

Ferris, J., Wynne, H., & Single, E. (1998). *Measuring problem gambling in Canada: Draft Final Report for the Inter-Provincial Task Force on Problem Gambling.* Edmonton, Alberta: Canadian Centre for Substance Abuse.

Fisher, S. (2000). Developing the DSM-IV-MR-J criteria to identify adolescent problem gambling in non-clinical populations. *Journal of Gambling Studies, 16,* 253–273.

Gambino, B., Fitzgerald, R., Shaffer, H., Renner, J., & Courtage, P. (1993). Perceived family history of problem gamblers and scores on SOGS. *Journal of Gambling Studies, 9,* 169–184.

Getty, H. A., Watson, J., & Frisch, G. R. (2000). A comparison of depression and styles of coping in male and female GA members and controls. *Journal of Gambling Studies, 16,* 377–391.

Goldstein, L., Manowitz, P., Nora, R., Swartzburg, M., & Carlton, P. L. (1985). Differential EEG activation and pathological gambling. *Biological Psychiatry, 20,* 1232–1234.

Gonzalez-Ibanez, A., Jimenez, S., & Aymami, M. N. (1999). Evaluacion y tratamiento cognitivo-conductual de jugadores patologicos de maquinas recreativas con premio. *Anuario de Psicologia, 30,* 111–125.

Govoni, R., Rupcich, N., & Frisch, G. R. (1996). Gambling behavior of adolescent gamblers. *Journal of Gambling Studies, 12,* 305–317.

Griffiths, M. (1990). The cognitive psychology of gambling. *Journal of Gambling Studies, 6,* 31–42.

Griffiths, M. (1995). *Adolescent gambling.* London: Routledge.

Grun, L., & McKeigue, P. (2000). Prevalence of excessive gambling before and after introduction of a national lottery in the United Kingdom: Another example of the single distribution theory. *Addiction, 95,* 959–66.

Gupta, R., & Derevensky, J. L. (1996). The relationship between gambling and video-game playing behavior in children and adolescents. *Journal of Gambling Studies, 12,* 375–394.

Gupta, R., & Derevensky, J. L. (1997). Familial and social influences in juvenile gambling. *Journal of Gambling Studies, 13,* 179–192.

Gupta, R., & Derevensky, J. L. (1998a). An empirical examination of Jacob's General Theory of Addictions: Do adolescent gamblers fit the theory? Journal of Gambling Studies. *Journal of Gambling Studies, 14,* 17–49.

Gupta, R., & Derevensky, J. L. (1998b). Adolescent gambling behavior: A prevalence study and examination of the correlates associated with problem gambling. *Journal of Gambling Studies, 14,* 319–345.

Gupta, R., & Derevensky, J. L. (2000). Adolescents with gambling problems: From research to treatment. *Journal of Gambling Studies, 16,* 315–342.

Harter, S. (1985). *The self-perception profile for children.* Denver, CO: University of Denver.

Jacobs, D. F. (1986). A general theory of addictions: A new theoretical model. *Journal of Gambling Behavior, 2,* 15–31.

Jacobs, D. F. (1988). Evidence for a common dissociative like reaction among addicts. *Journal of Gambling Behavior, 4,* 27–37.

Jacobs, D. F. (1993). A review of juvenile gambling in the United States. In W. R. Eadington & J. A. Cornelius (Eds.), *Gambling behavior and problem gambling* (pp. 431–441). Reno: University of Nevada.

Jacobs, D. F. (2000). Juvenile gambling in North America: An analysis of long term trends and future prospects. *Journal of Gambling Studies, 16,* 119–152.

Jacobs, D. F., Marston, A. R., Singer, R. D., Widaman, K., Litle, T., & Veizades, J. (1989). Children of problem gamblers. *Journal of Gambling Studies, 5,* 261–268.

Kuley, N. B., & Jacobs, D. F. (1988). The relationship between dissociative-like experiences and sensation seeking among social and problem gamblers. *Journal of Gambling Behavior, 4,* 197–207.

Ladouceur, R., Boudreault, N., Jacques, C., & Vitaro, F. (1999). Pathological gambling and related problems among adolescents. *Journal of Child & Adolescent Substance Abuse, 8,* 55–68.

Ladouceur, R., Dubé, D., & Bujold, A. (1994). Gambling among primary school students. *Journal of Gambling Studies, 10*, 363–370.

Ladouceur, R., & Mireault, C. (1988). Gambling behaviors among high school students in the Quebec area. *Journal of Gambling Behavior, 4*, 3–12.

Ladouceur, R., & Walker, M. (1996). A cognitive perspective on gambling. In P. M. Salkovskies (Ed.), *Trends in Cognitive and Behavioral Therapies* (pp. 89–120). UK: John Wiley and Sons.

Lesieur, H. R. (1984). *The chase.* Cambridge, MA: Schenkman.

Lesieur, H. R., & Rothschild, J. (1989). Children of Gamblers Anonymous members. *Journal of Gambling Behavior, 5*, 269–282.

Lopez-Ibor, J. J. (1988). The involvement of serotonin in psychiatric disorders and behaviour. *British Journal of Psychiatry, 153*, 26–39.

McCormick, R. A. (1994). The Importance of coping skill enhancement in the treatment of the pathological gambler. *Journal of Gambling Studies, 10*, 77–86.

Moreno, I., Saiz-Ruiz, J., & Lopez-Ibor, J. J. (1991). Serotonin and gambling dependence. *Human Psychopharmacology, 6*, 9–12.

National Research Council (1999). *Pathological gambling: A critical review.* Washington, DC: National Academy Press.

Nower, L., Gupta, R., & Derevensky, J. (2000, June). Youth gamblers and substance abusers: A comparison of stress-coping styles and risk-taking behaviors of two addicted adolescent populations. Paper presented at the 11th International Conference on Gambling and Risk–Taking Behavior, Las Vegas, NV.

Peacock, R. B., Day, P. A., & Peacock, T. D. (1999). Adolescent gambling on a Great Lakes Indian Reservation. *Journal of Human Behavior in the Social Environment, 21*, 5–17.

Powell, J., Hardoon, K., Derevensky, J. L. & Gupta, R. (1999). Gambling and risk-taking behavior among university students. *Substance Use and Misuse, 34*, 1167–1184.

Reynolds, W. M. (1987). *Reynolds Adolescent Depression Scale.* Champagne, IL: Psychological Assessment Resources.

Rosenthal, R. (1992). Pathological gambling. *Psychiatric Annals, 22*, 72–78.

Roy, A., de Jong, J., & Linnoila, M. (1989). Extraversion in pathological gamblers: Correlates with indexes of noradrenergic function. *Archives of General Psychiatry, 46*, 679–681.

Rugle, L., & Melamed, L. (1993). Neuropsychological assessment of attention problems in pathological gamblers. *Journal of Nervous and Mental Disease, 181*, 107–112.

Shaffer, H., & Gambino, B. (1989). The epistemology of 'addictive disease': Gambling as a predicament. *Journal of Gambling Behavior, 3*, 211–229.

Shaffer, H. J., & Hall, M. N. (1996). Estimating prevalence of adolescent gambling disorders: A quantitative synthesis and guide toward standard gambling nomenclature. *Journal of Gambling Studies, 12*, 193–214.

Steel, Z., & Blaszczynski, A. (1996). The factorial structure of pathological gambling. *Journal of Gambling Studies, 12*, 3–20.

Stinchfield, R. (2000). Gambling and correlates of gambling among Minnesota public school students. *Journal of Gambling Studies, 16*, 153–173.

Stinchfield, R., Cassuto, N., Winters, K., & Latimer, W. (1997). Prevalence of gambling among Minnesota public school students in 1992 and 1995. *Journal of Gambling Studies, 13*, 25–48.

Stinchfield, R. D., & Winters, K. C. (1998). Adolescent gambling: A review of prevalence, risk factors and health implications. *Annals of American Academy of Political and Social Science, 556*, 172–185.

Victorian Casino and Gaming Authority (1997). *Definition and incidence of pathological gambling including the socioeconomic distribution,* Melbourne, VIC: Victorian Casino and Gaming Authority.

Vitaro, F., Arseneault, L., & Tremblay, R. E. (1997). Dispositional predictors of problem gambling in male adolescents. *American Journal of Psychiatry, 154*, 1769–1770.

Vitaro, F., Arseneault, L., & Tremblay, R. E. (1999). Impulsivity predicts problem gambling in low SES adolescent males. *Addiction, 94*, 565–575.

Vitaro, F., Ladouceur, R., & Bujold, A. (1996). Predictive and concurrent correlates of gambling in early adolescent boys. *Journal of Early Adolescence, 16*, 211–228.

Volberg, R. (1993). *Gambling and problem gambling among adolescents in Washington State: Report to the Washington State Lottery.* Albany, NY: Gemini Research.

Volberg, R. (1996). *Gambling and problem gambling in New York: A ten year replication survey, 1986–1996: Report to the New York Council on Problem Gambling.* Albany, NY: Gemini Research.

Walker, M. (1992). *The psychology of gambling.* London: Pergamon Press.

Walker, M. (1998). On defining pathological gambling. *National Association of Gambling Studies Newsletter, 10*, 5–6.

Winters, K. C. (1992). Development of an adolescent alcohol and other drug abuse screening scale: Personal Experience Screening Questionnaire. *Addictive Behavior, 17*, 479–490.

Winters, K. C., Stinchfield, R. D., & Fulkerson, J. (1993). Toward a development of an adolescent gambling problem severity scale. *Journal of Gambling Studies, 9*, 63–84.

Winters, K. D., Stinchfield, R. D., & Kim, L. G. (1995). Monitoring adolescent gambling in Minnesota. *Journal of Gambling Studies, 11*, 165–183.

Wood, R. T. A., & Griffiths, M. D. (1998). The acquisition, development and maintenance of lottery and scratchcard gambling in adolescence. *Journal of Adolescence, 21*, 265–273.

Wynne, H., Smith, G., & Jacobs, D. F. (1996). *Adolescent gambling and problem gambling in Alberta.* Edmonton, Alberta: Alberta Alcohol and Drug Abuse Commission.

Zuckerman, M. (1994). *Behavioral expressions and biosocial bases of sensation seeking.* New York: Cambridge University Press.

Chapter 11

Prevention Efforts Toward Reducing Gambling Problems[1]

Jeffrey L. Derevensky, Ph.D., Rina Gupta, Ph.D.,
Laurie Dickson, M.A. and Anne-Elyse Deguire, M.Sc.

The National Research Council's (1999) seminal review of the scientific literature for the National Gambling Impact Study Commission noted a trend toward the proliferation of gambling venues, increased expenditures, and the seriousness of the adverse consequences for those individuals with a gambling problem. Current attempts at primary prevention of gambling problems have been limited at best (National Research Council, 1999), nevertheless, the need to reduce the prevalence and risks associated with gambling problems remains an important goal. While such primary prevention programs can be conceptualized for individuals of any age, the vast majority of primary prevention programs intended to prevent gambling problems have focused upon youth, with some being oriented for other particularly high-risk and vulnerable groups (e.g., elderly/seniors, minorities,

---

1. A large part of this review is based upon a report prepared by Derevensky, Gupta, Dickson, & Deguire (2001). *Prevention Efforts Toward Minimizing Gambling Problem* for the National Council for Problem Gambling, Center for Mental Health Services (CMHS) and the Substance Abuse and Mental Health Services Administration (SAMHSA), Washington, D.C.; papers by Dickson, Derevensky, & Gupta (2002). The prevention of youth gambling problems: A conceptual model. *Journal of Gambling Studies, 18*, 161–184; and Dickson, Derevensky & Gupta (2004). Harm minimization and youth gambling problems. *Journal of Research on Adolescence, 19*, 233–263.

individuals with low income, and those experiencing other impulse and additive disorders) (see Derevensky, Gupta, Dickson, & Deguire, 2001 for a list of prevention programs). This chapter summarizes the current literature on the prevention of gambling problems and harm minimization, highlights our current knowledge gaps, identifies issues of concern, presents a viable model for the development and evaluation of prevention programs, and provides recommendations for future directions. It is important to note at the outset that the current scientific knowledge concerning adolescent gambling behavior in general, and problematic gambling in specific, and its social impact is just beginning in earnest. As such, before *Best Practices* can be established, further basic and applied empirical and longitudinal research is necessary.

The Prevention of Youth Gambling

Much of the current primary prevention efforts have been aimed at school-age children. This is typical of primary prevention programs focused upon minimizing and/or preventing multiple mental health, antisocial, and risk-taking behaviors. Recent analyses has suggested that today's youth are at high risk for engaging in a multitude of risky behaviors including substance abuse, adolescent pregnancy, youth violence, school dropout (Bronfenbrenner, McClelland, Wethington, Moen, & Ceci, 1996; Weissberg, Wallberg, O'Brien, & Kuster, 2003) and gambling (National Research Council, 1999). Grasping the severity of the consequences associated with youth problem gambling is often difficult in light of the widespread attitude that youth have little readily available access to money and the perception that few have significant gambling or gambling-related problems. The fact that youth gamble has been well established (see the reviews and meta-analyses by Jacobs, 2000, in this volume; National Research Council, 1999; Shaffer & Hall, 1996, 2001). It is important to note that youth not only gamble for money with their peers and family members, but they have been shown to gamble in most forms of legalized and state sanctioned gambling in spite of legal restrictions and prohibitions. While most adolescents gamble in a socially acceptable manner with few apparent gambling related problems, as a group they have been shown to be particularly susceptible and at-risk for the development of serious gambling problems (Derevensky & Gupta, 1999; Derevensky, Gupta & Winters, 2003; Gupta & Derevensky, 2000; National Research Council, 1999).

Adolescent prevalence rates of problem gambling have been consistently reported to be between 4–8% (two to four times that of adults) (Gupta & Derevensky, 1998a; Jacobs, 2000; National Research Council, 1999; Shaffer & Hall, 1996, 2001), with another 10–15% of youth being at-risk for the development of a serious gambling problem (Derevensky & Gupta,

2000; Derevensky, Gupta & Winters, 2003; Gupta & Derevensky, 1998a; National Research Council, 1999; Shaffer & Hall, 1996). The rapid movement from social gambler to problem gambler (Gupta & Derevensky, 2000; Gupta & Derevensky, 1998a) and the induction of gambling as a rite of initiation into adulthood (Svendsen, 1998) points to the possibility that adolescents are particularly vulnerable.

Similar to adults, our current empirical knowledge of youth problem gambling includes a profile of the adolescent problem gambler that reflects the serious nature of gambling-related problems. (For a detailed summary of the current empirical knowledge of adolescent problem gamblers see the reviews by Derevensky & Gupta, 1999, 2000, 2004; Gupta & Derevensky, 2000; Hardoon & Derevensky, 2002; and Stinchfield, in this book). Increased efforts to understand the economic, social, familial and psychological costs of gambling, and the recognition of the adolescent population as being particularly at-risk for developing problem behaviors (Baer, MacLean, & Marlatt, 1998; Jessor, 1998; Luthar, Cicchetti, & Becker, 2000a) and gambling-related problems (Gupta & Derevensky, 1998a; Wynne, Smith, & Jacobs, 1996) amplifies the necessity for effective prevention initiatives targeting vulnerable populations (Dickson, Derevensky, & Gupta, 2002; National Research Council, 1999). While it has been noted that little progress has been made in understanding the efficacy of treatment of adolescent problem gambling, the characteristics of those seeking help (Gupta & Derevensky; 2000, in this book; Rugle, Derevensky, Gupta, Stinchfield & Winters, 2001), and that no scientifically validated *Best Practices* currently exists for the treatment of pathological gambling (Nathan, 2001), empirical knowledge of the prevention of this disorder and its translation into science-based prevention initiatives are particularly scarce (Dickson et al., 2002).

Within the past two decades there has been increased interest in general human development and the prevention of high-risk behaviors (Nation et al., 2003). This research, converging with the examination of causes and remedies for psychological disorders, *prevention science,* has formed the basis of many school-based prevention efforts (Coie et al., 1993; Greenberg et al., 2003). While our current knowledge of the efficacy of prevention of youth gambling problems is limited, the substantial literature on prevention of adolescent alcohol and substance abuse has a rich history of research, program development and implementation, and evaluation which can help to shape future directions for the prevention of gambling problems. As both a mental and a public health issue (see Korn & Shaffer, 1999 for a comprehensive review and the work by Messerlian, Derevensky & Gupta, 2003 for a public health perspective on youth gambling), the conceptualization of problem gambling, as another form of risk-taking behavior, and its adverse consequences substantiates the need for effective prevention initiatives.

Efforts to address adolescent risky lifestyles have traditionally been streamed into prevention programs aimed towards non-users (primary prevention), screening for potential problems (secondary prevention), and treatment (tertiary prevention) for those who have developed problems (e.g., alcohol use and abuse, substance abuse, smoking). In terms of primary prevention, the bulk of resources have been allocated toward initiatives with the goal of preventing or postponing the initial use of substances or activities such as gambling. However, the question of whether the traditional approach of promoting non-use as an adequate means of preventing problems has been increasingly raised (Beck, 1998; Brown & D'Emidio Caston, 1995; Cohen, 1993; Erickson, 1997; Gorman, 1998; Marlatt, 1998; Pouline & Elliott, 1997; Thombs & Briddick, 2000), especially in the field of alcohol use and gambling (Dickson, Derevensky & Gupta, 2004).

Although few reduction prevention initiatives currently exist for problem gambling, the increasing widespread use of the harm-reduction approach in the field of alcohol and substance abuse calls for an examination of the validity of harm-reduction as it relates specifically to gambling (for a historical overview of the development of harm-reduction see Erickson, 1999 and Marlatt, 1996). It has recently been advocated that initiatives move toward designing prevention strategies that target multiple risk behaviors based on theoretical and empirical evidence of common risk and protective factors across adolescent risky behaviors (Battistich, Schaps, Watson, & Solomon, 1996; Costello, Erkanli, Federman, & Angold, 1999; Galambos & Tilton-Weaver, 1998; Jessor, 1998; Loeber, Farrington, Stouthamer-Loeber, & Van Kammen, 1998) including problem gambling (Jacobs, 1998; Dickson et al., 2002, 2004; Gupta & Derevensky, 1998b). Considering that serious gambling problems result in far-reaching and long-lasting negative consequences and that gambling is largely promoted and easily accessible, the importance of primary prevention takes center stage in addressing this important issue. While prevention efforts are critical in protecting youth, adults and seniors from developing serious problems, the specific type of prevention approach that should be adopted remains unclear.

Researchers, treatment providers, educators, and policy makers would benefit from a conceptual examination of the harm-reduction paradigm for its application in the prevention of problem gambling and other risky behaviors. However, there currently remains insufficient empirical knowledge about how to promote the use of harm-reduction strategies. Furthermore, there are few, if any, program evaluations delineating the potential positive and/or negative outcomes resulting from the implementation of various harm-reduction *prevention* programs for the range of adolescent risky behaviors that have been realized (Ogborne & Birchmore-Timney, 1999; Poulin & Elliott, 1997; Thombs & Briddick, 2000).

Abstinence Versus Harm Reduction Approaches

There are two global paradigms under which particular prevention approaches can be classified, either *abstinence* or *harm-reduction* (the terms harm-reduction and harm minimization have often been used interchangeably). While these two approaches are not completely mutually exclusive, they are predicated upon different short-term goals and processes. The central question currently being asked is which form of prevention is best for targeting the issue of gambling problems?

Harm-reduction strategies (policy, program, intervention) seek to help individuals without demanding abstinence (Magham, 2001; Riley et al., 1999). Included in such an approach would be secondary prevention strategies, based upon the assumption that individuals cannot be prevented from engaging in particular risky behaviors (Baer, MacLean, & Marlatt, 1998; Cohen, 1993); tertiary prevention strategies (DiClemete, 1999); and a 'health movement' perspective (Denning & Little, 2001; Heather, Wodak, Nadelmann, & O'Hare, 1993; Messerlian et al., 2003).

While negative consequences of excessive gambling are evident (e.g., financial difficulties, depression, suicide ideation and attempts, health problems, academic problems, criminal and antisocial behavior, familial disruptions, peer difficulties, etc.) (Derevensky & Gupta, 2004; Stinchfield, in this volume), it still remains unclear as to whether the costs of legalized gambling outweigh their benefits. By default, most governments seem to have adopted a harm-minimization approach, such that policy efforts have been aimed at reducing or minimizing the negative impact of gambling while not limiting revenues or access for the general public.

Underage youth are, in general, prohibited access to government regulated forms of gambling and venues. While these laws are necessary, research clearly indicates that early gambling experiences mostly occur with non-regulated forms of gambling (e.g., playing cards for money, placing informal bets on sports events, wagering on games of skill or parents gambling for/and with their children (Gupta & Derevensky, 1998a; Jacobs, 2000, in this volume). This highlights both the paradox and the confusion as to which primary prevention approach to promote; abstinence or harm-reduction? If one were to advocate an abstinence approach, is it realistic to expect youth to stop gambling when between 70–80% of children and adolescents report having gambled during the past 12 months (Gupta & Derevensky, 1998a; Jacobs, 2000; National Research Council, 1999). Similar to adults, one could argue that it would be unrealistic to expect youth to stop gambling completely, especially since it is exceedingly difficult to regulate access to gambling activities organized amongst themselves (e.g., card betting, sports betting, wagering on personal games of skill, etc.). And while we remain concerned about the occurrence of serious gambling problems amongst youth, it is also recognized that many youth, like adults, are able to gamble without developing any significant gambling related problems. Nevertheless, the harm-reduction approach is also questionable because it assumes, as a basic tenet, that youth will gamble in spite of legal restrictions.

Research highlights that age of onset of gambling behavior represents a significant risk factor, with the younger the age of initiation being correlated with the development of gambling related problems (Dickson et al., 2004; Gupta & Derevensky, 1998a, Jacobs, 2000; National Research Council, 1999; Wynne et al., 1996). Thus, delaying the age of onset of gambling experiences would be fundamental in a successful prevention paradigm, consistent with an abstinence approach, and does not adhere to the principles of the harm-reduction model.

The harm-reduction approach, nonetheless, makes intuitive sense on other levels. As gambling has been historically part of our culture (Fleming, 1978) and is consistent with the expansion of gambling sites and types of games offered, the harm-minimization approach seems a sensible approach. Included under the principles of harm-minimization is the promotion of responsible behavior; teaching and informing youth about the facts and risks associated with gambling, changing erroneous cognitions, misperceptions, and beliefs, along with enhancing skills needed to maintain control when gambling. If these skills are encouraged and reinforced for youth through their formative years, it is plausible that they may be less vulnerable to the risks of a gambling problem once gaining legal access to gambling forums.

The application of the harm-reduction paradigm to a broad range of problem behaviors has not been without criticism. However, given that there are a number of socially and widely acceptable risk behaviors (e.g., alcohol consumption and gambling) where involvement in such activities can be viewed as lying on a continuum ranging from no—to significant psychological, social, physical, and financial harm to self and others, the utility of the harm-reduction approach as a means to prevent problem behavior remains promising.

Harm-Reduction for Problem Behaviors Associated with Socially Acceptable Risky Activities

Gambling as a Socially Acceptable Activity

The goal of harm-reduction to prevent problem behavior rather than the risky behavior itself appears appropriate for activities that are very much a social reality. There is ample reason to believe that involvement in risky behaviors can be approached responsibly, controlling the progression to problem behavior given that the majority of those youth who drink alcohol or gamble do not develop significant problems. Furthermore, research on the patterns of use (Gliksman & Smythe, 1982) and personal and social control mechanisms of various substance use (Boys et al.,1999; Dembo et al., 1981; Kandel, 1985) point to the possibility of achieving controlled involvement in risky behaviors, free from problematic involvement. There is evidence from studies using adults that substance users do in fact make rational choices, weighing the perceived positive gains versus risks of drug or alcohol use, and utilize informal control mechanisms of social networks (Cheung, Erickson, & Landau, 1991; Erikson, 1982; Murphy, Reinarman, & Waldorf, 1989). More research needs to be undertaken with adolescents to examine whether similar processes can be induced.

Research on risk and protective factors offer an important reminder that the cause of such variance results from the interaction of present risk and protective factors operating within complex person-environment-situation interactions. Thus, it can be argued that the continuum of harm is associated with a number of different risk profiles and that harm-reduction is a useful means to prevent normal adolescent gambling behavior to becoming increasingly problematic.

Harm-Reduction Prevention Programs

The strategies of harm-reduction prevention are similar to those associated with other approaches and are consistent with a public health framework (Messerlian et al., 2003). For example, school-based drug education programs and media campaigns are common strategies used regardless of prevention orientation (e.g., abstinence, harm-reduction). To date, universal harm-reduction programs have generally been primarily integrated in the form of school-based drug, alcohol and smoking education and prevention programs. There exist a greater variety of strategies employed in terms of selective prevention, given the variety of at-risk populations that selective programs may target (e.g., street youth at high-risk for drug and alcohol abuse, or entire schools at high-risk for a multiplicity of problems due to socio-cultural factors).

The components of universal harm-reduction prevention programs have the specific objectives of modifying positive attitudes towards risky behaviors, making informed choices about engaging in risky behavior (e.g., by raising awareness of risk factors which may lead to excessive use) and efficient decision-making. It is expected that once an individual has adequate awareness and knowledge about risky activities and have developed good decision-making skills, they can make appropriate decisions about whether they need to avoid alcohol, tobacco, and illegal drugs completely, how they will be careful if choosing to experiment with risky activities, and when they should seek help for a problem (Beck, 1998).

Resilient Youth

Empirical research focused upon resilient youth, in general, supports a positive profile that includes problem solving skills (the ability to think abstractly and generate and implement solutions to cognitive and social problems), social competence (encompassing the qualities of flexibility, communication skills, concern for others, and pro-social behaviors), autonomy (self-efficacy and self control), and a sense of purpose and future (exhibited in success orientation, motivation, and optimism) (Brown, D'Emidio-Caston, & Benard, 2001). Evidence of resiliency in children (e.g., Garmezy, 1985; Rutter, 1987; Werner, 1986) has expanded the prevention field from a risk-prevention framework to one that includes both risk-prevention and the promotion of protective factors. Masten, Best and Garmezy (1990) have suggested that protective factors can serve to mediate or buffer the effects of individual vulnerabilities or environmental adversity so that the adaptational trajectory is more positive than if the protective factors are not at work. Protective factors, in and of themselves, do not necessarily promote resiliency. If the strength or number of risk factors outweigh the impact of protective factors, the chances that poor outcomes will ensue increases.

Studies have examined the effects of a large number of risk and protective factors associated with excessive alcohol and substance abuse (see Derevensky et al., 2001; Dickson, Derevensky & Gupta, 2003). Such risk and protective factors can be grouped into a number of domains. In their conceptual model, Bournstein, Zweig and Gardner (1999) illustrate that each of these domains interact with the individual, who processes, interprets, and responds to various factors, based upon unique characteristics brought to the situation. The Centre for Substance Abuse Prevention has incorporated this model, as a conceptual framework for targeting high-risk groups and their potential outcomes.

Protective and risk factors have been shown to interact such that protective factors reduce the strength of the relation of the stressor and their outcomes. There are numerous examples as to how protective factors influence positive outcomes. For example, the effects of positive school experiences have been shown to moderate the effects of family conflict, which in turn decreases the association between family conflict and several adolescent problem behaviors (e.g., pathological gambling, alcohol and substance abuse, suicide, and delinquency) (Jessor, Van Den Bos, Vanderryn, Costa & Turbin, 1995).

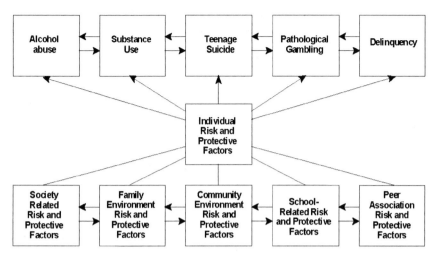

Figure 1. *A conceptual model for understanding the domains of risk and protective factors that influence an individual's behavior.* (adapted from *Understanding Substance Abuse Prevention: Toward 21st Century Primer on Effective Programs* (Bournstein, Zweig, & Gardner, 1999). Centre for Substance Abuse Prevention (CSAP) & Substance Abuse and Mental Health Services Administration (SAMHSA).

In an attempt to conceptualize our current state of knowledge concerning the risk factors associated with problem gambling, a similar paradigm was created by Dickson et al. (2002) based upon our current knowledge of youth with severe gambling problems. Within the individual domain, poor impulse control, high sensation-seeking, unconventionality, poor psychological functioning, low self-esteem, early and persistent problem behaviors and early initiation are commonly found. Common risk factors in the family domain include familial history of substance abuse, parental attitudes, and modeling of deviant behavior. Within the peer domain, social expectancies and reinforcement by peer groups are common risk factors across addictions. Although some research has been undertaken to identify risk factors of problem adolescent gambling (see Derevensky & Gupta, 2000; Dickson et al., 2003; Griffiths & Wood, 2000; Gupta & Derevensky, 2000 for reviews) there are few studies which have examined protective mechanisms, or more generally, resiliency for youth with respect to problem gambling. In a recent study by Dickson et al. (2003), after examining a wide number of variables, family cohesion and school connectedness were found to serve as protective factors for preventing gambling problems. Protective factors that have been examined across other youthful risky behaviors and addictions generally fall into the three categories: care and support, dispositional attributes such as positive and high expectations, and opportunities for participation (Werner, 1989). These characteristics appear to describe each domain that fosters resiliency in youth.

Review of Current Prevention Programs

Few primary prevention programs for problem gambling currently exist. Of those that are currently being implemented (although implementation is quite sporadic), most developed for youth have no science-based underlying principles, have failed to account for risk and protective factors, and few have been systematically evaluated (see Derevensky et al., 2001 for a comprehensive list of programs). The majority of these programs can be defined as primary and/or universal preventive efforts aimed at reducing the incidence of problem gambling. Several programs explicitly identified factors associated with the development of problem gambling but these factors were not always defined as a risk or a protective factor, nor were there many programs that pointed to the scientific validity of such factors.

Commonalities and Differences Amongst Programs

Prevention programs to reduce the incidence of gambling problems for youth generally incorporate a universal model aimed at raising awareness concerning issues related to problem gambling. Most programs have not been systematically evaluated as to their efficacy in achieving their explicit or implicit goals and many are not based upon current knowledge of risk or protective factors, falling far short of models and standards associated with *Best Practices*. Most programs conceptualize gambling as an addiction, foster a harm-reduction model and encourage responsible gambling. Some programs, however, stress the importance of abstinence. This distinction probably lies within the specific population targeted. Programs targeted toward populations where the prevalence of gambling and other addiction and/or mental health problems is high (e.g., First Nations; Native Americans), suggest prevention programs might encourage abstinence over harm minimization, taking a tertiary approach in their prevention efforts.

Since the objectives of the majority of current programs are to raise awareness, most present information relevant to gambling, problem gambling, motivations to gamble, warning signs, consequences associated with excessive gambling, and how and where to get the help for an individual with a gambling problem. Several curriculums go a little further than merely presenting factual information; encouraging the development of interpersonal skills enabling youth to better cope with stressful life events, techniques to improve self-esteem, and suggestions for resisting peer pressure.

A number of programs place greater emphasis on the mathematical aspect of gambling including teaching students about the odds and probabilities associated with games of chance, while others emphasize issues related to erroneous cognitions and thoughts.

A Conceptual Framework for Harm-Reduction Prevention

An examination of the commonalities of risk and protective factors for problem gambling and other addictions provides ample evidence to suggest that gambling may similarly be incorporated into more general addiction and adolescent risk behavior prevention programs. Current research efforts (Battistich, Schaps, Watson, & Solomon, 1996; Costello et al., 1999; Galambos & Tilton-Weaver, 1998; Loeber et al., 1998) suggest a more general mental health prevention program that addresses a number of adolescent risky behaviors (e.g., substance abuse, gambling, risky driving, truancy, and risky sexual activity). More recent science-based programs such as the Centre for Substance Abuse Prevention's Eight Model Programs (Brounstein et al., 1999) provide evidence that prevention programs for risky behaviors are indeed effective. Dickson et al. (2002) has suggested that there is empirical and clinical evidence which points to the need to examine similarities and differences amongst addictive behaviors, the need to analyze multiple risk and protective factors, and the importance of understanding the coping mechanisms of individuals engaging in risky behaviors.

Despite the complexities of using the risk-protective factor model (see Coie et al., 1993), Dickson et al. (2002) proposed this model to establish the theoretical basis of harm-reduction as it is predicated upon science-based prevention principles. This model has empirical validity in understanding current trends in adolescent risk behavior theory (Jessor, 1998). As well, its role in empirically-supported theory of intentional behavioral change (DiClemente, 1999) which has been used to understand the *initiation* of health-protective behaviors and health-risk behaviors such as gambling, as well as its potential to *modify* problem behaviors such as alcoholism and problem gambling (DiClemente, Delahanty & Schlundt, in this volume; DiClemente, Story & Murray, 2000).

Dickson et al.'s (2002, 2003) adaptation of Jessor's (1998) model views problem gambling within a risky behavior paradigm. This conceptual framework is predicated upon a theoretical foundation for general mental health prevention programs that fosters resiliency. Risk and protective factors operate *interactively*, in and across a number of domains (biology, social environment, perceived environment, personality and behavior). The risk and protective factors represented in Figure 2 have been previously identified

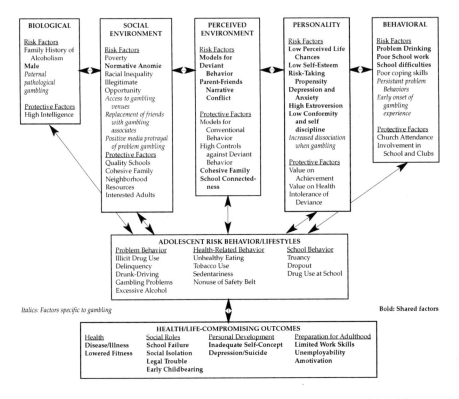

Figure 2. Adapted from Jessor's (1998) and Dickson et al.'s (2002) revision of the adolescent risk behaviour model with youth gambling risk factors incorporated (Dickson et al., 2003).

from empirical research. This model provides flexibility, permitting an incorporation of current research on risk and resilience. Problem gambling has been included into this framework based upon a growing body of empirical research. Unique risk factors (indicated in Italics), based upon current research findings (see Derevensky & Gupta, 2004), including paternal pathological gambling, access to gambling venues, depression and anxiety, high extroversion, low conformity and self-discipline, poor coping skills and adaptive behavior, persistent problem behaviors and early onset of gambling experiences have been incorporated. Problem adolescent gambling also shares a number of common risk factors with other health compromising behaviors (indicated in bold font). These include being male, normative anomie, models for deviant behavior, parent-friends normative conflict, low self-esteem, high risk-taking propensity, poor school work and school difficulties. The remaining risk factors in this model are those that have either not been studied or have not been found to be risk factors for problem gambling but have been found to be antecedents for other adolescent risk behaviors. The illustration of numerous possible risk behavior antecedents, risk behaviors, and health-compromising outcomes in this model clearly points to the need for multifaceted approaches to prevention.

Recommendations and New Directions

There is little doubt that the proposed model requires further testing and refinement. Yet all prevention programs require testing for effectiveness *prior* to their widespread implementation and require ongoing evaluation for program refinement. The lack of empirical testing of the effectiveness of the current prevention programs is of considerable concern. Viewing risk and protective factors in light of the domains in which they operate provides a means to specify program goals (targeting specific factors), to establish outcome evaluation criteria, and to assess effectiveness of prevention programs. A number of evaluations of drug and alcohol programs are incorporated in this model, and in doing so, have acquired additional understanding about how the effects of specific risk and protective factors work. Similar information gained from existing gambling prevention programs can be useful to refine and improve such programs.

Research in the field of gambling is relatively new. Yet, the scientific standards expected from this field need to be no less rigorous. It is necessary to ensure that scientifically validated prevention program evaluations meet the highest scientific standards as advocated by the Center for Substance Abuse Prevention (2001). The established criteria adopted to determine the credibility of evaluations include theory-driven findings, high fidelity implementation, quality of sampling design, the use of appropriate psychometric evaluation measures, appropriateness of data collection and analysis techniques, and addressing plausible alternative hypotheses concerning program effects, integrity, and utility (Brounstein et al., 1999; Center for Substance Abuse Prevention, 2001). Current scientific data concerning program effectiveness is either limited at best or non-existent for the current gambling prevention programs.

Findings from the field of adolescent alcohol and substance abuse suggest that no one single approach to prevention appears to be uniformly successful (Baer, MacLean, & Marlatt, 1998). As such, a combination of strategies seems to work best toward the goal of nurturing resilience. The Center for Substance Abuse Prevention (2001) has outlined a number of strategies that can be combined in the development of school, family and community prevention programs that target each area that affects youth functioning. These strategies include information dissemination, prevention education (critical life and social skills), offering alternative activities, problem identification and referral, community-based processes (training community members and agencies in substance use and gambling education and prevention) and active lobbying for policy modifications or additions that aim to reduce risk factors and enhance protective factors. It is important to note that a number of guiding principles, including the appropriate timing of the intervention (to occur in a child's life when they will have maximal impact) and socio-cultural relevance (norms, cultural beliefs and practices) to matching a prevention program with a target population need to be considered (Nation et al., 2003).

It is crucial for programs to adjust the strategies and material of prevention programs to the developmental level of the individual receiving the intervention. As such, developmental research should form the basis of prevention strategies. Prevention programs also need to bear in mind that coping strategies and social, academic, employment and economic pressures may change (Eisenberg, Fabes, & Guthrie, 1997) and ensure that materials and outcome measures are congruent with current knowledge about coping and adaptive behaviors at different ages.

Prevention and Social Policy

Prevention programs, in a global way, represent a form of social policy. This is particularly important within the context of the debate between harm-reduction versus abstinence. It has been argued that the strength of prevention programs that address problem gambling issues are highly dependent upon clarity in the articulation of responsible social policies and ensure that they reflect research based findings on resilience and effective program evaluations. Current policies that reflect the predominant attitude that gambling has few negative consequences and is merely a form of entertainment leaves little credence to effective abstinence gambling prevention initiatives. Changing widespread attitudes about problem gambling will empower prevention efforts to encourage individuals to make healthy decisions about gambling and other potentially health-compromising behaviors.

Social policies concerning problem gambling are relatively scarce. Furthermore, the lack of parental concern (Ladouceur, Jacques, Ferland, & Giroux, 1998), and ineffective gambling law enforcement, in particular, the selling of lottery and scratch tickets to youth (Shaffer & Zinberg, 1994; Felsher, Derevensky & Gupta, 2003) is of considerable concern. Current research on substance abuse prevention suggests that programs may be more effective if prevention services incorporate students' perceptions and attitudes (Brown & D'Emidio, 1995; Gorman, 1998). While there is preliminary research to suggest that perceptions of skill and luck can be modified for gambling activities (Baboushkin, Derevensky, & Gupta, 1999), there is little evidence and empirical support that attitudes toward gambling can be modified and have long-lasting changes. Much needed basic and applied research funding is required to help identify common and unique risk and protective factors for gambling problems and those similar to other addictive behaviors. In addition, longitudinal research to examine the natural history of pathological gambling from childhood to adolescence through later adulthood is required.

Concluding Remarks

Only recently have health professionals, educators and public policy makers acknowledged the need for prevention of problem gambling. In light of the scarcity of empirical knowledge about the prevention of this disorder, the similarities between adolescent problem gambling and other risk behaviors, particularly alcohol and substance abuse, have been examined and found to be informative in the conceptualization of the future direction of gambling prevention programs. It is important to note that while some of these risk factors are consistent with individuals with delinquent and antisocial behaviors, and that delinquents have a higher risk for problem gambling (Magoon, Gupta & Derevensky, in press; Westphal, Rush, Stevens, & Johnson, 1998), further empirical research is necessary before definitive conclusions can be drawn concerning the comparability between these groups. As well, a review of the current literature found that most pathological gambling prevention programs lack a strong theoretical orientation and they have been implemented without being empirically evaluated. This is of serious concern as such programs may in fact be promoting gambling behavior. Finally, most existing programs are school-based programs aimed at children and adolescents. This should not be misconstrued to suggest that only youth remain high risk for the development of serious pathological gambling programs or that such behaviors can not occur at any age.

We have attempted to illustrate the importance of using a conceptual model as the foundation for prevention efforts and have argued that research, development of prevention programs, and their acceptability into school-based curriculum and community programs requires much needed basic and applied research. There is a solid and growing empirical base indicating that well-designed, appropriately implemented school-based prevention can positively influence multiple social, heath, and academic outcomes (Greenberg, Weisberg et al., 2003). Despite our limited knowledge of the role of protective factors in gambling problems, there is ample research to suggest that direct and moderator effects of protective factors can be used to guide the development of future prevention and intervention efforts to help minimize risk behaviors. Dickson et al.'s (2002) adaptation of Jessor's (1998) risk behavior model provides a promising framework from which to begin the much needed development of effective, science-based prevention initiatives for minimizing and ensuring a harm-reduction approach for problem gambling among youth as well as other selected groups.

There is a strong belief that competence and health-promotion programs are best initiated before students are pressured to experiment with risky behaviors. Early intervention prevention programs which follow adolescents through high school will likely result in fewer youth with gambling problems. Socio-cultural factors also remain crucial in developing effective programs. Prevention programming will need to account for the changing forms and opportunities for gambling. Ultimately, school-based initiatives may have to examine the commonalities amongst multiple risky behaviors before educators become inundated with the implementation of prevention programs for risky behaviors and have little time for the educational curriculum.

References

Baboushkin, H., Derevensky, J. L., & Gupta, R. (1999, June). *Modifying children's perception of the amount of skill and luck involved in gambling activities.* Paper presented at the annual meeting of the National Council on Problem Gambling, Detroit.

Baer, J. MacLean, M. and Marlatt, G. (1998). Linking etiology and treatment for adolescent substance abuse: Toward a better match. In R. Jessor. *New perspectives on adolescent risk behavior.* Cambridge, UK: Cambridge University Press.

Battistich, V., Schaps, E., Watson, M., & Solomon, D. (1996). Prevention effects of the Child Development Project: Early findings from an ongoing multisite demonstration trial. *Journal of Adolescent Research, 11,* 12–35.

Beck, J. (1998). 100 Years of "Just say no" versus "Just say know." Reevaluating drug education goals for the coming century. *Evaluation Review, 22,* 15–45.

Bournstein, P. J., Zweig, J. M., & Gardner, S. E. (1999). *Understanding substance abuse prevention—toward the 21st century: A primer on effective programs.* Rockville: U.S. Department of Health and Human Services, Substance Abuse and Mental Health Services Administration, Center for Substance Abuse Prevention, Division of Knowledge Development and Evaluation.

Boys, A., Marsden, J., Griffiths, P., Fountain, J., Stillwell, G. & Strang, J. (1999). Substance use among young people: the relationship between perceived functions and intentions. *Addiction, 94,* 1043–1050.

Bronfenbrenner, U., McClelland, P., Wethington, E., Moen, P., & Ceci, S. (1996). *The state of Americans: This generation and the next.* NY: Free Press.

Brown, J. H., & D'Emidio-Caston, M. (1995). On becoming 'at risk' through drug education: How symbolic policies and their practices affect students. *Evaluation Review, 19,* 451–492.

Brown, J. H., D'Emidio-Caston, M., & Benard, B. (2001). *Resilience education*. Thousand Oaks: Corwin Press.

Center for Substance Abuse Prevention (2001). *Principles of substance abuse prevention* (DHHS Publication No. SMA 01–3507). Rockville, MD: National Clearinghouse for Alcohol and Drug Information.

Cheung, Y. W., Erickson, P. G., & Landau, T. (1991). Experience of crack use: Findings from a community-based sample in Toronto. *Journal of Drug Issues, 21*, 121–140.

Cohen, J. (1993). Achieving a reduction in drug-related harm through education. In N. Heather, A. Wodak, E. Nadelmann, P. O'Hare (Eds.), *Psychoactive drugs and harm reduction: From faith to science*. London: Whurr Publishers Ltd.

Coie, J., Watt, N., West, S., Hawkins, J., Asarnow, J., Markman, H., Ramey, S., Shure, M., & Long, B. (1993). The science of prevention. *American Psychologist, 48*, 1013–1022.

Costello, E. J., Erkanli, A., Federman, E., & Angold, A. (1999). Development of psychiatric comorbidity with substance abuse in adolescents: Effects of timing and sex. *Journal of Clinical Child Psychology, 28*, 298–311.

Dembo, R., Babst, D. V., Burgos, W. & Schmeidler, J. (1981). Survival orientation and the drug use experiences of a sample of inner city junior high school youths. *The International Journal of the Addictions, 16*, 1031–1047.

Denning, P. & Little, J. (2001). Harm reduction in mental health: The emerging work of harm reduction psychotherapy. *Harm Reduction Communication, 11*, 7–10.

Derevensky, J. L., & Gupta, R. (1999, June). *Youth gambling problems: Prevalence, clinical treatment, and social policy issues*. Paper presented at the annual meeting of the national council on problem gambling, Detroit.

Derevensky, J. L., & Gupta, R. (2000). Prevalence estimates of adolescent gambling: A comparison of SOGS-RA, DSM-IV-J, and the GA 20 Questions. *Journal of Gambling Studies, 16*, 227–252.

Derevensky, J., & Gupta, R. (2004). Adolescents with gambling problems: A review of our current knowledge. *e-Gambling: The Electronic Journal of Gambling Issues, 10*, 119–140.

Derevensky, J., Gupta, R., Dickson, L., & Deguire, A-E. (2001). *Prevention efforts toward minimizing gambling problems*. Paper prepared for the National Council on Problem Gambling, Center for Mental Health Services (CMS) and the Substance abuse and Mental Health Services Administration (SAMHSA), Washington, D.C.

Derevensky, J. L, Gupta, R., & Emond, M. (1995, August). *Locus of control, video game playing, and gambling behavior in children*. Poster presented at the annual meeting of the American Psychological Association, New York City.

Derevensky, J. L., Gupta, R., & Winters, K. (2003). Prevalence rates of youth gambling problems: Are the current rates inflated? *Journal of Gambling Studies, 19*, 405–425.

Dickson, L., Derevensky, J. L., & Gupta, R. (2002). The prevention of youth gambling problems: A conceptual model. *Journal of Gambling Studies, 18*, 161–184.

Dickson, L., Derevensky, J. L., & Gupta, R. (2003). *Youth gambling problems: The identification of risk and protective factors*. Report prepared for the Ontario Problem Gambling Research Centre, Guelph, Ontario, Canada.

Dickson, L., Derevensky, J. L., & Gupta, R. (2004). Harm reduction for the prevention of youth gambling problems: Lessons learned from adolescent high-risk prevention programs. *Journal of Adolescent Research, 19*, 233–263.

DiClemente, C. C. (1999). Prevention and harm reduction for chemical dependency: A process perspective. *Clinical Psychology Review, 19*, 173–186.

DiClemente, C. C., Story, M., & Murray, K. (2000). On a roll: The process of initiation and cessation of problem gambling among adolescents. *Journal of Gambling Studies, 16*, 289–313.

Eisenberg, N., Fabes, R., & Guthrie, I. (1997). Coping with stress: Roles of regulation and development. In S. A. Wolchik, I. N. Sandler, et al. (Eds.), *Handbook of children's coping: Linking theory and intervention. Issues in clinical child psychology.* (pp.41–70). New York: Plenum Press.

Erickson, P. G. (1997). Reducing the harm of adolescent substance use. *Canadian Medical Association Journal, 156,* 1386–1393.

Erickson, P. G. (1999). Introduction: The three phases of harm reduction. An examination of emerging concepts, methodologies, and critiques. *Substance Use & Misuse, 34,* 1–7.

Erikson, E. H. (1982). *The life cycle completed: A review.* New York: Norton.

Felsher, J., Derevensky, J. L., & Gupta, R. (2003). Parental influences and social modeling of youth lottery participation. *Journal of Community and Applied Social Psychology, 13,* 361–377.

Fleming, A. M. (1978). *Something for nothing: A history of gambling.* New York: Delacorte Press.

Galambos, N. L., & Tilton-Weaver, L.C. (1998). Multiple risk behavior in adolescents and young adults. *Health Review, 10,* 9–20.

Garmezy, N. (1985). The NIMH-Israeli high-risk study: Commendations, comments, and cautions. *Schizophrenia Bulletin, 11,* 349–353.

Gliksman, L., & Smythe, P. C. (1982). Adolescent involvement with alcohol: A cross-sectional study. *Journal of Studies on Alcohol, 43,* 370–379.

Gorman, D. M. (1998). The irrelevance of evidence in the development of school-based drug prevention policy, 1986–1996. *Evaluation Review, 22,* 118–146.

Greenberg, M. T., Weissberg, R. P., O'Brien, M. U., Zins, J. E., Fredericks, L., Resnik, H., et al. (2003). Enhancing school-based prevention and youth development through coordinated social, emotional, and academic learning. *American Psychologist, 58,* 466–474.

Griffiths, M. D., & Wood, R., T. (2000). Risk factors in adolescence: The case of gambling, video-game playing, and the internet. *Journal of Gambling Studies, 16,* 199–226.

Gupta, R., & Derevensky, J. (1998a). Adolescent gambling behavior: A prevalence study and examination of the correlates associated with excessive gambling. *Journal of Gambling Studies, 14,* 319–345.

Gupta, R., & Derevensky, J. (1998b). An empirical examination of Jacobs' General Theory of Addictions: Do adolescent gamblers fit the theory? *Journal of Gambling Studies, 14,* 17–49.

Gupta, R., & Derevensky, J. (2000). Adolescents with gambling problems: From research to treatment. *Journal of Gambling Studies, 16,* 315–342.

Hardoon, K., & Derevensky, J. (2002). Child and adolescent gambling behavior: Our current knowledge. *Clinical Child Psychology and Psychiatry, 7,* 263–281.

Heather, N., Wodak, A., Nadelmann, E., & O'Hare, P. (1993). *Psychoactive drugs and harm reduction: From faith to science.* London: Whurr Publishers Ltd.

Jacobs, D. F. (2000). Juvenile gambling in North America: An analysis of long term trends and future prospects. *Journal of Gambling Studies, 16,* 119–152.

Jessor, R. (1998). *New perspectives on adolescent risk behavior.* In R. Jessor (Ed.), *New perspectives on adolescent risk behavior.* Cambridge, UK: Cambridge University Press.

Jessor, R., Van Den Bos, J., Vanderryn, J., Costa, F. M., & Turbin, M. S. (1995). Protective factors in adolescent problem behavior: Moderator effects and developmental change. *Developmental Psychology, 31,* 923–933.

Kandel, D. B. (1985). On processes of peer influences in adolescent drug use: A developmental perspective. *Advances in Alcohol and Substance Abuse, 4,* 139–163.

Korn, D., & Shaffer, H. (1999). Gambling and the health of the public: Adopting a public health perspective. *Journal of Gambling Studies, 15,* 289–365.

Ladouceur, R., Jacques, C., Ferland, F., & Giroux, I. (1998). Parents' attitudes and knowledge regarding gambling among youths. *Journal of Gambling Studies, 14,* 83–90.

Loeber, R., Farrington, D., Stouthamer-Loeber, M., & Van Kammen, W. (1998). Multiple risk factors for multi-problem boys: Co-occurrence of delinquency, substance use, attention deficit, conduct problems, physical aggression, covert behavior, depressed mood, and shy/withdrawn behavior. In R. Jessor (Ed.), *New perspectives on adolescent risk behavior*. Cambridge, UK: Cambridge University Press.

Luthar, S. S., Cicchetti, D., & Becker, B. (2000a). The construct of resilience: A critical evaluation and guidelines for future work. *Child Development, 71,* 543–562.

Magoon, M., Gupta, R., & Derevensky, J. L (in press). Juvenile delinquency and adolescent gambling: Implications for the juvenile justice system. *Criminal Justice and Behavior*.

Mangham, C. (2001). Harm reduction or reducing harm? *Canadian Medical Assoication Journal, 164,* 173.

Marlatt, G. A. (1996). Harm reduction: Come as you are. *Addictive Behaviors, 21,* 779–788.

Marlatt, G. A. (1998). Basic principles and strategies of harm reduction. In G. A. Marlatt, (Ed.), *Harm reduction: Pragmatic strategies for managing high-risk behaviors* (pp. 49–66). New York: The Guilford Press.

Masten, A., Best, K., & Garmezy, N. (1990). Resilience and development: Contributions from the study of children who overcome adversity. *Development and Psychopathology, 2,* 425–444.

Messerlian, C., Derevensky, J. L., & Gupta, R. (2003). *Youth gambling problems: A public health framework*. Unpublished manuscript, McGill University, Montreal, QC, Canada.

Murphy, S. B., Reinarman, C. & Waldorf, D. (1989). An 11-year follow-up of a network of cocaine users. *British Journal of Addiction, 84,* 427–436.

Nathan, P. (2001, December). *Best practices for the treatment of gambling disorders: Too soon?* Paper presented at the annual Division on Addictions, Harvard Medical School conference, Las Vegas.

Nation, M., Crusto, C., Wandersman, A., Kumpfer, K. L., Seybolt, D., Morrissey-Kane, E., et al. (2003). *American Psychologist, 58,* 449–456.

National Gambling Impact Study Commission (1999). National Gambling Impact Study Commission: Final Report. Chicago: National Opinion Research Center.

National Research Council (1999). *Pathological gambling: A critical review*. Washington, D. C.: National Academy Press.

Ogborne, A. C., & Birchmore-Timney, C. (1999). A framework for the evaluation of activities and programs with harm-reduction objectives. *Substance Use & Misuse, 34,* 69–82.

Poulin, C., & Elliott, D. (1997). Alcohol, tobacco and cannabis use among Nova Scotia adolescents: Implications for prevention and harm reduction. *Canadian Medical Association Journal, 156,* 1387–1393.

Riley, D., Sawka, E., Conley, P., Hewitt, D., Mitic, W., Poulin, C., Room, R., Single, E., & Topp, J. (1999). Harm reduction: Concepts and practice—a policy discussion paper. *Substance Use & Misuse, 34,* 9–24.

Rugle, L., Derevensky, J., Gupta, R., Stinchfield, R. & Winters, K. (2001). *The treatment of problem and pathological gamblers*. Paper prepared for the National Council for Problem Gambling, Center for Mental Health Services (CMS) and the Substance Abuse and Mental Health Services Administration (SAMHSA), Washington, D.C.

Rutter, M. (1987). Psychosocial resilience and protective mechanism. *American Journal of Orthopsychiatry, 57,* 316–331.

Shaffer, H. J., & Hall, M. N. (1996). Estimating the prevalence of adolescent gambling disorders: A quantitative synthesis and guide toward standard gambling nomenclature. *Journal of Gambling Studies, 12,* 193–214.

Shaffer, H. J., & Hall, M. N. (2001). Updating and refining prevalence estimates of disordered gambling behavior in the United States and Canada. *Canadian Journal of Public Health, 92*, 168–172.

Shaffer, H. J., & Zinberg, N. E. (1994). *The emergence of youthful addiction: The prevalence of under-age lottery use and the impact of gambling.* Technical Report for the Massachusetts Council in Compulsive Gambling (011394–100).

Svendsen, R. (1998). *Gambling among older Minnesotans.* Prepared for the National Research Council Committee on the Social and Economic Impact of Pathological Gambling. Minnesota: Minnesota Institute of Public Health.

Thombs, D., & Briddick, W. (2000). Readiness to change among at-risk Greek student drinkers. *Journal of College Student Development, 41*, 313–322.

Weissberg, R., Walberg, H., O'Brien, M., & Kuster, C. (2003). *Long-term trends in the well-being of children and youth.* Washington, DC: Child Welfare League of America Press.

Werner, E. E. (1986). Resilient offspring of alcoholics: A longitudinal study from birth to age 18. *Journal of Studies on Alcohol, 47*, 34–40.

Werner, E. E. (1989). High risk children in young adulthood: A longitudinal study from birth to 32 years. *American Journal of Orthopsychiatry, 59*, 72–81.

Westphal, J. R., Rush, J. A., Stevens, A. L., & Johnson, L. J. (1998). *Pathological gambling among Louisiana students: Grades six through twelve.* Paper presented at the American Psychiatric Association Annual Meeting. Toronto, Canada.

Wynne, H. J., Smith, G. J., & Jacobs, D. F. (1996). *Adolescent gambling and problem gambling in Alberta.* Alberta, Canada: Alberta Alcohol and Drug Abuse Commission.

Chapter 12

Youth Gambling Problems:
A Need for Responsible Social Policy

Jeffrey L. Derevensky, Ph.D., Rina Gupta, Ph.D.,
Carmen Messerlian, M.Sc. and Meredith Gillespie, B.A.

Games of chance have been popular throughout time. Beginning around 3000 B.C. Egyptian popular forms of gambling included astragals, primero (an early card game found in Europe) and wagering on chariot races (Caltabiano, 2003). Egyptian and Middle Eastern archeological sites have revealed historical accounts of the pervasiveness of gambling in ancient cultures (Ashton, 1968). While gambling in general remained a popular pursuit, the negative effects associated with excessive problem gambling were also documented. Plato suggested that a demon named *Theuth* created dice (astragals or knucklebones as they were originally named) and early reports indicate that King Richard the Lion-Hearted, who led the crusade in 1190, issued orders restricting gambling with dice to his troops. Gambling problems were not isolated only to the common man but to royalty as well. King Henry VIII is reported to have lost the largest and most famous church bells in England at that time-the Jesus bells that hung in St. Paul's Cathedral-in a game of dice (Fleming, 1978).

The history of gambling on an international level has passed through a number of cycles from prohibition to widespread proliferation (Rose, 2003a). Gambling has gone from being associated with sin, criminal behavior, and corruption to its current position as a form of socially acceptable entertainment. Gambling revenues have emerged as an important source of funds for governments, charities, and businesses. The changing landscape of gambling throughout the world seems to suggest that the pendulum between abstinence and widespread acceptance may never swing back to prohibition or to a more restrictive position. More and more countries have either introduced gambling or permitted the establishment of gambling in their jurisdictions.

Until relatively recently, gambling problems have not been viewed as a public health problem (Korn & Shaffer, 1999) or public policy issue but rather as a personal or individual problem (Whyte, 2003). A new surge of research has expanded our knowledge of gambling problems and its societal impact, with legislators being forced to carefully examine the social and financial costs associated with gambling expansion and regulation as well as assessing the accrued financial benefits (National Institute of Economics and Industry Research, 2003).

The prevailing attitudes of government legislators and the public at large appears to suggest that new gaming venues, new forms of gambling (e.g., new technologies in the form of interactive lotteries, Internet gambling and telephone wagering), and the proliferation of current forms of gambling (e.g., casinos, electronic gambling machines, lotteries) will continue to expand rapidly. While a number of social policy experts have suggested that at some point in time there will be a saturation point, the gambling industry continues to expand worldwide at an unprecedented rate with revenues far exceeding all forms of the entertainment industry (e.g., music, movies, theatre, etc.) combined. The anti-lobbying groups appear to have been minor impediments and irritants to slowing the growth of specific forms of gambling. While there have been some notable exceptions for the prohibition of gambling (e.g., Turkey where a new Muslim government banned gambling; the public outcry helped remove video lottery terminals and electronic gambling machines from South Carolina; and there is a movement to reduce the number of electronic gambling machines in several Australian states), the anti-gambling movement appears to have done little to curtail the continued expansion of gambling in spite of the empirical evidence documenting some of the social and personal costs.

Currently, gambling is not viewed negatively but rather as a legitimate, socially acceptable form of entertainment. Over 85% of Americans report having gambled at least once during their lifetime and 65% report gambling during the past year (National Research Council, 1999), with somewhat similar results being reported in Canada (Azmier, 2000), Australia (Productivity Commission, 1999), and New Zealand (Abbott, 2001). Nevertheless, gambling remains a highly contentious social policy issue throughout the world [see the reports from the U.S. National Gambling Study Impact Commission (NORC, 1999), Canada West Foundation (Azmier,

2001), Canadian Tax Foundation Report (Vaillancourt & Roy, 2000), the U.K. Gambling Review Report (2001), the Australian Productivity Commission Report (1999), the National Centre for the Study of Gambling, South Africa Report (Collins & Barr, 2001), and those from New Zealand (Abbott, 2001)]. While the perspective is slowly changing that gambling is not necessarily a harmless, innocuous behavior with few negative consequences, most adults support their continued opportunity to gamble and perceive it to be considerably less harmful than other potentially additive behaviors and harmful social activities (Azmier, 2000).

The legitimacy of gambling has often been tied to the perceived public good associated with its revenues (Preston, Bernhard, Hunter & Bybee, 1998). Some of America's best-known universities including Harvard, Yale, Princeton, William and Mary, Dartmouth, Rutgers, and the University of Pennsylvania have historically acquired operating funds through the proceeds generated from lotteries. This early tradition continues, with many state and national lotteries promoting their products by reporting that a proportion of the proceeds are used for needed educational initiatives and social service programs. In other jurisdictions, gambling revenues are partially or totally used for charitable purposes.

Gambling remains somewhat unique from other public policy issues as it cuts across a number of other policy domains including social, economic, public health, criminal and justice policy (Wynne, 1998). As a public health policy issue, gambling has been growing in importance. Korn and Shaffer (1999) have made a very strong argument for viewing gambling within a public health framework by examining it from a population health and human ecology perspective. They have suggested that disordered gambling may not only be problematic in and of itself, but also may be a gateway to alcohol and substance abuse, depression, anxiety and other significant mental health disorders.

Gambling, once perceived as an activity primarily relegated to adults, has become a popular form of entertainment for adolescents (National Research Council, 1999). While in most jurisdictions legislative statutes prohibit children and adolescents from participating in legalized forms of gambling due to age restrictions, their resourcefulness enables many youth to engage in both regulated legal forms of gambling and those non-regulated gambling activities. Research has revealed that upwards of 80% of adolescents have engaged in some form of gambling (see the reviews by Jacobs, in this volume; National Research Council, 1999, and the meta-analysis by Shaffer & Hall, 1996), with most best described as social gamblers having few gambling-related problems. Yet, there remains ample evidence that between 4–8% of adolescents have a very serious gambling problem with another 10–15% at-risk for the development of a gambling. While difficulties in the measurement of adolescent pathological and disordered gambling exist (see Derevensky & Gupta in this volume, and Derevensky, Gupta & Winters, 2003 for a comprehensive examination of this issue), the National Research Council report concluded that "the proportion of pathological gamblers among adolescents in the United States could be more than three times that of adults (5.0% versus 1.5%)" (National Research Council, 1999, p.89). In the U.S. and Canada, these prevalence estimates indicate that approximately 15.3 million 12–17 year olds have been gambling, while 2.2 million are likely experiencing serious gambling related problems. Trends between 1984–2002 seem to indicate a continued increase in the proportion of youth who report gambling within the past year and those who report some gambling related problems (Jacobs, in this volume).

Our prevailing social policies, often established by default, appear predicated upon a harm minimization model (see Dickson, Derevensky & Gupta, 2004 for a more comprehensive discussion). Yet the development of effective social policy needs to be both reflective and directive of the social context from which it is derived. As such, good social policies should reflect the current status of gambling while simultaneously projecting its future; it must be sensitive to its historical context, yet must exist within the prevailing ideological, social, economic and political values (Hall, Kagan & Zigler, 1996); and such policies must also be considerate of broader cultural and religious influences and differences. The escalation of government supported (and owned) gambling is an enormous social experiment for which we currently do not have sufficient and reliable data to predict the long-term social costs (Derevensky, Gupta, Hardoon, Dickson & Deguire, 2003).

The social costs of gambling are often difficult to quantify, with some suggesting that the economic and social costs have either been largely understated or ignored (Henriksson, 1996). Assessing the social costs and benefits of gambling has created considerable debate among social scientists and economists (see the special issue of the *Journal of Gambling Studies*, 2003, vol.19). Given methodological difficulties in assessing and adequately describing the social costs associated with gambling, and the significant source of revenues for governments, expansion has continued at a rapid rate. Nevertheless, the National Research Council (1999) has highlighted the need to pay special attention to high-risk, vulnerable groups, with adolescents being one such identified group.

There has been ample empirical research which has revealed that excessive gambling among adolescents has been associated with increased alcohol and substance abuse disorders (Hardoon, Derevensky & Gupta, 2002; Winters & Anderson, 2000; Winters, Anderson, Leitten, & Botzet, in this volume), higher rates of depressive symptomatology, higher rates of anxiety, and increased suicide ideation and attempts (Gupta & Derevensky,

1998a; Ste-Marie, Derevensky & Gupta, 2003), increased delinquency and criminal behavior (Magoon, Gupta & Derevensky, in press), disruption of familial relationships, poor academic performance (Derevensky & Gupta, 2004), and poor general health (Marshall & Wynne, 2003; Potenza, Fiellen, Heninger, Rounsaville & Mazure, 2002) (A comprehensive discussion of the correlates associated with adolescent excessive gambling problems can be found in this volume by Stinchfield). Clearly, the negative consequences borne by youth experiencing gambling problems are serious and the damage can be long lasting and devastating to the individual afflicted, their peers and family.

The pro-gambling and anti-gambling groups have been engaged in a long-running struggle for control over public policy toward gambling (Sauer, 2001). Such changes in public policy in the United States has been documented and applied to a number of political economy models. In applying such a model, Sauer (2001) contends that larger governments, which in turn require greater revenues to operate, have prompted gambling expansion. Gambling revenues have become increasingly significant to governments and are often perceived as being a form of voluntary taxation. Consequently, Sauer has suggested that ultimately such changes in social policy directions, accompanied by stricter regulation, would necessitate significant cuts in government expenditures and/or increased non-gambling revenues. However, given the climate of huge government deficits the need for revenues remain, with gambling expansion not likely to be curtailed.

Public policy, as a representation of societal values, aims to significantly reduce social, emotional, mental and physical health problems related to a wide-range of societal issues through both the promotion of wellness and the recognition of appreciable risk. Such efforts may emanate through the initiation of prevention programs (i.e., programmatic policies) and/or through the adoption of formal laws and regulations, and the establishment of regulatory oversight bodies. Yet, the regulatory agencies providing the oversight for gambling are sometimes intricately linked to the beneficiaries of gaming revenue. Such government bodies are often charged with the responsibilities associated with a duty-of-care while simultaneously being directly or indirectly responsible for maintaining or increasing revenues. This is particularly true in jurisdictions where governments are the recipients of the proceeds of gambling revenues, own the gambling venues, and those individuals responsible reporting directly to the Directors/Ministers of Finance.

Policy-makers and legislators need to adopt a multidimensional perspective, viewing the issues from a systemic perspective. Accordingly, policy recommendations must incorporate multiple domains of functioning (e.g., physical, social, interpersonal, cognitive, environmental, and psychological domains), due to the strong interdependencies that exist between them (Cowen & Durlak, 2000). Effective social policies should reflect the bi-directionality of influence between individuals and their community; supporting policy recommendations that indirectly target the individual through their improvement of the community at large. A multidisciplinary effort is required in order to make such multi-component policies feasible (Levant, Tolan & Dodgen, 2002). Such efforts can take the form of programmatic and regulatory policies.

Programmatic Policies

Programmatic policies encompass a public commitment to prevention through funding, implementation and institutionalization of prevention practices (Pentz, 2000). Through community education, training and the provision of support services, these practices seek to improve the environment and increase the skills of individuals within a community. There is considerable need for policy to support more investments in science-based prevention activities (see chapter by Derevensky et al. in this book), as opposed to relying on the therapeutic-restorative initiatives that are currently at the core of the mental health system. A strong foundation of evidence attests to the efficacy of both wellness enhancement and risk-reduction initiatives, as both approaches offer equitable and efficient distribution of services to a larger portion of the population (Cowen & Durlak, 2000). Although they differ substantially in their respective objectives, the strategies implemented and their target populations, both approaches are complimentary. Policies that support strategies aimed at promoting competence are rare, compared to those that seek to reduce negative behaviors through risk-reduction efforts. Nevertheless, both modes of prevention are mutually deserving of a far greater allocation of resources than has been provided to date.

Regulatory Policies

In contrast to programmatic policies, regulatory policies seek to more broadly reduce risks within a community by restricting access to a product or service (e.g., tobacco, alcohol or gambling). Through legislated increases in price or taxation, minimum-age requirements, prohibition of certain types of products, and mandatory training of sales staff and servers, these policies aim to deter youth from participating in high-risk activities. However, the effectiveness of such policies is certainly conditional upon adherence to the prevailing regulatory policies and current statutes. Their enforcement, however, is also significantly contingent upon the acceptance of the implemented practices/regulations within the community and the perceived severity of problems associated with a particular behavior. This may account for the ease with which underage youth purchase lottery tickets in spite of legal prohibitions (Felsher, Derevensky & Gupta, 2003).

Youth Gambling Within the Context of Adolescent Risky Behaviors

On a global level, gambling behavior amongst adolescents may be viewed as one form of risky behavior. Similar to experimentation with alcohol, drugs, and unprotected sexual behavior, most adolescents perceive gambling as a form of entertainment and excitement with few potential negative consequences. From a developmental perspective, adolescence is marked by significant physiological, cognitive and emotional changes, feelings of insecurity, an increase in risk-related behaviors, and a desire for greater independence and autonomy. Given their proclivity for risk-taking, their perceived invulnerability, their lack of recognition that gambling can result in problems, adolescents remain a high-risk group for a gambling problem and multiplicity of health-related problems (Derevensky, Gupta & Winters, 2003; National Research Council, 1999).

As a society we need to explore proactive social policies that will help limit the prevalence of pathological gambling. As such, an examination of social policies designed to limit adolescent risky behaviors may be appropriate. Given that adolescent alcohol consumption has many similarities to gambling behavior, an examination of the existing social policies and their effects may prove useful in guiding the development and framework for policies focused upon youth gambling.

Alcohol Control Policies: An Example

A number of alcohol social policies have been instituted in order to limit youth alcohol consumption and minimize alcohol-related problems (e.g., traffic accidents resulting from driving while intoxicated, binge drinking, poor school performance, teenage alcoholism) by directly restricting alcohol marketing, how it is sold, and places where alcohol may be consumed. Policy-related legislation with respect to alcohol consumption appears to have had significant effects in reducing health-related behaviors (Cowen & Durlak, 2000; Wandersman & Florin, 2003; U.S. Department of Health and Human Services, 2000).

Legal drinking age and age-identification policies. The age at which youth are permitted to legally consume alcohol has been shown to be related to alcohol consumption and accident rates. Following the 1984 federal legislation raising the legal drinking age in the United States from age 18 to 21, alcohol consumption was found to have decreased considerably. It is estimated that 250,000 fewer young adults were drinking heavily, with alcohol-related motor vehicle fatalities involving young people having decreased by 26% (O'Malley & Wagenaar, 1991).

The enforcement of age-identification policies plays an essential role in the adherence to legal drinking age legislation. Such policies include written guidelines found in establishments selling alcohol thereby providing employees with pertinent information regarding the inspection of identification of customers attempting to purchase alcohol. These guidelines mandate that employees refuse the sale of alcohol to customers failing to present valid age identification. Furthermore, by providing detailed instructions of identification inspection procedures, employees are better able to detect the presence of false documents under the existing guidelines. Licensing or law enforcement authorities may perform compliance checks in order to ensure that alcohol is not being sold to underage youth. Strict administrative penalties, including monetary fines and/or a revocation of an establishment's alcohol license are applied against those who have violated regulations. When compliance checks were performed, sales of alcohol to underage youth were found to have decreased substantially (from 60–80% to 25–30%) (Lewis et al., 1996; Preusser, Williams, & Weinstein, 1994).

Alcohol prices and taxation. As youth generally have limited access to money, price increases and heavy taxation have been shown to significantly restrict the accessibility and availability of alcohol (Cowen & Durlak, 2000). Higher taxes and prices of alcohol led to a reduction in alcohol consumption (U.S. Department of Health and Human Services, 2000), and have been linked to lower incidences of alcohol-related fatalities. However, there is some concern that college males still remain high-risk for binge drinking (U.S. Department of Health and Human Services, 2000).

Responsible beverage service training polices (RBST). The educational training of managers, servers and retailers concerning strategies and legal liabilities have been used to prevent the sale of alcohol to intoxicated adults and underage youth (often mandated by local or provincial/state law). It provides the opportunity for such individuals to acquire pertinent knowledge about alcohol policies enforced within the community, as well as to gain the skills necessary to comply with such regulations.

Drunk-driving penalties. Drinking under the influence (DUI) penalties have been shown to reduce drinking and binge-drinking among both underage and older students (U.S. Department of Health and Human Services, 2000).

Alcohol advertising. Restrictions of alcohol advertising and alcohol sponsorship of community events may limit exposure to alcohol messages outside the home. Policies may restrict both the availability and the location of alcohol advertising within a community. Similarly, they may prohibit the distribution of alcohol promotional items at events where youth are in attendance. Survey research on alcohol advertising and young people has reliably demonstrated a small but significant relationship between exposure to and awareness of alcohol advertising and drinking beliefs and behaviors (U.S. Department of Health and Human Services, 2000). The incremental effect of this relationship over time, with persistent exposure, may be significant. Some communities have regulated where alcohol advertising can be displayed. For example, the city of Oakland, California, by statute, prohibits alcohol advertisements on billboards in residential areas, near schools, within three blocks of recreation centers, churches, and licensed day care facilities. As a result, only 70 of the city's 1,450 billboards are available for alcohol advertisements (Scenic America, 2003).

Social access policies. While underage youth may obtain alcohol from parents, siblings, friends and other adults, various policies have been enacted limiting access to alcohol in public places. Restrictions of the use of alcohol at parks, beaches and other public spaces have been enacted. Such restrictions may range from complete prohibition to specified times when alcohol may be used in demarcated drinking areas. Alcohol restrictions at community events have also been shown to limit consumption.

Social host liability legislation may further act as a strong deterrent to providers of alcohol, as there is a salient risk that legal proceedings will occur if injury or death results from supplying alcohol to an underage youth. As a result, adults who serve or provide alcohol to persons under the legal drinking age can be held legally liable for their behavior and the well-being of those individuals. These laws may deter parents from hosting underage parties where alcohol is served and/or from purchasing alcohol for their children. A national survey conducted by Wagenaar, Harwood, Toomey, Denk, and Zander (2000) suggests that 83% of adults support policies that impose monetary penalties on adults who supply alcohol to underage youth.

Programmatic policies. Unlike regulatory policies, programmatic policies aim to institutionalize prevention education in order to reduce levels of alcohol consumption in youth. These policies may include formalizing prevention program funding in participating schools or communities (e.g., continued allocation of resources), or formalizing procedures to ensure the integrity of program implementation (e.g., teacher training in prevention) and have been shown to yield positive results (Pentz, 2000).

Social Policies Affecting Youth Gambling

Gambling behavior has been shown to begin earlier than most other potentially addictive behaviors including tobacco, alcohol, and drug use (Gupta & Derevensky, 1996, 1998b). Given that there are few observable signs of gambling dependence among children, these problems have not been as readily noticed compared to other addictions (e.g., alcohol or substance abuse) (Arcuri, Lester & Smith, 1985; Hardoon & Derevensky, 2002; Lesieur & Klein, 1987). Currently, gambling is advertised widely, relatively easily accessible to youth, and often found in places that are perceived to be glamorous and exciting (e.g., bars, casinos). Gambling also provides opportunities for socializing, be it positive or negative (Stinchfield & Winters, 1998). Although betting in casinos, on electronic gaming machines and lotteries, in general, are prohibited for adolescents (age restrictions and statutes differ between countries, states and provinces), the enforcement of these laws is becoming increasingly difficult (Moore & Ohtsuka, 1997) and almost non-existent in many jurisdictions.

Gambling is an Emerging Public Health Issue

Given the pervasiveness of the problems associated with youth gambling problems and the concomitant mental health, social, economic, educational and legal problems, there is a need to clearly identify the social, economic and familial costs associated with youth gambling. We need a better understanding of the effects of accessibility and availability of gaming venues on future gambling behaviors and to determine whether all forms of gambling are equally problematic. Specific research needs to focus on gambling advertisements and their relationship to the onset and maintenance of adolescent gambling and problem gambling. Adequate funds must be made available to help youth currently experiencing severe gambling and gambling-related behaviors and their families to develop systematic evaluations of treatment approached to help establish *Best Practices* for working with these youth (Nathan, 2001) and ways to encourage youth with severe gambling problems to seek professional assistance (see Derevensky, Gupta & Winters, 2003). A public health approach should take into consideration the necessary balance among health, social, and economic costs and benefits when formulating a responsible gambling policy and strategy (Korn & Shaffer, 1999; Messerlian, Derevensky & Gupta, 2003).

The Development of Responsible Social Policies

As problem gambling cuts across a number of different policy domains, a multidimensional approach is required to develop responsible social policies. By necessity this will incorporate legislative, judicial, educational and social aspects. While some of these initiatives and recommendations will need to be similar to policies currently in place regarding alcohol and drug use, others may be specific and unique to gambling.

The Need for Prevention Initiatives Incorporating a Harm Minimization Strategy

Despite some controversy over whether abstinence versus harm-minimization should be used in prevention programs (see Dickson, Derevensky & Gupta, 2004 for a review of this literature), there is little doubt that most youth gamble amongst themselves, with family members, and on government regulated gambling. Still further, most jurisdictions have multiple forms of government regulated gambling subject to age restrictions (this varies depending upon the type of gambling activity. For example, lottery purchases usually have lower age limits than casino playing whereas bingo may have no restrictions). The reality remains that legalized, regulated forms of gambling have become mainstream and widely accepted as a socially acceptable form of entertainment (Azmier, 1999). As such, similar to alcohol use, preparing youth to engage in this behavior in a responsible manner, when age appropriate, is important.

A review of the literature revealed that relatively few gambling prevention or sensitization programs exist and those programs that do exist lack empirical validity as to their effectiveness (Derevensky, Gupta, Dickson & Deguire in this volume). Programs incorporating science-based problem gambling prevention need to be funded, developed and evaluated as to their efficacy in order to help establish model programs. Such prevention initiatives must begin early in the child's elementary school years and should include competency building skills, enhancement of effective coping and adaptive behaviors, must emphasize changing attitudes, increase knowledge related to gambling, help modify erroneous cognitions, strengthen problem solving skills, and enhance coping and adaptive skills. Given the wide age range of youth that these programs need to target, different developmentally appropriate programs are required (Derevensky, Gupta, Dickson & Deguire, 2003).

Technological Advances and Social Policy Implications

Unlike most other adolescent high-risk behaviors, technological advances have made a wide variety of gambling venues highly attractive to adolescents.

Today's youth, having spent their formative years on personal computers and playing interactive video-games, appear particularly susceptible to the lure of some of the new gambling venues and technologies (e.g., Internet gambling, slot machines incorporating video-game graphics and technology, VLTs, computer-based lottery games, interactive television games, and telephone wagering) (Griffiths & Wood, 2000). It is predicted that participation in Internet gambling will continue to significantly increase as (a) it is easily accessible, (b) it has the potential to offer visually stimulating effects similar to video games, slot machines and VLTs, (c) the event frequency can be rapid, (d) many of these games are widely advertised on Internet servers through pop-up windows, (e) many sites provide incentives to attract new customers, and (f) such sites are actively exploring alternative methods for transferring of funds for wagering (Griffiths & Wood, 2000; Messerlian, Byrne & Derevensky, 2004).

Given the increasing popularity, accessibility and familiarity of the Internet, this represents another venue for potential problems for adolescents. There is little if any security verifying the age of the user. As most Internet gambling websites are housed in off-shore operations, there is little regulation (Kelley, Todosichuk & Azmier, 2001). Many websites offer free games, free practice sites, and financial rewards and incentives (often referred to as *perks*), available to anyone with access to a computer and Internet service provider. These sites now offer a multitude of casino type games including blackjack, roulette, slots, poker, virtually identical to real casinos while incorporating sophisticated graphics. Such sites also offer sports betting, another attractive activity for adolescents. With new sites appearing daily, researchers suspect that the distinction between *gambling* and *gaming* (this term is used to denote playing games on the computer, not the new terminology used by the industry to refer to gambling) may become blurred by the on-line gambling industry (Messerlian et al., 2004). Some preliminary data suggests that a large number of adolescents report playing on the practice sites (not for real money), with even more youth experiencing gambling problems reporting doing so (Hardoon, Derevensky & Gupta, 2002). Such practice sites expose youth to adult forms of gambling, encouraging them to practice and perhaps move toward wagering money. Internet casino sites (often referred to as *properties*) also have reward, loyalty programs which may be enticing to youth. Such programs include earning redeemable *comp* points through playing (Peak Entertainment which owns five sites enables players to earn comp points interchangeably on all their sites); high initial deposit bonuses (with some sites including 100% match bonus dollars); returning player bonuses of up to $20 per month; *Refer-A-Friend* bonuses as high as $50; 10% bonuses for wire transfers of funds, certified check and money orders; and some sites even provide "Bettor's Insurance" programs which returns 10% of net gaming losses (Gambling Online, 2003).

While little is currently known about the number of young people actually accessing gambling via Internet sites there is ample evidence to suggest this is a highly viable venue for youth gambling. Research by Willms and Corbett (2003) has suggested that upwards of 48% of youth age 15 are currently playing a variety of games (non-gambling games) on the Internet. In a recent study, Hardoon et al. (2002) found that 25% of adolescents with serious gambling problems and 20% of those at-risk for a gambling problem reported playing on-line gambling type games using *practice sites.* The use of the Internet may present a special danger for individuals at high-risk for developing a gambling problem (Messerlian et al., 2004).

While technological advances may be a cause for concern, nevertheless, it may also provide innovative and exciting ways of presenting prevention programs for youth through web-based initiatives and on-line treatment. For example, the University of Toronto (YouthBet.net), the Louisiana Department of Health and Hospitals (thegamble.org) and the North American Training Institute (WannaBet.org) all provide on-line gambling sensitization and prevention programs designed for adolescents.

Advertising

The advertising and glamorization of gambling in the media, movies and television is of significant concern. The use of highly visible, branded products or personalities endorsing gambling is problematic. For example, the Virginia State Lottery has advertising campaigns associated with NASCAR racing (a highly popular sport for adolescent and young adult males), several states have used *Betty Boop* (a cartoon character) with their lottery scratch tickets with opportunities to win leather jackets and other promotional material as well as money, while other promotions include the opportunity to win motorcycles, exotic vacations and *Cash-for-Life* (Derevensky, Gupta, Hardoon, Dickson & Deguire 2003). James Bond, the sophisticated and debonair secret agent in films, is often found in exotic casinos and gaming venues.

Adolescents have been shown to be particularly observant of casino and lottery advertisements. They have been shown to be more prone to purchase scratch-tickets when advertised and placed on checkout counters of local convenience stores (Derevensky & Gupta, 2001; Felsher et al., 2003). As such, government regulatory bodies need to establish strict advertising guidelines to discourage extravagant or misleading claims about gambling and opportunities to win. Interestingly, state lottery corporations in the United States are exempt from the federal truth-in advertising regulations.

Specific licensed products particularly attractive to underage populations, including *South Park, Betty Boop,* and the *World Wrestling Federation* licensed products should be prohibited from being associated with gambling.

Advertising campaigns if used properly can form a major part of a prevention campaign. Advertisements geared toward informing and sensitizing adolescents to addictive behaviors may actually be beneficial (Byrne, Dickson, Derevensky, Gupta & Lussier, 2004; Earle, 2000). Advertising designed to raise awareness that youth gambling can become problematic can and should be implemented. The Connecticut State Lottery in collaboration with the Connecticut Council on Problem Gambling has developed an impressive television public service announcement highlighting the potential problems associated with sports betting by adolescents. Other states have developed similar programs; many which need to be evaluated for their effectiveness (see Byrne et al., 2004 for a comprehensive discussion). More regulatory bodies are encouraged to work with prevention specialists to develop such programs using multiple medium.

Age Restrictions

As a general rule, most regulated forms of gambling have legal, minimum age restrictions. Nevertheless, there exists considerable variability in legislative regulation of gambling aimed at adolescents. For example, while casino entry in many jurisdictions is relegated to individuals age 21 in the United States, within Canada the entry age is 18 or older depending upon the jurisdiction and the type of game (e.g., some provinces have higher age minimums for casinos than other regulated activities). In the U.K. there are no age restrictions on fruit machine playing (small wager slot machines). Special exemptions often exist in many jurisdictions for bingo (thought to be a family activity and not contributing to gambling problems). Lottery purchases are generally perceived to be less problematic, thus having a younger age requirement for purchases. Rose (2003b) has noted that in spite of adverse political and moral pressure, those few legislators who have looked at lowering the legal minimum age to gamble have been dissuaded given their conclusions that revenues would not increase substantially. Yet, while there is evidence that the amount wagered by underage individuals may be relatively insignificant from the industry's perspective, it is nevertheless considerable and can result in problematic behavior (Derevensky & Gupta, 2004; Gupta & Derevensky, 1998a; National Research Council, 1999).

Research has revealed that early onset of gambling results in gambling problems (Gupta & Derevensky, 1998b; Wynne, Smith & Jacobs, 1996) and that adult pathological gamblers report engaging in both regulated and unregulated forms of gambling quite early (Productivity Commission, 1999). There also remains concern that early gambling behavior begins at home, with many youth wagering money on card games with parents (Gupta & Derevensky, 1997). Some have argued that by raising the minimum age to 21, early onset of gambling, especially in term of organized, government regulated gambling may be raised.

Prices

One of the concerns about lottery purchases for youth is the low cost of tickets. In many jurisdictions in North America the cost for purchasing a lottery draw ticket (e.g., *6/49, Select 7*, etc.) is $1.00, with tickets for scratch cards and pull-tabs ranging between .50-$20.00. At the lower end, the costs are generally affordable for even young adolescents. Most casinos have no entry admission fees and slot machine playing can be as little as .05 per spin. Raising the cost per ticket and the cost of playing a slot machine may have a discouraging effect on adolescents. Further research and exploration concerning pricing is warranted.

Responsible Training Programs

While many casinos have responsible gaming programs, few lottery and bingo vendors have participated in such programs. Those dispersing lottery tickets, bingo cards, as well as employees in the casino industry require greater knowledge of the risks associated with youth problem gambling. Such individuals must also be held legally responsible when permitting underage youth from gambling.

Penalties Associated with Underage Gambling

There is evidence that while legislative statutes exist, underage adolescents have little difficulty in gaining access to these venues (Felsher et al., 2003; Jacobs, 2000, in this volume). When consulting lottery officials, none deny the fact that few, if any, vendors have been fined or had their licenses temporarily or permanently revoked for permitting underage purchases. Casino operators have taken the issue more seriously as fines levied for underage gambling have been significant in the United States and Canada. The failure to enforce current statutes can be accounted for by both the perceived loss of revenues, the belief that certain forms of gambling are relatively innocuous, and that there is a general perception that pathological gambling is an adult phenomenon. While few adolescents have experienced serious gambling related problems resulting from excessive lottery playing, it has been argued that this may well be a gateway behavior to more serious forms of gambling (Derevensky & Gupta, 2001; Shaffer & Zinberg, 1994).

Availability of Gambling Venues

There is a growing recognition that easy accessibility to gambling venues leads to increased gambling. Historically, in North America, one had to travel to Nevada or Atlantic City to gamble. Today virtually all States and Provinces run a lottery, with many having casinos. Within Canada, 8 Provinces operate 38,652 legal, government owned Video Lottery Terminals, generating annual revenues over $2.64 billion (KPMG, 2003). These machines, generally relegated to establishments serving alcohol or racetracks, appear almost everywhere with establishments often advertising themselves as *Mini Casinos*. Their availability in low-income areas and near schools remains highly problematic. Given that there is a financial incentive to have patrons play these machines with very little, if any, enforcement of underage playing, there is little adherence to current legislative statutes.

Regulatory Bodies

Regulatory bodies need an arms-length approach to monitor gambling, set and establish rules and guidelines, develop responsible social policies, and establish strict enforcement of statutes and policies. Such regulatory bodies need to work closely with both the gaming industry and researchers in developing sound principles and policies. Periodic commissions to review national policies on gambling while beneficial are not entirely sufficient. Policies need to be implemented that promote responsible gambling, adopt harm minimization approaches, govern advertising, facilitate the dissemination of pertinent material, and have input in the establishment of funds for research, treatment facilities and prevention activities. Applicants for a gambling license, including governmental agencies, must adopt a clear mission statement concerning their policy on pathological gambling and the allocation of funds for dealing with problem gamblers and their families. The creation of a dedicated fund for the development and ongoing support of problem gambling research, public awareness, prevention, education and treatment programs needs to be established by those governmental bodies and or private entities profiting from gambling revenues.

Regulatory bodies need to be active and sensitive to emerging social issues related to problem gambling. Such social issues may result from technological advances, changing patterns of behavior, and advances in our knowledge. Regulatory bodies must maintain as their primary responsibility to protect the public.

Information Dissemination

Major advancements continue to be made in our understanding of the correlates and risk factors associated with adolescent problem gambling (see Derevensky & Gupta, 2004; Dickson et al., 2004; Stinchfield, in this volume). The establishment of a national or international clearinghouse for research and materials will help disseminate new findings. Such a clearinghouse would have as its mandate to distribute information concerning *Best Practices* in the field of gambling prevention and treatment. Government gaming commissions and regulatory bodies in collaboration with organizations designated to help problem gamblers should produce and distribute educational material, produce warning signs on gambling machines, empirically examine responsible gaming features on electronic gambling machines, and make available information concerning the probabilities associated with different types of gambling activities.

Concluding Remarks

Problem gambling is governed by a complex set of interrelating factors, causes, and determinants. It is the interplay of the multiple factors and causes that likely determine one's propensity to develop a gambling-related problem (Blaszczynski, 1999; Derevensky, Gupta, Hardoon, Dickson & Deguire, 2003; Jacobs, 1986). Viewing gambling behavior from an ecological, public health policy perspective necessitates moving beyond merely offering problem gamblers treatment and counselling (Messerlian et al., 2003).

Research in the field of youth gambling still remains in its infancy and more basic and applied research is needed to help identify common and unique risk and protective factors for gambling problems and other addictive behaviors; longitudinal research is necessary to examine the natural history of pathological gambling from childhood to adolescence through later adulthood; molecular, genetic and neuropsychological research is necessary to help account for changes in gambling progression; research assessing whether certain gambling activities may become a gateway to subsequent gambling problems is required; and the development and / or refinement of current instruments used to assess adolescent gambling severity is warranted (Derevensky, Gupta, Hardoon et al., 2003).

Educational institutions have the potential to strongly influence the health of our youth and represent an ideal setting in which to implement health promotion and problem gambling prevention strategies. Some school practices may unwittingly be promoting gambling through the organizing of fundraising activities including lottery/raffle draws, casino nights, and permitting card playing. Clear school policies, analogous to those in place for drug and alcohol use, must be written concerning youth gambling.

There is a need to develop social policies that balance public health interests with the economic gains of governments and industry, and the entertainment value received by the consumer. Public policy development may be a cost-effective and socially responsible way of reducing the burden of gambling disorders and related problems, while simultaneously protecting the public. Through public education, research, and policy advocacy, governments can establish sensible public policies on the regulation, growth and expansion of gambling products, activities and venues.

From a social policy perspective, legislative and regulatory bodies have the mandate to determine suitable forms of gambling, to raise the legal age for government regulated forms of gambling, and have the ability to enforce current statutes. Many other more visible adolescent problems have prompted significant social policy recommendations (e.g., cigarette smoking, alcohol and substance use and abuse, increased rates of suicide). Issues surrounding youth gambling problems have been greatly ignored. Only recently have health professionals, educators and public policy makers acknowledged the need for the prevention of problem gambling. In light of the scarcity of empirical knowledge about the prevention of this disorder, the similarities between adolescent problem gambling and other risk behaviors, particularly alcohol and substance abuse, can be informative in the conceptualization of the future direction of gambling prevention programs, social policy development, and should be made a priority for legislators.

The field of youth gambling is relatively new and as a result there currently are significant gaps in our knowledge. A better understanding of the influence of advertising and the effects of accessibility and availability of gaming venues on future gambling behaviors needs further exploration. Adolescent pathological gamblers, like their adult counterpart, continue to chase their losses, have a preoccupation with gambling, have an impaired ability to stop gambling in spite of repeated attempts and their desire to do so, and frequently get involved in delinquent criminal behavior to support their gambling. This behavior continues independent of the accompanying negative consequences and ensuing problems. Stricter enforcement of current statutes and innovative way of protecting our youth are necessary.

With the acceptance of gambling as a socially acceptable form of entertainment, the lure of gambling for adolescents and the widespread proliferation of gambling venues the social impact and potential negative consequences appear to have been largely ignored or discounted. Youth gambling remains an important social and public policy issue that will continue to grow. Regulatory boards and government officials are well advised to draw upon the lessons learned from the field of alcohol research and to take this issue seriously as it requires our immediate attention, concern and efforts.

References

Abbott, M. W. (2001). *What do we know about gambling and problem gambling in New Zealand? Report # 7 of the New Zealand Gaming Survey.* Wellington, New Zealand: The Department of Internal Affairs.

Arcuri, A. F., Lester, D., & Smith, F. O. (1985). Shaping adolescent gambling behavior. *Adolescence, 20,* 935–938.

Ashton, J. (1968). *The history of gambling in England.* New York: Burt Franklin.

Australian Productivity Commission. (1999). *Australia's gambling industries.* Canberra; Commonwealth of Australia.

Azmier, J. (2000). *Gambling in Canada: Triumph, tragedy, or tradeoff. Canadian gambling behavior and attitudes.* Calgary, AB: Canada West Foundation.

Azmier, J. (2001). *Gambling in Canada: An overview.* Calgary: Canada West Foundation.

Blaszczynski, A. (1999). Pathological gambling and obsessive compulsive spectrum disorders. *Psychological Reports, 84,* 107–113.

Byrne, A., Dickson, L., Derevensky, J., Gupta, R., & Lussier, I. (2004). *An examination of social marketing campaigns for the prevention of youth problem gambling.* Unpublished manuscript, McGill University, Quebec, Canada.

Caltabiano, N. J. (2003). From antiquity to Australia: A brief account of gambling. *eCOMMUNITY: International Journal of Mental Health & Addiction, 1.*

Collins, P., & Barr, G. (2001). *Gambling and problem gambling in South Africa: A national study.* National Center for the Study of Gambling, South Africa.

Cowen, E. L., & Durlak, J. A. (2000). Social policy and prevention in mental health. *Development and Psychopathology, 12,* 815–834.

Derevensky, J., & Gupta, R. (2001). Le problème de jeu touché aussi les jeunes. *Psychologie Québec, 18,* 23–27.

Derevensky, J., & Gupta, R. (2004). Adolescents with gambling problems: A review of our current knowledge. e-Gambling: The Electronic Journal of Gambling Issues, 10, 119–140.

Derevensky, J., Gupta, R., Hardoon, K., Dickson, L., & Deguire, A-E. (2003). Youth gambling: Some social policy issues. In G. Reith (Ed.), *Gambling: Who wins? Who loses?* NY: Prometheus Books.

Derevensky, J., Gupta, R., & Winters, K. (2003). Prevalence rates of youth gambling problems: Are the current rates inflated? *Journal of Gambling Studies, 19,* 405–425.

Dickson, L., Derevensky, J., & Gupta, R. (2004). Harm reduction for the prevention of youth gambling problems: Lessons learned from adolescent high-risk prevention programs. *Journal of Adolescent Research, 19,* 233–263.

Earle, R. (2000).*The art of cause marketing: How to use advertising to change personal behavior and public policy.* Chicago: NTC Business Books.

Felsher, J., Derevensky, J. & Gupta, R. (2003). Parental influences and social modeling of youth lottery participation. *Journal of Community and Applied Social Psychology, 13,* 361–377.

Fleming, A. (1978). *Something for nothing: A history of gambling.* New York: Delacorte Press.

Gambling Online (2003). Top rewards program: Peak Entertainment. *Gambling Online, The Yearbook Edition, 36.*

Griffiths, M., & Wood, R. (2000). Risk factors in adolescence: The case of gambling, video-game playing, and the internet. *Journal of Gambling Studies, 16,* 199–225.

Gupta, R., & Derevensky, J. L. (1996). The relationship between gambling and video-game playing behaviour in children and adolescents. *Journal of Gambling Studies, 12,* 375–394.

Gupta, R., & Derevensky, J. L. (1997). Familial and social influences on juvenile gambling behavior. *Journal of Gambling Studies, 13,* 179–192.

Gupta, R., & Derevensky, J. (1998a). Adolescent gambling behavior: A prevalence study and examination of the correlates associated with excessive gambling. *Journal of Gambling Studies, 14,* 319–345.

Gupta, R., & Derevensky, J. (1998b). An empirical examination of Jacobs' General Theory of Addictions: Do adolescent gamblers fit the theory? *Journal of Gambling Studies, 14,* 17–49.

Hall, N., Kagan, S., & Zigler, E. (1996). The changing nature of child and family policy: An overview. In E. Zigler, S. L. Kagan, & N. Hall (Eds.), *Children, families and government: Preparing for the twenty-first century.* Boston: Cambridge University Press.

Hardoon, K., & Derevensky, J. (2002). Child and adolescent gambling behavior: Our current knowledge. *Clinical Child Psychology and Psychiatry, 7,* 263–281.

Hardoon, K., Derevensky, J., & Gupta, R. (2002). *An examination of the influence of familial, emotional, conduct and cognitive problems, and hyperactivity upon youth risk-taking and adolescent gambling problems.* Guelph, Ontario: Ontario Problem Gambling Research Centre.

Henriksson, L. E. (1996). Hardly a quick fix: Casino gambling in Canada. *Canadian Public Policy, 22,* 116–128.

Jacobs, D. F. (1986). A General Theory of Addictions: A new theoretical model. *Journal of Gambling Behavior, 2,* 15–31.

Jacobs, D. F. (2000). Juvenile gambling in North America: An analysis of long term trends and future prospects. *Journal of Gambling Studies, 16,* 119–152.

Kelley, R., Todosichuk, P., & Azmier, J. J. (2001). *Gambling@home: Internet gambling in Canada* (Gambling in Canada Research Report No. 15). Calgary, AB: Canada West Foundation.

Korn, D., & Shaffer, H. (1999). Gambling and the health of the public: Adopting a public health perspective. *Journal of Gambling Studies, 15,* 289–365.

KPMG (2003). *Canadian gaming highlights.* Toronto: KPMG reports.

Lesieur, H. R., & Klein, R. (1987). Pathological gambling among high school students. *Addictive Behaviors, 12,* 129–135.

Levant, R. F., Tolan, P., & Dodgen, D. (2002). New directions in children's mental health: Psychology's role. *Professional Psychology: Research and Practice, 33,* 115–124.

Lewis, R. K., Paine-Andrews, A., Fawcett, S. B., Francisco, V. T., Richter, K. P., Copple, B, et al. (1996). Evaluating the effects of a community coalition's efforts to reduce illegal sales of alcohol and tobacco products to minors. *Journal of Community Health, 21,* 429–436.

Magoon, M., Gupta, R., & Derevensky, J. (in press). Juvenile delinquency and adolescent gambling: Implications for the juvenile justice system. *Criminal Justice and Behavior.*

Marshall, K., & Wynne, H. (2003). Fighting the odds. *Statistics Canada Perspectives, December,* 5–13.

Messerlian, C., Derevensky, J., & Gupta, R. (2003). *A new way forward: A public health approach to youth problem gambling.* Paper presented at the annual meeting of the National Council on Problem Gambling, Louisville, June.

Messerlian, C., Byrnes, A., & Derevensky, J. (2004). Gambling, youth and the Internet: Should we be concerned? *The Canadian Child and Adolescent Psychiatry Review, 13,* 12–15.

Moore, S. M., & Ohtsuka, K. (1997). Gambling activities of young Australians: Developing a model of behavior. *Journal of Gambling Studies, 13,* 207–236.

Nathan, P. (2001, December). *Best practices for the treatment of gambling disorders: Too soon.* Paper presented at the annual Harvard-National Centre for Responsible Gambling Conference, Las Vegas.

National Institute of Economic and Industry Research (2003, July). *The economic impact of gambling: A report for the Casino Community Benefit Fund.* New South Wales: Department of Gaming and Racing.

National Opinion Research Center (1999). *Gambling impact and behavior study: Report to the National Gambling Impact Study Commission.* Chicago, IL: National Opinion Research Center at the University of Chicago.

National Research Council (1999). *Pathological gambling: A critical review.* Washington, DC.: National Academy Press.

O'Malley, P. M., & Wagenaar, A. C. (1991). Effects of minimum drinking age laws on alcohol use, related behaviors and traffic crash involvement among American youth: 1976–1987. *Journal of Studies on Alcohol, 52,* 568–579.

Pentz, M. A. (2000). Institutionalizing community-based prevention through policy change. *Journal of Community Psychology, 28,* 257–270.

Potenza, M. N., Fiellin, D. A., Heninger, G. R., Rounsaville, B. J., & Mazure, C. M. (2002). Gambling: An addictive behavior with health and primary care implications. *Journal of General Internal Medicine, 17,* 721–732.

Preston, F., Bernhard, B. J., Hunter, R., & Bybee, S. (1998). Gambling as stigmatized behavior: Regional relabeling and the law. *The Annals of the American Academy of Social Scientists, 556,* 186–196.

Preusser, D. F., Williams, A. F., & Weinstein, H. B. (1994). Policing underage alcohol sales. *Journal of Safety Research, 25,* 127–133.

Rose, I. N. (2003a). Gambling and the law: The new millennium. In G. Reith (Ed.), *Gambling: Who wins? Who loses?* Amherst, New York: Prometheus Books.

Rose, I. N. (2003b). *Legislative activity and inactivity.* Costa Mesa, CA: Gambling and the Law.

Sauer, R. D. (2001). The political economy of gambling regulation. *Managerial and Decision Economics, 22,* 5–15

Scenic America (2003). Alcohol billboards: Assistance for communities in adopting ordinances. Accessed online on 12/18/03 at: http://www.scenic.org/fact11.htm.

Shaffer, H. J., & Hall, M. M. (1996). Estimating the prevalence of adolescent gambling disorders: A quantitative synthesis and guide toward standard gambling nomenclature. *Journal of Gambling Studies, 12,* 193–214.

Shaffer, H. J., & Zinberg, N. E. (1994). *The emergence of youthful addiction: The prevalence of underage lottery use and the impact of gambling.* Technical report for the Massachusetts Council in Compulsive Gambling (011394–100).

Ste-Marie, Gupta, R., & Derevensky, J. (2002). Anxiety and social stress related to adolescent gambling behavior. *International Gambling Studies, 2,* 123–141.

Stinchfield, R., & Winters, K. C. (1998). Gambling and problem gambling among youth. *Annals of the American Academy of Political and Social Sciences, 556,* 172–185.

United States Department of Health and Human Services (June, 2000). *Tenth Special Report to U.S. Congress on Alcohol and Health: Highlights from Current Research.*

Vaillancourt, F., & Roy, A. (2000). *Gambling and governments in Canada, 1969–1998: How much? Who pays? What payoff. Special Studies in Taxation and Public Finance, No. 2.* Toronto: Canadian Tax Foundation.

Wagenaar, A.C., Harwood, E. M., Toomey, T. L., Denk, C. E., & Zander, K. M. (2000). Public opinion on alcohol policies in the United States: Results from a national survey. *Journal of Public Health Policy, 21,* 303–327.

Wandersman, A., & Florin, P. (2003). Community interventions and effective prevention. *American Psychologist, 58,* 441–448.

Whyte, K. (2003). A public policy response to problem gambling. In G. Reith (Ed.), *Gambling: Who wins? Who loses?* New York: Prometheus Books.

Willms, J. D., & Corbett, B. A. (2003). Tech and teens: Access and use. *Canadian Social Trends, 69,* 15–20.

Winters, K. C., & Anderson, N. (2000). Gambling involvement and drug use among adolescents. *Journal of Gambling Studies, 16,* 175–198.

Wynne, H. (1998). *Adult gambling and problem gambling in Alberta.* A report prepared for the Alberta Alcohol and Drug Abuse Commission. Edmonton, AB: Wynne Resources Ltd.

Wynne, H., Smith, G., & Jacobs, D. (1996). *Adolescent gambling and problem gambling in Alberta.* A report prepared for the Alberta Alcohol and Drug Abuse Commission. Edmonton, AB: Wynne Resources Ltd.

Index